THE HANDBOOK OF
CANCER IMMUNOLOGY

THE HANDBOOK OF CANCER IMMUNOLOGY

Volume 1

Basic Cancer-Related Immunology

THE HANDBOOK OF CANCER IMMUNOLOGY

Edited by

Harold Waters

Smithsonian Science
Information Exchange

RC 268.3
H 35
v. 1
1978

Garland STPM Press
New York & London

342400

To cancer researchers, treaters and administrators,
professionals all, who should make it a point to live and
die with a few cancer patients yearly, and who should be
creative and anarchistic enough to recognize the unique
spores that probably float by daily

Copyright © 1978 by Garland STPM Press.
A division of Garland Publishing, Inc.

All rights reserved. No part of this work covered by the copyright
hereon may be reproduced or used in any form or by any means—graphic,
electronic, or mechanical, including photocopying, recording, taping,
or information storage and retrieval systems—without permission of
the publisher.

15   14   13   12   11   10   9 8 7   6   5   4   3   2   1

Library of Congress Cataloging in Publication Data
Main entry under title:

Basic cancer-related immunology.

(The Handbook of cancer immunology; v. 1)
Includes bibliographical references and index.
1. Tumors—Immunological aspects. 2. Immunology.
3. Cancer—Immunological aspects. I. Waters, Harold,
1942–   II. Series. [DNLM: 1. Neoplasms—Immunology
—Handbooks. QZ200 H235 v. 1]
RC268.3.H35 vol. 1 [QR188.6] 616.9′94′079 s
ISBN 0-8240-9864-1   [616.9′94′079]   76-52693

Printed in the United States of America

CONTENTS

PREFACE

Surgery became the first answer to the problem of cancer probably not all that long after Galen noticed the crab-like resemblance of a breast tumor. Then came radiotherapy. And about ten years or so ago, chemotherapy emerged as the expected final solution to the problem of human cancer At that time it was anticipated that a new miracle drug was just around the corner, but to everyone's disappointment such has failed to materialize, though there are a number of good drugs that sometimes work and sometimes don't.

More recently, the disciplines of immunology and immunotherapy have been touted as *the* answer. The rationale is sound: shore up the body's own defenses and reject neoplastic cells like a mismatched organ transplant. Unfortunately, the art is currently only slightly more sophisticated and clinically reproducible than hitting cancer cells over the head with a ballpeen hammer.

In this series we attempt to bring the body knowledge of cancer-related immunology nose to nose with the body dogma. We would like to help retard the premature ossification of immunology into the long bones of dogma, which of course does not preclude being dogmatic. We would also like to show that cancer immunology has more to offer than just the promise of nonspecific immune stimulation. These studies on immunology as a science are presented in order to help clarify the basic biology of cancer cells, the role and biological function of cell surface markers, and the interactions between cells—normal and normal, normal and neoplastic, and even neoplastic and neoplastic.

This volume deals with the basics of current, cancer–related immunobiology starting off with the frontiers of immunology and the challenging question: does ontogeny still recapitulate phylogeny? Then we ask about the effects of aging and the role of genetic control on the immune system.

There is a serious need to know a great deal more about the commuter traffic patterns of lymphoid cells and what meaningful experiences they have during their travels and travails. These are addressed and available information reviewed.

Evidence for organ specificity of defenses against tumors is presented in a provocative, well-written chapter that demonstrates how we have only started to scratch the surface in our knowledge of exactly how and how exactly the immune system functions. Focussing more finely into the black box we find that the functional role of cell surface immunoglobulins, although much studied in recent years, is also just now beginning to come into view.

Finally we address the questions of whether immunity facilitates metastases or whether these reconnoitering cells are just tougher and foxier than their primary tumor counterparts. The last chapter in this volume turns the coin on edge and suggests that cell-mediated immunosuppressive effects of irradiation may result in the phenotypic expression of important somatic mutations in T cells.

Throughout the series we have made use of overlapping chapters, more in some areas than others. This approach is the same used in holding anything of value and interest to the light and rotating it through several planes to, for the moment, catch its essence—to figure it out.

Harold Waters
Washington, D.C.
January 1978

CHAPTER 1

ON THE FRONTIERS OF IMMUNOLOGY

Vilas V. Likhite

Harvard Medical School
Boston, Massachusetts 02115

The field of immunology has made significant progress, augmenting considerably the knowledge of host responses toward neoplasia and leading to the present frontiers.

Introduction

In the present era, scientists find themselves in the midst of enormous efforts to delineate the nature of those responses conferred by the tumor-bearing host and which appear to parallel the various intricacies of immune responses that can be either beneficial or deleterious to the host. The path to these efforts was set down by Gross (49), who, in 1943, suggested that the host immune response was displayed in the destruction of tumor cells transplanted into presensitized mice. However, these suggestions remained neglected until 1953, when Foley (40) provided more conclusive data supporting Gross' claims. Subsequent work by Gorer (47) and Kidd and Toolan (60) revealed that lymphocytes and histiocytes were the effectors against tumor cells and that necrobiosis of both tumor cells and effectors occurred following close interaction. The precedence for tumor-specific antigens had been provided by Rous (101), but not identified and developed until much later through efforts by both virologists and animal biologists, when the concept of virions and/or tumor-specific transplantation antigens was demonstrated to be of considerable importance in the initiation of the host defenses. Thereafter, the impetus for continuous and creative efforts in cancer immunology was provided by the theories of immunosurveillance, so ably developed by Burnet (16) and championed by Thomas (116). Data supporting these concepts were provided by the following findings (65): (a) increased incidence of neoplasms in immunodeficiency and autoimmune diseases; (b) negative influence of immunosuppressive substances on rate of development and extent of metastatic spread of malignancies; (c) the immunosuppressive effects of carcinogens; and (d) the high incidence of tumors in the recipients of kidney transplants during immunosuppressive therapy. However, arguments against these mechanisms have been suggested by Prehn (94), who pointed out that if the above concepts were true, then: (i) tumors that had escaped the surveillance mechanisms would be weakly antigenic or nonantigenic, yet tumor-specific antigens have been detected on most tumor cells; (ii) tumors developing in an unpoliced environment should be strongly antigenic, but they rarely express new antigens; (iii) tumors transplanted across a histocompatibility barrier to thymectomized skin-grafted animals were rejected, whereas the skin was accepted; and (iv) transplantation of syngeneic tumor cells into homografts of skin in experimental animals resulted in the rejection of the skin but not the tumor. The true value of these concepts has been that they have motivated the scientific world into formulating imaginative ideas of experimentation providing vast amounts of knowledge. These motivations have included the disciples of tumor virology and immunology and their parallel efforts have led to the identification of host immune defenses and have thereby effected the study of coordinated and chronological events in the host-tumor relationships.

Organization of the Lymphoid System by Function

Fortunately, the discipline of immunology has already borne witness to a vast amount of information with the precedent having been set by microbiologists, parasitologists, biochemists, and, of course, classical immunologists. Initially these investigators devoted their efforts to the understanding of the many facets of the humoral immune responses and therefore their observations appear to be more complete than those involving cell-mediated immunity. The comprehensive knowledge relating to components of the cell-mediated immune responses has come forward through the efforts of microbiologists and transplantation immunologists. Their endeavors have led to a modeling of the precursor lymphoid system developed through the efforts of Miller (72), Glick (46), and Cooper and Good (25). This organization has benefited from observations by clinical immunologists, who recognized and characterized the paralleling functional anomalies found in immunodeficiency syndromes of children.

Generally speaking, two functionally distinct populations of lymphocytes are involved in the organization of the lymphoid system (see Fig. 1). One cellular component of lymphoid tissue was found to be dependent on the thymus for its development and responded to antigenic stimulation by the expression of the cell-mediated immune response and has therefore been categorized as the thymus-dependent lymphoid system. The second functionally distinct population of small lymphocytes expressed response to antigenic stimulation with the production of humoral antibody and was therefore called the humoral immune response. The cell-mediated immune response (delayed hypersensitivity, allograft rejection, tumor and parasitic immunity, etc.) was found to involve the participation of macrophages and thymus-dependent lymphocytes, but not circulating antibody (cell-bound antibody appears to be present in the cells participating in the cell-mediated reactions). Yet one could classify a factor of the cell-mediated immune response as being dependent on circulating reagenic antibody and basophils and mast cells, which are involved in effecting the immediate hypersensitivity response. This response dif-

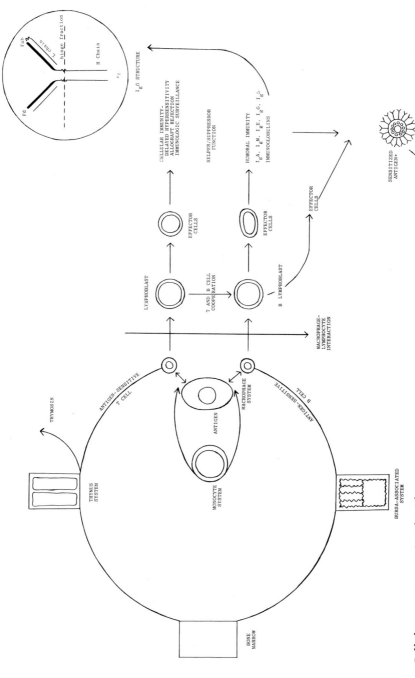

Fig. 1. Cellular events associated with adaptive immunity.

fered from the delayed hypersensitivity response in that it was manifested from within minutes to hours, following contact with the sensitizing antigen, as compared to the delayed hypersensitivity response, which
reached a peak at 24 to 72 hours. Antigenic stimulation has been observed
to elicit within the sensitized host either one, both, or all three types of
immune responses, depending, of course, on the nature of the antigen and
the capabilities of the host. The lymphocytes of the thymus-dependent
lymphoid tissue are called T lymphocytes, whereas those of the
immunoglobulin-producing lymphoid tissue are called B lymphocytes. T
lymphocytes are found in the thymus-dependent lymphoid areas, including the middle and deep cortical ("paracortex") areas of lymph nodes, the
periarteriolar sheaths of the malpighian body of the spleen, and the inter-
nodular space of the gut-associated lymphoid organs (88). B lymphocytes
are located in the nodules and medulla of the lymph nodes, the peripheral
layer of the splenic malphigian body, the perifollicular areas and red pulp
of the spleen, and the nodules of the gut-associated lymphoid system.

Cellular Mechanisms Associated with Induction of the Immune Response

Although the precise pathways of the interaction between the
precursors of the antibody producing thymus-independent B lymphocyte
involved in the humoral response and the thymus-dependent T lymphocyte involved in delayed hypersensitivity (or cell-mediated) immune response have not been thoroughly delineated, there has been no doubt that
these two classes of small lymphocytes, cytologically indistinguishable
from each other at their resting state, participate with the macrophages in
the interactions and processes that constitute the immune response. As
the B lymphocytes and their progeny secrete antigen-specific antibody
molecules and the antigen-combining sites of the surface receptors of the
B lymphocytes that are responsible for their secretion (48, 99) have been
defined, their specificities are well understood. The range of specific
chemical configurations (presented to these cells) against which antibodies can be produced has remained very large, and has resulted in the
observation of extensive variations within B lymphocyte cell receptors
(IgG). As previously mentioned, the humoral immune response to antigen
has been found to consist of at least three phases which may merge into
each other, yet merit being defined as distinct from each other. The inductive, or latent, phase consists of the time between antigenic challenge and
first appearance of antibody, whereas the productive, or logarithmic,
phase describes the rapid increase of circulating antibodies. The circulating antibody levels then reach a plateau—the stationary phase of antibody

production. The nature of response toward first sensitization (primary immune response versus subsequent sensitization (secondary immune response) is characterized by the stationary phase, which reaches a higher level, for a longer time interval, with subsequent sensitizations.

On entering antibody-forming tissue, the antigen interacts with the three functionally different cells—mononuclear phagocyte and T dependent and B independent lymphocyte. The order of interaction remains unclear, although the rank seems determined by means of the specific antigen configurations which lock on the specific determinants present on these cells [Fig. 1]. Following introduction in antibody-forming tissue, the antigen is initially confronted by mononuclear phagocytic cells of the reticuloendothelial system (48). These phagocytes can be either the circulating blood monocyte, the tissue macrophage, or both. The precise nature of the intervention of the macrophage between the antigen and antigen-sensitive lymphocyte remains unclear, but has been progressively characterized. Macrophages are involved in both primary and secondary immune responses, although the extent of participation in each phase may vary (37, 81). Most likely, there are a number of mechanisms by which macrophages help to activate antigen-sensitive lymphocytes. For example, antigen may be presented in an appropriate stimulating form or soluble factors may be elaborated in order to achieve lymphocyte activation (38). This has been evidenced by the gathering of lymphocytes around macrophages to which antigen has bound (following introduction of antigen) and the formation of lymphoreticular islands in the antibody-forming tissue. Thus, the retention of antigen on the surface membranes of the macrophage would allow for contact between it and the lymphocytes continuously moving in the neighborhood (20, 70). At this time, antigen bound to macrophages may be either transferred directly to lymphocytes or processed prior to transfer (103, 120). Direct macrophage-lymphocyte interaction appears to depend on reactions between cell surface receptors that are products of the major histocompatibility gene complex and may involve the Ir gene product (10).

Ingestion of antigen or its retention on the membrane of a reticuloendothelial cell may be enhanced by opsonizing antibody coating target particle or antibody cytophilic to the macrophage (10, 68). Prior to active sensitization of the lymphocyte to the antigen, the macrophage may process the antigen into immunogenic units to which endogenous RNA becomes attached. This antigen-RNA complex may be presented to the pre-committed, to-be-sensitized, lymphocyte (39, 86). This complex has been observed to behave as an adjuvant. Additional evidence for the role of this RNA complex is the finding that the IgM antibody produced by the lymph node cells has allotype markers which are peculiar to the macrophage donor (8). Furthermore, additional supportive evidence for the role of an instructive macrophage RNA has come from work in which nonimmune rabbit spleen cells have been converted by the RNA of lymphoid cells from immunized rabbits to produce both IgM and IgG antibody of the immunized animals' Fc allotype (9). RNA can be employed to induce lymphoid cells to produce a specific migration-inhibiting factor (85). However, immunologic specificity seems to develop during lymphoid differentiation beyond a stem-cell stage (80). Macrophages can become specifically cytotoxic to target cells by means of a factor released specifically by sensitized lymphocytes which subsequently may become bound to the macrophages (34, 69) or they may become armed following interaction with T lymphocytes (35).

The antigens that stimulate antibody responses may be divided into broad functional classes, depending on the lymphocyte class involved—T-cell-dependent and T-cell-independent antigens. T-cell-independent antibody responses to these antigens by B cells are dependent on a harmonious, positive regulatory influence or the helper effect of T cells. Generally, T-cell-independent antigens are polymeric molecules with repeating subunits such as lipopolysaccharide flagellin and polyvinyl pyrrolidone, whereas T-cell-dependent antigens appear to be complex multideterminant antigens such as heterologous erythrocytes and hapten-protein conjugates (36). For some antigens, at least two types of lymphoid cells must interact for antibody production to occur. T lymphocytes may cooperate in antibody production by presenting antigens to B lymphocytes in a form suitable to induce optimum antibody formation (30). In addition to this helper function in humoral antibody production, T lymphocytes may also have a suppressor role that controls the rate of antibody production (43). Suppressor T lymphocytes may function through the release of a soluble factor (115). The antigenically stimulated small lymphocyte with immunoglobulin-producing potential evolves through a series of differentiation and proliferative steps to a mature plasma cell. It passes through a phase in which it appears as a primitive blast cell, when during its metamorphoses it produces IgM and then IgG antibodies. This cell may then mature into plasma cell, where it is restricted to produce IgG. Cells producing IgM and IgG may arise from the same or separate precursor cells (50, 112, 113) following a phenomenon described as IgM–IgG switch.

It appears that the switchover from production of IgM to IgG antibody occurs because of a feedback control mechanism that is dependent on the synthesis of a critical level of IgG antibody (119). Lymphocytes carry distinct markers on their cell surfaces which may combine with specific antigen, thus triggering further immunologic development of the lymphocyte (99). Human peripheral blood B lymphocytes may carry surface determinants of either IgA, IgM, or IgG immunoglobulins (12). The im-

munoglobulin receptors on B lymphocytes in the marrow carry mostly
IgM, whereas those in the peripheral blood carry mostly IgG (1). Following sensitization and prior to production of immunoglobulin by the B
lymphocyte, the immunoglobulin that is randomly dispersed on the cell
surface becomes aggregated over one pole of the cell, undergoing a phenomenon called "capping" (114). This cap is divided by the cell by means
of pinocytosis, after which there is regeneration of the surface immunoglobulin. Although immunoglobulins on B cells have been well studied,
the T lymphocytes may also have surface receptors which appear to be
similar to C_3 and IgM, but in smaller quantities than in the B cells (98).
They also have receptors for adrenergic sensitivity—α-adrenergic receptors may stimulate, whereas β-adrenergic inhibit blast transformation in
vitro. They also have receptors for histamine and prostaglandins of the E
series.

Secondary Immune Response

A secondary immune response occurs when lymphoid tissue is
reexposed to an antigen with which it has had a previous immune encounter. This phase has a shorter induction phase, and there is also a
rapid production of more antibody (mostly IgG) than before. The cells
participating in the secondary immune response are the progeny of cells
sensitized to the antigen during the previous exposure. Generally speaking, the circulating lymphocytes found in the peripheral blood may be
any one of five functionally specific cell types: (a) the uncommitted but
immunologically competent lymphocyte of the immunoglobulin-producing system; (b) the uncommitted but immunologically competent lymphocyte of the thymus-dependent system; (c) the memory cell of the immunoglobulin-producing system; (d) the memory cell of the thymus-dependent system; and (e) the effector cell of the thymus-dependent system.

Cell-Mediated Immunity: Thymus-Dependent
Lymphoid System and Its Reaction

Information on the specificity of T lymphocyte was initially limited to results of functional analysis (89), but as a consequence of studies
of the T lymphocyte receptors there has been considerable knowledge
regarding the restricted range of specificity of these cells, notably the
recognition of histocompatability antigens (109) and the regulatory
functions of the immune response (18). In directing these reactions, the T
cell takes part in precise types of interactions with other cells by means of

recognition of the surface markets of the target cell. This concept of the restricted nature of the range of specific responses mounted by the T cell was first developed as a result of studies of delayed hypersensitivity and contact reactivity (42). T-lymphocyte-dependent responses and their pro-liferation and production of migration inhibition factor (MIF) (29, 91) develop principally in response to protein and polypeptide antigens in contrast to responses following immunization with polyvalent haptens and polysaccharides. As previously mentioned, T lymphocytes have been shown to exert both positive regulatory effects (helper T cells) and nega-tive regulatory effects (suppressor T cells) in the antibody responses (44, 75).

A feature of immune responses to thymus-dependent antigens is that they are controlled in an antigen-specific manner by the operation of major histocompatibility complex (MHC) genes of higher vertebrates (10). The regulatory action of these immune response (Ir) genes has been dem-onstrated through the study of structurally simple antigens regulating not only positive but also specific suppressor responses (31). The role of these genes in the control of immune responses to individual thymus-dependent antigens is significant in that a major function of T lympho-cytes appears to be to recognize and react with MHC gene products of the same and other species (109). An example is the acceptance or prompt rejection of tissue or organ transplants (107), controlled by the specific immune-response genes—genes which regulate mixed lymphocyte reac-tivity and genes which code for a class of membrane glycoproteins. Among the characteristics of the reactivity of T lymphocytes with MHC gene products are: (a) reaction towards the membrane antigens encoded by individual allogeneic MHC heplotype (123); and, (b) heterogeneous functions of the T cell population and the surface antigens that they express (21).

T lymphocytes of different functional classes tend to differ from each other in their recognition of MHC-encoded antigens, whereby one popula-tion of T lymphocytes (killer T cells) may contain cells that lyse al-logeneic, xenogeneic, or modified syngeneic target cells (5, 21). The other principal T cell population reactive with MHC antigens recognizes anti-gens coded for the I region of the MHC and accounts for the mixed lym-phocyte reaction and the graft-versus-host reaction. It can also play a regulatory role in amplifying the immune response that leads to the ap-pearance of killer T cells (102). Thus, the population has the highly specialized capacity to recognize or to be activated by MHC gene products or both, with their ability to react to protein antigens being regulated by the Ir genes encoded in the MHC.

The above findings raise a question as to whether the capacity to recognize thymus-dependent antigens and MHC gene products is a characteristic of a clone of T cell population (or independent T cell populations). The clonal theory is supported by the finding that distinct T cell classes are responsible for effecting the cytotoxic and mixed lymphocyte responses. Contrary evidence is provided by the findings that lymphocytes from nonimmunized donors are reactive with all the alloantigens and xenoantigens controlled by the MHC region, modified autologous antigens (virus-infected cells or tumor cells) for which syngeneic killer T cells have been identified, and all the numerous thymus-dependent antigens. However, Simonsen (108) and Heber-Katz and Wilson (51) have proposed that the same clones of T cells that are reactive to the MHC gene products may also be reactive with thymus-dependent antigens. In order to reconcile these differences, one must follow the work of Zinkernagel and Doherty (124) and Shearer, Rehn, et al. (106), who demonstrated that MHC gene products do participate in the specificity of T lymphocyte responses mediated principally towards non-MHC antigens. These excellent studies examined the specificity of T-lymphocyte-effected lysis of syngeneic target cells which were modified either by chemicals or virus infection and showed that the modified membrane antigens of these target cells could express their killer activity when the target cells were of the same MHC type as the killer cells. Thus, the sensitizing cell and the target cell (as well as the killer T cell) had to share similar MHC configurations, which suggested that the same determinants (i.e., MHC gene products and thymus-dependent antigen) must be used for both primary sensitizing and secondary killer responses. However, additional experiments have also indicated that the MHC restriction required similarity between the sensitizing cell and target cell, rather than similarity between the target and killer cells.

Evidence suggesting the involvement of MHC gene products in sensitization and elicitation of T lymphocyte responses to conventional antigens has been supported by studies revealing an activation of T lymphocytes by macrophages that had been minimally exposed to antigen and a subsequent cooperation between T and B lymphocytes. It also appears that the antigen-processing macrophage and the immunogen-receptive T lymphocyte have similarities in their MHC-I region determinants (100), an event that appears to be of further importance in the primary and secondary B-cell-dependent antibody responses (59, 73). Several lines of evidence now suggest that collaboration for both systems is restricted by a requirement that the macrophage, or B cell, participating in the primary response be similar in its I region. Collaboration between primed T and B cells has led to a similar conclusion—namely, that the interacting cells must be obtained from donors which are similar in the region of MHC. However, collaboration is not restricted by this locus (90).

Thus, responsiveness to the well-recognized thymus-dependent antigens requires the recognition of the antigen in the context of an appropriate gene product. This responsiveness is associated with two of the principal types of antigens for which T cells appear to be specific. A function of these Ir genes may be to induce molecular associations of antigen and MHC gene products on the macrophage or B cell (or both) to produce an immunogen. An additional function may be expressed within T lymphocytes as a part of the system through which either thymus-dependent antigen or MHC gene product is recognized on the cell surface.

T lymphocytes may exert critical regulatory controls on the immune response of B lymphocytes and of other T lymphocytes. Separate classes of T cells can mediate the positive helper and the negative suppressor cell functions (22). The regulatory action exerted by T cells appears to be more complex than the more simple negative or positive control of antibody responses in general, and involves the selective action of T lymphocytes, together with antigen, on clones of responding and proliferating cells with distinctive functional phenotypes. Some of the phenomena that reflect these fine regulating activities of T lymphocytes on B lymphocyte differentiation can be cited as follows: (i) the stimulation of antibody responses of IgG, as compared to IgM (95); (ii) the selection of precursor cells that secrete a given class or subclass of immunoglobulin and even its allotype variants (52); (iii) the increase in the affinity of antibody during the immune response (45); (iv) the selective activation of a clonally restricted hapten-specific antibody which is dependent on the thymus-dependent carrier molecule to which the hapten is conjugated (23); (v) the expression of the idiotypes on antibody molecules specific for complementary determinants present on the same carrier molecule (82); and (vi) the selection of precursors of antibody-forming cells which produce hapten-specific antibody of a net charge opposite to that of the carrier molecule forming the hapten-carrier conjugate (105). It has also been observed that the specificity of the regulatory activity by the T lymphocyte indicates that the individual helper T lymphocyte expresses three different kinds of specificity: capacity to recognize thymus-dependent antigens, MHC gene products, and membrane markers reflecting cell immunoglobulin potential. Undoubtedly as the data become less circumstantial and more complete, one can begin to decide for oneself which mechanism remains principal in consideration of the antigen employed for experimentation.

Role of Cytophilic Antibody in Cell-Mediated Immune Responses

As stated previously, delayed hypersensitivity and humoral immunity are two functionally distinct immune responses. A single antigen can elicit either one or both types of responses following administration in the mammalian host. Although it has been succinctly clarified that circulating antibody does not seem to participate in cell-mediated immune reactions, it may not be without a humoral component. The surface membranes of specifically sensitized small lymphocytes may carry antibodies that allow them to recognize and react with the specific antigen to which they have become immune. These antibodies appear to have a high affinity for the lymphocyte and could be released on direct contact with antigen. The macrophages that participate in the delayed hypersensitivity reaction possess surface receptors to cytophilic antibody which could also play a role in the recognition and binding of antigen at a reaction site (15).

Molecular Mediators of Cellular Immune Induction

Following antigenic stimulation, T lymphocytes will produce and release a number of soluble factors, called lymphokines, that are believed to play a significant role in cellular immune reactions (92). B lymphocytes may also have the capacity to produce some of these factors (with identical physiochemical characteristics)—namely, migration inhibitory factor, monocyte chemotactic factor, leucocyte inhibitory factor, and interferon. These lymphokines are cell-free soluble factors which are generated during interaction of sensitized lymphocytes and antigen, but which by themselves are expressed without immune specificity (33). They can also be released following nonspecific mitogenic stimulation. Many of these substances are proteins (110) of 30,000 to 60,000 molecular weight and exhibit the capacity to confer delayed hypersensitivity skin reactions in the skin of experimental animals.

1. MIGRATION INHIBITORY FACTOR (MIF). The original observations of Rich and Lewis (96) have been extended to develop an assay system for in vitro correlation of delayed hypersensitivity (96) involving MIF which has been known to mediate an inhibition of macrophage migration from antigenic site and may also activate them. MIF is obtained from the supernatants of lymphocytes cultured with antigens for periods of about 7 days and has been found to be a glycoprotein (guinea pig) with a molecular weight of about 50,000, and lacks species-specificity (41). It appears to be produced by sensitized lymphocytes in vivo after reaction with specific antigen (11). The MIF then functions to immobilize macrophages at the site of the reaction. The inhibition of human leukocyte migration has been studied as an in vitro correlate of in vivo delayed hypersensitivity (28). In addition, RNA extracted from immune-specific lymph nodes has been observed to transfer inhibition of migration to cells from an unsensitized host (117) and may also initiate antibody production.

2. LYMPHOTOXIN. Lymphocytes stimulated *in vitro* by antigen phytohemagglutinin, or allogeneic lymphocytes can produce a nonspecific lymphocytotoxin that is toxic to target cells and can be assayed by means of exposing mitomycin treated cell lines to supernatants of PHLA-stimulated lymphocytes thought to contain lymphocytotoxin (111).

3. TRANSFER FACTOR. In man, it is possible to transfer tuberculin or streptococcal sensitivity from one individual to another with injections of viable leukocytes (62) or whole blood (76) or extracts of hypersensitive leukocytes. This nonimmunogenic active agent, originating probably in a small lymphocyte (initially described by Lawrence) has now been referred to as the "transfer factor." The transfer factor has the capacity to confer delayed hypersensitivity and allograft rejection ability without the capacity to confer production of antibodies. It can act across species barriers, with sensitivity persisting up to two years. In addition, it has the ability *in vitro* to induce lymphocyte transformation to specific antigens in previously unsensitized lymphocytes (76).

Amongst its properties are: (i) it is dialyzable; (ii) its molecular weight is less than 10,000; (iii) it is unaffected by DNAase, RNAase, and trypsin; (iv) it is stable at $-20°C$; and (v) it is a nonprotein and an RNA-like substance consisting of polynucleotides and polypeptides. Effectivity depends on the ability of the recipient of a transfer factor to possess the capacity to produce a specific immune response. It is degraded by RNAase III, which will degrade double-stranded RNA, suggesting that transfer factor consists of mainly a double-stranded RNA polynucleotide (93). Also, in higher animals, transfer factor may have an active nondialyzable fraction with a molecular weight of 150,000 (14).

4. INTERFERON. Following antigenic, nonspecific mitogenic or viral stimulation, human lymphocytes will produce interferon. Interferon has been observed to have several effects in addition to its antiviral activities. These include an ability to enhance phagocytosis and cytotoxicity by sensitized lymphocytes. It will also inhibit mitosis and the colony-stimulating factor (71).

5. CHEMOTACTIC FACTOR. Chemotactic factors for both monocytes and polymorphonuclear leucocytes have been found in the supernatants of antigen-stimulated lymphocyte cultures (121). These factors are distinct from each other and from MIF.

6. PROSTAGLANDINS. Stimulation of human lymphocytes with antigens or nonspecific mitogens in culture will lead to formation and release of prostaglandin E, a fatty acid precursor most likely derived from cell membrane phospholipid and may (in high concentrations) effect a feedback inhibition (PGE_2) of the immune response (32).

7. THYMOSIN. A purified extract of the thymus has been characterized by the ability of the serum tested to modify rosette-forming cells present in the spleen of adult thymectomized mice (6). It is present in serum and maintains a well-functioning T-dependent lymphocyte-mediated immunity.

Immunoglobulin

Since 1938, when Tiselius and Kabat demonstrated that antibodies were predominantly gammaglobulins, mainly five classes of immunoglobulins have been recognized—IgG, IgA, IgM, IgD, and IgE, in order of descending concentration in serum. The fundamental structure of immunoglobulins has been found to consist of a pair of identical polypeptide chains containing approximately 200 amino acids (light chains), linked by disulfide bonds to a pair of larger polypeptide chains of about 450 amino acids called heavy chains (H-chains) (see Fig. 1). Of these chains, about one-half of the amino acids on the terminal reactive portion are interchangeable, whereas the remaining sequences appear to be constant.

Generally speaking, antibody molecules are bivalent, which allows for antibodies to crosslink with two antigenic groups and subsequently results in clumping or agglutination, a process that enables the clearing of antigen in the blood stream. Besides variation in each antibody molecule that determines its specificity for the antigen, additional differences are present in the common, or Fc, region, which has allowed for the formal classification of immunoglobulins.

IgG (γ-G, β_2-globulin, 7S-γ-globulin, and complement-fixing γ-globulin) represents the most common form of antibody molecule in man, comprising about 70% of the total γ-globulin pool. Its structure has been regarded as a prototype for other forms of immunoglobulin. It consists of the usual four-polypeptide-chain structure, with two light chains and two heavy chains. The light chains have been antigenically differentiated into kappa (κ) and lambda (λ) chains, and the heavy chains called the gamma (γ) chain. The chain has been characterized as four antigenic types which differentiate the γ G into four subclasses—namely, IgG_1, IgG_2, IgG_3, and IgG_4, according to the descending order of concentration. IgG$_1$ consists of about 70% of the total IgG pool and fixes complement along with IgG$_3$ (8%). IgG$_2$ represents 18% of the total IgG pool and weakly fixes complement, whereas IgG$_4$ (4%) does not fix complement. In the common region of the γ chain is a portion of the molecule which is altered after the Fab regions have reacted with antigen, and this alteration in shape activates the complement pathway.

IgA (γ-A or β2A-globulin) is called the secretory immunoglobulin and is found predominantly in salivary and gastrointestinal secretions. Following its synthesis, it is attached to an additional protein called transport, or T, protein, produced by the mucosal cell and attached during its secretory transport. It protects this immunoglobulin against denaturation. IgA reflects about 10% of the total γ-globulin pool.

IgM (m.w. 900,000) has a heavy chain that represents a pentamer of 5-γ-G subunits attached by disulfide bonds to terminal Fc fragments. IgM is the first class to be formed after immunization and remains within the circulation, being unable to pass the vascular barrier. They fix complement and appear to be 700 to 1000 times more efficient than IgG in agglutinating and lysing. The antibodies to ABO blood groups are reflected in this immunoglobulin.

IgD (δ chain) is present in trace qualities and its function has been poorly defined.

IgE (ε) has been distinguished from IgA by its antigenically different heavy chain. It has a significant role in allergic diseases, where sensitizing γ-E coats Fc receptors on basophils and mast cells with their Fc portion and stimulates release of vasoactive amines and lipids, resulting in allergic reactions.

Immediate Hypersensitivity and Reagin Allergy Reactions

Immediate hypersensitivity and reagin-mediated allergic reactions differ from humoral immunity reactions in that cells are involved in their effective reactions; they differ from delayed hypersensitivity responses in that circulating antibody and basophils or mast cells participate in effecting this reaction, which occurs within minutes to hours, as compared to days for the delayed hypersensitivity reactions. It was initially observed by Portier and Richet, during their attempts at developing immunity to sea anemone toxins in dogs, that on second injection of the toxin the dogs became violently ill and frequently died abruptly, and thereafter the increased susceptibility was named anaphylaxis. Subsequently, Arthus found that intradermal injection of antigen into previously immunized animals produced local inflammation and necrosis at the site of antigen administration—whence named the Arthus Reaction, of which the systemic version is called serum sickness.

As the actual interaction of antibody and its corresponding antigen is usually beneficial to the host, some additional amplifying or mediating mechanism is needed to effect the harmful action on the host. There have been several effector systems delineated (see Fig. 1), and the common denominator of these diverse effector mechanisms is that the Fc portion of the antibody molecule is usually the focal point of participation, either alone or together with effector cells such as macrophages, granulocytes, and mast cells. Of these, the best understood is the one associated with reagin-mediated allergy (83). The single most serious disease included in the category is asthma, with a more common condition being allergic rhinitis. By the early 1920s, Prausnitz and Kausner demonstrated that the skin reactivity to antigen could be demonstrated from patient to patient with serum; the active principle was called reagin, which was subsequently characterized as IgE by the Ishizakas and by Bennich and Johansson. Hypersensitivity reactions have been classified by Gells and Coombs into four categories based on the nature of the antibody or effector cell, the nature of the antigen, and the time course of the reaction. Generally speaking, reagin-mediated allergy is considered as Class I, and reactions involving other types of immunoglobulins are considered Class II when the antigen is cell-bound, or Class III when the antigen is soluble and tissue damage is caused by deposition antigen-antibody complexes. The Class IV reactions are those of the cell-mediated type, commonly considered to be the delayed-hypersensitivity type.

A number of laboratory models have been developed for the study of reagenic antibodies and the reactions they initiate. This knowledge has arrived through helminthic infestations and *Bordetella pertussis* antigens, which are potent stimuli for production of IgE antibodies (118). Usually, serum IgE levels are elevated early during the primary sensitization and cannot be boosted following reinjection (77). Thymus-dependent lymphocytes and specific helper T cells in cooperation may be essential for synthesis although thymectomy results in increased production of IgE. The anaphylactic state induced by active sensitization of the host by antigen is called *active anaphylaxis* and that obtained by administration of antibody, *passive anaphylaxis*. In active anaphylaxis, the first injection of antigen is called the sensitizing injection, and the second the shocking dose. The route of administration of the sensitizing injection can vary, whereas the shocking dose must be administered intravenously in order to observe consistent results, although a larger amount of antigen administered by means of subcutaneous or intracutaneous injection (or inhalation) can elicit the same results (83). Subthreshold injections may result in desensitization of the response to the specific antigen. In passive anaphylaxis, antibody is administered to the host and followed by a shocking dose of antigen 24 to 48 hours later (63). Sometimes antigen may be administered initially, followed by an intraveous injection of antibody, with the same resultant reaction, called *reversed passive anaphylaxis*. Cutaneous anaphylaxis can be observed when the local skin site is sensitized by an intracutaneous injection of antibody (or antigen and antibody) and the mixture of antigen and dye injected intravenously 3 to 6 hours later. The reaction is called *passive cutaneous anaphylaxis (PCA)* if antibody is injected before the antigen and *reversed PCA* if the antigen is injected before the antibody. These reactions are dependent on the presence of basophils and mast cells having antigen-specific IgE bound to specific receptors on their membrane surfaces (56). Upon exposure to sensitizing antigen, these cells release much of their stored pharmacological mediators of anaphylaxis (especially histamine), which cause localized increases in capillary permeability and smooth muscle contraction.

Scientists have begun to divide anaphylactic reactions into two operational subgroups: cytotropic and aggregate (55, 57). In cytotropic antibody-mediated anaphylaxis, antibodies sensitize primary target cells so that subsequent interaction with antigen discharges chemical mediators from the target cell, which affect capillary permeability, smooth muscle contraction, and so on, at secondary sites. An antibody derived from the same species is referred to as homocytotropic and that from a different species, heterocytotropic. There are both heat-stable (IGa) and heat-labile (IgE) antibodies for basophils and mast cells (7, 54). Aggregate anaphylaxis does not require a latent period between the administration of antibody and challenge with antigen (as sensitization is not involved), but nevertheless the resultant effects are due to release of the same mediators. For example, an aggregate system can activate the complement cascade and its effective subunits (as discussed below).

The Pharmacological Mediators of Anaphylaxis

The classic mediator of anaphylaxis is the highly potent histamine molecule, which is found as an ion exchange resin to the anionic polymers in the granules of mast cells and basophils (7). Following reaction (during mediator release) with sensitizing antigen, the membranes of these cells develop invaginations which fuse with the perigranular membrane surrounding the mediator-containing granules. Subsequently, the granule contents come into direct contact with the extracellular milieu and the cationic mediators are released into the medium in exchange for Na^+ and K^+ ions. The reaction is generally over in a matter of seconds and minutes and is self-limiting, although the cells rarely give up all their stored mediators and, at this time, the cells undergo a period during which they are not capable of further release of mediators. In addition to histamine, the mast cell may contain serotonin, which is also released during the reaction and has pharmacological properties similar to those of histamine (7). A third mediator of anaphylaxis, eosinophile chemotactic factor (ECF–A), also released in parallel to histamine, has a molecular weight below 1000 (peptide linkages are present) and is relatively specific for chemotactic activity for eosinophiles (4). Slow-releasing substance of anaphylaxis (SRS–A) may not be present in the cell granules in the preformed state, but may be produced prior to release by either a basophil or another polymorphonuclear leucocyte (7). It binds strongly to albumin (pure properties are thus difficult to obtain), but is relatively soluble in polar organic solvents in the presence of base. The contractions caused by this lipid-like material are characteristically slower in onset (4).

Plasma Kinins

Kraut, Frey, and Werle (4) were the first to demonstrate that there was hypotension following intravenous injection of pancreatic extract in dogs; the active principle was called kallikrein. Subsequent studies revealed that kallikrein reacted with plasma α-globulin, called kininogen, to form a smooth muscle stimulation by means of a substance called kallidin. Trypsin and some snake venoms also released a similar hypotensive, smooth muscle contracting substance called bradykinin (kalladin I), nonapeptide lacking the amino acid lysine and kalladin I [decapeptide = kalladin I + lysine]. In addition, plasmin, a fibrinolytic agent, also has been observed to have kinin-forming abilities and permeability-producing globulin (PF/dil) has similar actions. These agents, in addition to increasing permeability and smooth muscle stimulation, also initiate vasodilation and migration of leukocytes, and stimulate pain fibers.

Eosinophils in Anaphylaxis

There is ample evidence that eosinophils appear in the wake of anaphylactic reactions, and other forms of immediate hypersensitivity and concomitant eosinophilia are reflected by such hosts (87). These cells tend to aggregate at sites where antigen-antibody complexes form, and may be responsible for their clearance (67) by means of phagocytosis. They have been found to ingest bacteria as well as granules released from basophils and mast cells (122) and may also handle the released mediators such as histamine (7).

Immediate-hypersensitivity reactions differ from delayed-hypersensitivity reactions in that they are visible within minutes to a few hours and are initiated primarily by humoral reagenic antibodies produced by B lymphocytes in cooperation with T lymphocytes, as compared to the delayed-hypersensitivity reaction, which is mediated by T lymphocytes and visible within hours to 1 to 2 days or more. The immediate-hypersensitivity reactions have been further classified by means of the effector mechanism involved. Immediate-hypersensitivity reactions requiring antibody alone are quite rare, but can occur in clinical situations such as insulin therapy in diabetes mellitus and Factor VIII therapy in hemophilia A. They can also occur following antibody reactions in which the complement cascade has been activated. The enzymatic activity of $C_{\overline{42}}$ on C_3 produces a low-molecular-weight fragment called anaphylatoxin that can mimic the symptoms of anaphylaxis. Activation of the alternate pathway can also be initiated by aggregated immunoglobulins IgG_{1-4}, IgA, and IgE and the initiation site resides on the Fab position of the immunoglobulin molecule. There are several effector systems discussed hereafter and they serve as a means of classifying immediate hypersensitivity reactions (66).

Reactions Requiring Only Antibody

Immediate-hypersensitivity reactions involving antibody exclusively are rare; such are those involved with anti-insulin and antifactor VIII antibodies which have been known to result in the depletion of the active molecule.

Reactions Requiring Antibody and Complement

During the study of lytic properties of antisera, it was discovered that both a specific antibody and complementary nonspecific factors found in fresh serum were required for cell lysis. These factors are called the complement system, one major function of which is to mediate cell lysis in immediate-type hypersensitivity. The classical complement system consists of nine separate components (C_1 through C_9), which, following activation, interact sequentially with one another in a cascade fashion similar in principle to the coagulation sequence. The numbers do not follow the order of their activation; C_4 is out of sequence, being activated

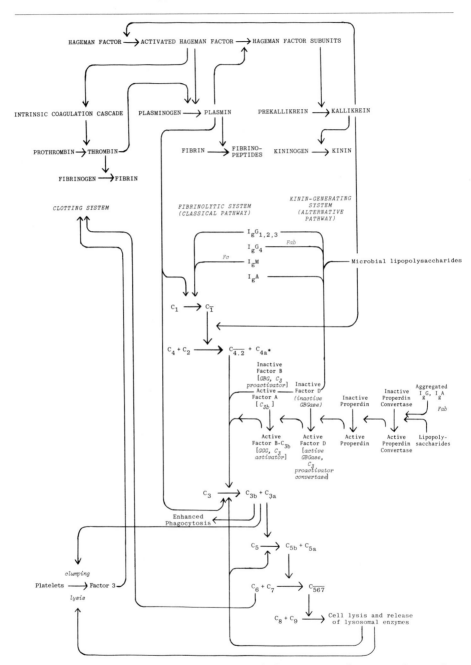

Fig. 2. Complement activation: Primary and alternating pathways and coagulation, fibrinolytic, and kinin-generating interactions.

second. Therefore the activation sequence is C_1, C_4, C_2, C_3, C_5, C_6, C_7, C_8, C_9 (see Fig. 2). In general, the activation of the components of the complement system involves enzymatic cleavage of each component into two fragments—the larger of the two fragments joins the activated preceding component, generating a new enzymatic activity that pursues cleavage of the next component. The smaller fragments are biologically active and contain important inflammatory activities. The first component of the complement system consists of three separate proteins, C_{1q}, C_{1r}, and C_{1s}, held together in a trimolar complex by calcium. Activation of the C_1 complex involves binding of C_{1q} subunit to at least two adjacent Fc portions of immunoglobulin molecules. The C_{1q} binding induces C_{1r} to activate C_{1s}. A single molecule of IgM or at least two closely placed IgG_1 or IgG_3 molecules can provide the Fc portions, whereas IgG_4 cannot activate C_1.

The Complement Cascade

"Complement" is a term employed in a system of factors occurring in normal serum that are activated by antigen-antibody interaction and subsequently mediate a number of biologically significant consequences. It is a heat-labile serum cofactor associated with immune hemolysis and bactericidal reactions. Since the original identification of C_3 as βic-globulin by Müller-Eberhard (78), the great majority of complement components and their inhibitors and alternate pathways of their activation have been determined. In addition to the previously mentioned interactions, this system has been thought to be more important in vivo in the facilitation of phagocytosis and exhibits degrees of involvement in other plasma enzyme cascades, such as the blood-clotting system. Generally speaking, the factors associated with the lysis of antibody-coated erythrocytes by the "classical" pathway are called the 9 complement components (consisting of 11 individual proteins) and have been given numbers designated as C_1–C_9. The immunochemical properties of the 9 numbered components are seen in Figure 2, which gives a general scheme in regard to the cascade of complement activation.

The first component of complement C_1 is a macromolecular complex held together by calcium ions which, if chelated by EDTA, break into three subcomponents, C_{1q}, C_{1r}, and C_{1s}. It appears that this molecule contains six subunits made up of three different types of polypeptide chains (a part of each being sensitive to collagen) and carries the binding site for fixed antibody. There is a central subunit joined by connecting strands to the six terminal subunits resembling flower heads, where the antibody-binding sites may be located. C_{1q} in the presence of EDTA can precipitate aggregated γ-globulin and soluble immune complexes and may also bind

IgG. In man, it binds with IgM, IgG_1, IgG_3, and IgG_2 (according to intensity) and does not react with IgG_4, IgA, IgD, or IgE. C_{1r} can act proteolytically with C_{1s} to activate it, a reaction that can be inhibited by the $C_{\overline{1}}$-inhibitor and also Ca^{++}. C_{1s} carries the proenzyme site which, on activation, is converted to $C_{\overline{1}}$, the enzyme that subsequently acts on C_4 and then on C_2. The reaction between C_1 and immunoglobulins appears to occur at some site in the third domain of heavy chain and two closely adjacent IgG molecules, or with a single IgM molecule.

It appears that C_4 is the primary substrate of $C_{\overline{1}}$ with resultant fragments C_{4a} and C_{4b}. C_{4a} is split off and the remaining major fragment C_{4b} has an activated binding site capable of combining with receptors on cell membranes (by hydrophobic binding) or IgG molecules, or on other C_4 molecules during its short nascent stage. In the presence of Mg^{++}, C_2 will bind to activated C_4 in the absence of $C_{\overline{1}}$, but the binding is reversible and not associated with splitting of C_2. However, if $C_{\overline{1}}$ is present, then splitting of C_2 occurs and the larger fragment C_{2b} remains attached to C_4, thereby forming the second complement enzyme—C_3 convertase, or C_{42}. The biological activity of the other C_2 fragments formed—one having molecular weight of 60,000—resembles that of kinins. C_{42} is unstable, with a half-life of 7 minutes, and C_2 elutes in inactive form, leaving C_4 bound at the complement-fixation site, where it can react with further C_2 to generate $C_{\overline{42}}$. Once $C_{\overline{3}}$ convertase is generated at the complement-fixation site, there is no further requirement for C_1.

C_3 is the bulk component of complement that can be removed by absorption with yeast (a phenomenon related to the alternate pathway to be discussed later). $C_{\overline{42}}$ action on C_3 splits a small fragment C_{3a} (m.w. 7,000), which has chemotactic and anaphylotoxic activity. The larger portion C_{3b} has a binding site analogous to that described for C_4, and becomes attached to cell membrane. The fixation of C_{3b} at the complement-fixation site brings about biologically important consequences, mainly the C_3 adherence reactions and the feedback alternate pathway. C_{3b} which is liberated and is rapidly broken down into serum βiA globulin, C_{3c}, C_{3b}, βic globulin, and C_{3d} (Ig_2D globulin). These are called A and D determinants of C_3.

Both $C_{\overline{42}}$ and C_{3b} and C_5, C_6, C_7 are required at the complement-fixation site for the generation of the heat-stable intermediate. The final component after the reaction of C_7 is the trimolecular complex $C_{\overline{567}}$, which binds to membranes. C_5 is the first component to react; C_{5a} (m.w., 15,000) is split off, which has the biological activity of naphylotoxin and chemotactic factor. The large fragment C_{5b} binds to the complement-fixation site. C_6 is the first component to be bound and gives rise to $C_{\overline{56}}$. C_7 is the last to react and binds membrane only minimally, but is primarily a chemotactic factor. The binding of C_8 and C_9 are required to mediate lysis. It appears that

C_8 is the major factor in the production of lysis. Both C_8 and C_9 are bound to the complement-fixing site—C_8 binds to $C_{\overline{567}}$ and C_9 to C_8. Lysis can be prevented by keeping the temperature at $0°$ C., suggesting that additional steps are involved to complete lysis which is on lipid aspects of the membrane, suggesting involvement of phospholipidase activity (26, 66).

Alternate Pathway of Complement Activation

Just as there are two pathways in the coagulation sequence, there are also two pathways for activation of the complement sequence: the classical pathway and the alternate pathway. The alternate pathway is the properidin system (see Fig. 2). Although many questions remain unanswered, the end result is an enzyme that is distinct from C_{42}, but continues the activation of C_3 and then the subsequent classical cascade (66), thereby bypassing the C_{142} of the classical cascade. Activation of the alternate pathway can be initiated by aggregated immunoglobulin $IgG_{1,2,3,4}$, IgA, and IgE and also by bacterial endotoxins, their cell walls, and polysaccharides such as insulin.

Complement and Inflammation

In addition to its lytic function, the activation of the complement cascade plays a very important role in the inflammatory process. As mentioned before, activation of C_3 and C_5 and, most likely C_4 (also C_2), leads to cleaving of the native protein molecule into two parts, of which one proceeds to be involved in the sequential activation of the cascade and ultimate cytolysis; the other fragments are capable of initiating and participating in the inflammatory process. The active molecules produced during C_3 and C_5 activation are C_{3a} and C_{5a}, which are low-molecular-weight compounds called anaphylatoxins that can contract smooth muscle and increase vascular permeability by means of release of vasoactive amines from mast cells. They are also chemotactic in that they attract polymorphonuclear leukocytes to the site of anaphylatoxin production. Cleavage of C_2 and/or C_4 leads to the liberation of a kinin-like moeity that contracts smooth muscle and increases vascular permeability by bypassing histamine release. C_{567} also has chemotactic factor and allows for not only participation in antibody-effected injury, but also antibody-directed inflammatory reactions. In addition to complement, there are also other enzyme effector systems which amplify inflammatory reactions. These are found in the clotting system and include the fibrinolytic (plasmin) system and the kinin system. It has been known for some time that the addition of immune complexes to blood or plasma can activate the clotting system, initiated by the clumping and adherence of platelets to C_{3b} in the immune complex and secondary release of platelet factor 3. In addition, activation of C_6 can also promote clotting. Activation of the Hageman Factor (Factor VII) initiates not only the intrinsic coagulation sequence, but also the plasmin system, which polymerizes fibrin into vasoactive fibrinopeptides, and activated Hageman Factor into fragments that activate the kinin system, which then reflects increased vascular permeability, chemotaxis of polymorphonuclear leukocytes, pain, and production of Fragment Kf (making C_1 efficient in the production of C_{42}) and can also initiate the complement cascade and generate anaphylatoxin from C_3. C_1 esterase inhibition can not only control the complementary system, but also results in the inhibition of plasmin, kinin generation, thrombin, and activated Factor VII.

Reactions Requiring Antibody and Macrophage

Not all antigen-antibody reactions (i.e., most immune hemolytic anemias) initiate the complement cascade. The antibodies in most immune hemolytic anemias are of the IgG class, and when bound to the red blood cell membrane are too widely separated to activate C_1. Nonetheless, these erythrocytes are destroyed by effector cells of the reticuloendothelial system—namely, macrophages which may be coated cytophilic antibodies (not to be confused with homocytotropic IgE antibodies). The erythrocytes are held in intimate contact with the reticuloendothelial by the antibody-laden macrophage, whereby they can be phagocytized and destroyed. There is additional evidence that lymphocytes can also serve as the effector cell with similar modes of action.

Reactions Requiring Antibody and Mast Cells

Mast cells contain metachromatic granules which are reservoirs for histamine, serotonin, and other vasoactive substances, allowing for an important effector mechanism in immediate hypersentivity. These chemical mediators increase vascular permeability, contract smooth muscle, and also activate Factor VII, hence, the intrinsic pathway of coagulation. Although several mechanisms exist for the release of these mediators, the most important involve mast cell cytotropic IgE antibodies; these, following reaction to the sensitizing antigen, attach to the membrane by their Fc receptors and disrupt the mast cell membrane (with subsequent release of the mediators).

Reactions Requiring Antibody, Complement, and Mast Cells

Anaphylaxis is divided into either the cytotropic IgE-dependent reaction or an aggregate-complement-dependent type mediated by means of the C_{3a} and C_{5a} anaphylatoxins, which can also provoke mast cells into releasing their vasoactive amines by reacting with distinct membrane rocoptors. In some species, platelets (which are reservoirs of vasoactive amines) can mediate these reactions by clumping about immune complexes or platelet lysis. It is certain that particulate immune complexes with C_{3b} promote immune adherence of the platelets onto the complexes, which can in turn result in release of the vasoactive substances without lysis of closely associated "innocent bystander" platelets. [See Fig. 2.]

Reactions Requiring Antibody, Complement, and Polymorphonuclear Leukocytes

The essential role of polymorphonuclear leukocytes in immediate hypersensitivity reactions is illustrated in experimental glomerulone-phritis with the antibody reacting with the glomerular basement membrane. The severity of the reaction is directly proportional to the number of polymorphonuclear leukocytes accumulating within the glomerulus, and the reaction can be delayed by depleting these effector cells and replenishing their transfusion into the host. Activation of the complement cascade is the major mechanism in this entity with participation of C_{3a}, C_{5a}, and C_{567}, which are chemotactic for the polymorphonuclear leukocytes. Following aggregation on the glomerular basement membrane, these effector cells will release enzymes (such as protease and peroxidases) within their lysozomes; effecting glomerular injury and subsequent attempts to phagocytoze the membrane-bound antibody results also in the stripping away of the endothelial lining from the intimate glomerular capillaries. In addition, activation of the clotting system can also play an important part in this type of glomerular injury.

Reactions Requiring Immune Complexes

Immediate hypersensitivity reactions associated with immune complexes often result in injury to cells and tissues which do not possess antigenic determinants but are actually innocent bystanders. The immune complexes are produced when there is an excess of antigen and, following antigen-antibody reaction during this entity, the circulating insoluble or soluble immune complexes are either cleared by the reticuloendothelial system or remain to injure, directly or indirectly, cells or tissue that happen to be in their vicinity. The vast amount of data pertaining to this system has been made available through the association of these mechanisms with the destruction of platelets and/or red blood cells. Two aspects of complement activation need to be considered in order to consider the mechanism of red blood cell or platelet destruction—first, the distinction between the fluid phase and membrane-bound activation, and, secondly, the erythrocyte and platelet membrane receptors that interact with C_{3b} to promote their immune adherence to immune complexes containing C_{3b}, the closely adherent cells being susceptible to clearing by the reticuloendothelial system. Some activated complement components may exist either freely or bound to receptors on membranes, or as antibody in the fluid phase. Activated C_{567} can exist in the fluid phase and can attach to nearby bystander cells, whereafter C_{567} forms a nidus (at this site) for C_8 and C_9 uptake and the consequential lysis of these innocent bystanders.

The mechanism of immune complex-induced tissue injury appears to be more complex than that of cells. Among the pertinent prerequisites that must be satisfied for mediation of tissue injury is the size of the immune complexes themselves. For example, large immune complexes (as seen in situations of antibody excess) are readily phagocytozed by the reticuloendothelial system and do not circulate freely, thereby preventing the opportunity for deposition in the tissue. On the other hand, although small-molecular-weight immune complexes (less than 19S) which are dictated by conditions of antigen excess persist in the circulation, they are just too small to be deposited in the tissue. Thus, they must not only be of a certain size to initiate injury to bystander tissue, but may need to contain a certain immunoglobulin type such as IgG or IgE (depending on the nature of the antigen) and their subsequent mediators to effect their injury. It seems that immune complex deposits occur during a limited time period when there is an equivalence balance of a ratio between circulating antigen and antibody. Early during antibody production, when antigen is in excess, the complexes are small, whereas later on, during the period of antibody excess, the resultant large immune complexes are cleared by the reticuloendothelial system. The glomerular deposition of immune complexes can actually result in injury, even when there is deficiency of complement and polymorphonuclear leukocytes.

Other Types of Immunologic Reactions

1. IMMUNOLOGIC TOLERANCE. Immunologic tolerance has been defined as the state of nonreactivity to an antigen that would ordinarily result in an immunological response. Here the tolerance is specific for the test antigen and is actively acquired, whereas that which is present normally for the antigenic determinants of the challenged subject's own tissue (one's immune apparatus) is in a state of tolerance to one's own tissue. The induction of tolerance was first attempted experimentally in fetuses and neonatal animals, an approach prompted by the observation by Owen (84) that dizygotic twin calves could possess two genetically distinct blood group types, their own and their twin's. In these instances, it was observed that anastomotic placental vessels allowed for in utero exchange of blood cells and that erythropoietic stem cells passed between the fraternal twins and produced two genetically distinct red blood cells in each twin resulting in mosaicism and each twin becoming a chimera (19). This exchange of cells may have occurred at a time in embryonic life when the body would accept foreign antigens as self-antigens, thereby allowing for their continued existence in the adult.

Potentially self-reactive T lymphocytes may be rendered tolerant to self-antigens due to the presence in the serum of soluble self-antigens in tolerogenic form (24). These can perhaps react with receptors on the cell surface of the lymphocytes and block them. Similar states can be mediated by antigen-antibody complexes, assuming that they involve self-antigens (2). Suppressor T lymphocytes may also prevent auto-antibody formation and could act in addition to the mechanism of specific deletion or destruction of clones of cells that might be capable of anti-self-immune reactions to preserve self-tolerance (17). In order that tolerance continue to be active, the antigen must persist within the body and, therefore, is most effectively maintained with cellular antigens where the antigen-bearing cells continue to divide, providing a continual source of antigen. Tolerance can be induced by overwhelming the immune capacity of adult animals with large amounts of antigen (58), as well as by means of administrations of subimmunogenic amounts of antigen (27, 79). These can be passed by marrow, leukocytes, and spleen cells administered in early life and result in the acceptance of skin grafts from which the donor cells were procured (13). An interesting reaction occurs in women with choriocarcinoma, a malignancy of the placental cells which are F_1 to their spouses'. Here the patients retain skin grafts from their husbands for prolonged periods of time (97).

The cellular basis for tolerance has been undefined, although the macrophage has been implicated by the finding that soluble antigen produces tolerance more readily than aggregated antigen. The difference may result from the fact that aggregated antigen is cleared more readily by the macrophage and that the soluble antigen may bypass the macrophage and cause the lymphoid cells to initiate tolerance. The finding that fetuses and newborn animals reflect a greater susceptibility to the induction of tolerance may be due to their immature lymphoid systems, along with poorly functioning reticuloendothelial systems which allow antigen more direct access to lymphoid cells in the neonate (74). Specific immunologic tolerance can be induced by overloading trapping mechanisms with particulate antigens, thereby effecting reticuloendothelial blockades. Immunosuppressive drugs can produce tolerance when administered to experimental animals and man (64, 104).

2. IMMUNE DEVIATION.

Usually antigenic stimulation may evoke a cell-mediated immune response, a humoral immune response, or both. However, in one experimental situation, administration of antigen can elicit humoral antibody production and can suppress delayed hypersensitivity reaction to that antigen following resensitization with the same antigen. The selective depression is called immune deviation (3). The antigen must be capable of inducing both humoral and cell-mediated immune responses, and during the second injection, the antigen is administered usually in complete Freund's adjuvant. Asherson suggests that animals may not be completely tolerant of particulate antigens of their own tissue (a state of immune deviation to them), which may reduce the danger of autoimmune disease while allowing for humoral antibody response to exogenous antigens that resemble normal tissue.

3. IMMUNOLOGIC ENHANCEMENT.

Both cell-mediated and humoral immune responses are responsible for allograft rejection, although the cell-mediated reaction predominates and the reactions evoked are toward the histocompatibility antigens present on the cell surface membranes. Preimmunization of a graft recipient with donor tissue will arouse both responses. The cellular reaction subsides first, and if donor tissue is transplanted, it may thereafter be accepted in the presence of circulating antibody. This successful take or delay is labeled immunological enhancement. Although the mechanisms remain unclear, the antibody could prevent the release of graft antigens or block access to them by sensitized cells (53). The antisera, which can be passively transferred, can be of syngeneic, allogeneic, or xenogeneic origin.

4. ALLOGENEIC INHIBITION.

Generally speaking, antigenic structures on cell surfaces may affect the growth of cells coming into contact with each other. Antigenic similarity favors growth, while antigenic dissimilarity inhibits growth—hence, the term allogeneic inhibition. It is best explained in murine systems where parental strain cells will react against F_1 hybrid cells, whereas the F_1 hybrid cells will also inhibit the growth of parental cells and are thought to be a nonimmunologic surveillance mechanism (61).

Conclusion

The continued understanding of the basics of the homeostatic interactions within the internal milieu of the immune responses has led to observations of somewhat similar findings within host-tumor relationships. These observations have resulted from the presence of cell surface antigens on tumor cells that are somewhat dissimilar to self and therefore are capable of inducing within the host some, if not all, of the predescribed intricacies associated with the host immune defenses and their attempts at controlling the tumor. As we will see shortly, the nature of the response represents an extremely fragile balance that is dependent on the capacity of the host to confer a destructive response toward the tumor versus one that may actually be beneficial to the tumor, by rendering it unrecognizable as non-self, as well as the immune capacities of the host. Of renewed importance is the documentation of the cell-mediated immune response as that being the most beneficial to the host in tumor cell destruction. It has been well established that immunostimulant adjuvants, such as live BCG, *Corynebacterium parvum,* and *Bordetella pertussis,* by their innate capacities as immunopotentiators, are capable of stimulating the host cell-mediated immune response either nonspecifically or specifically, when administered together with (tumor) antigens into the host. The subsequent response has been observed to be beneficial to the host in dealing with its tumor burden without being deleterious to the host. The next decade will most likely witness much progress in cancer control, which will depend on a multidisciplinary approach and on an intimate combination of available diagnostic and therapeutic methods at each stage of patient care. All aspects of immunology, as it relates to cancer, should have an adjunctive role to play in the various aspects of detection, treatment, and control of cancer. This will include a role for these modalities of the immune response in early diagnosis, identification, and assessment of the patient's disease, as well as evaluation and selection of chemotherapeutic agents which can be concomitantly employed in a synergistic manner. Additional benefits will also be provided by evaluation of short- and long-term consequences of excision therapy, appropriate regulation of body defense mechanisms, and preventative therapy, as long as the basic requirements and observations pertaining to host immune defenses as observed in experimental animals parallel those observed in the human host.

REFERENCES

1. Abdon, N. I., and Abdon, N. I. 1973. Immunoglobulin receptors on human lymphocytes. III. Comparative study of human bone marrow and blood B cells: Role of IgM receptors. *Clin. Exp. Immunol.* 13:45–54.

2. Allison, A. C. 1974. Interactions of T and B lymphocytes in self-tolerance and autoimmunity, in D. H. Katz and B. Benacerraf (eds.), *Immunological Tolerance: Mechanisms and Potential Therapeutic Applications.* Academic Press, New York.

3. Asherson, G. L. 1967. Antigen-mediated depression of delayed hypersensitivity. *Brit. Med. Bull.* 23:24–29.

4. Austen, K. F. 1971. Histamine and other mediators of allergic reactions, in M. Samter (ed.), *Immunological Diseases,* pp. 332–355. Little, Brown, Boston.

5. Bach, F. H., Bach, M. L., and Sondel, P. M. 1976. Differential function of major histocompatability complex antigens in T-lymphocyte activation. *Nature* 259:273–274.

6. Bach, J.-P., Dardenne, M., Papiernik, M., *et al.* 1972. Evidence for a serum factor secreted by the human thymus. *Lancet* Oct.–Dec.:1056–1058.

7. Bach, M. L. 1975. Reagin allergy, in B. A. Thomas (ed.), *Immunology,* pp. 19–32. Kalamazoo, Mich.: The Upjohn Co.

8. Bell, C., and Dray, S. 1970. Conversion of nonimmune spleen cells by ribonucleic acid of lymphoid cells from an immunized rabbit to produce γM antibody of foreign light-chain allotype. *J. Immunol.* 103:1196–1221.

9. Bell, C., and Dray, S. 1971. Conversion of nonimmune rabbit spleen cells by ribonucleic acid of lymphoid cells from an immunized rabbit to produce IgM and IgG antibody heavy-chain allotype. *J. Immunol.* 107:83–95.

10. Benacerraf, B., and McDevitt, H. O. 1972. Histocompatability-linked immune response genes. *Science* 175:273–279.

11. Bennet, B., and Bloom, B. R. 1968. Reactions *in vivo* and *in vitro* produced by a soluble substance associated with delayed-type hypersensitivity. *Proc. Natl. Acad. Sci.* 59:756–762.

12. Bert, G., Massaro, A. L., Di Cossano, D. L., *et al.* 1969. Electrophoretic study of immunoglobulins and immunoglobulin subunits on the surface of peripheral blood lymphocytes. *Immunology* 17:1–6.

13. Billingham, R. E., Brent, L., and Medawar, P. B. 1955. Acquired tolerance of skin homografts. *Ann. N.Y. Acad. Sci.* 59:409–416.

14. Bloom, B. R. 1973. Does transfer factor act specifically or as an immunological adjuvant? *N.E.J.M.* 288:908–909.

15. Boyden, S. V. 1964. Cytophilic antibody in guinea pigs with delayed hypersensitivity. *Immunology* 7:474–483.

16. Burnet, F. M. 1957. Cancer—A biological approach. *Brit. Med. J.* 779:841–847.

17. Burnet, F. M. 1969. *The Clonal Retention Theory of Acquired Immunity.* Cambridge Univ. Press, Cambridge, England.

18. Burnet, F. M. 1972. "Self-recognition" in colonial marine forms and flowering plants in relation to the evolution of immunity. *Nature* 232:230–235.

19. Burnet, F. M., and Fenner, F. 1949. *The Production of Antibodies.* Macmillan, London.

20. Calkins, C. E., and Golarb, E. S. 1972. Direct demonstration of lymphocyte-macrophage cooperation in the absence of physical contact between the two cell types. *Cell. Immunol.* 5:579–586.

21. Cantor, H., and Boyse, E. A. 1975. Functional subclasses of T lymphocytes bearing different Ly antigens. *J. Exp. Med.* 141:1376–1389.

22. Cantor, H., Shen, F. W., and Boyse, E. A. 1976. Separation of helper T cells from suppressor T cells expressing different Ly components. *J. Exp. Med.* 143:1391–1401.

23. Civin, C., Levin, H., Williamson, A., and Schlossman, S. 1976. The effects of antigen dose and adjuvant on the antibody response; amplification of restricted B cell clones. *J. Immunol.* 116:1400–1406.

24. Cohen, I. R., and Wekerle, H. 1973. Regulation of autosensitization. The immune activation and specific inhibition of self-recognizing thymus-derived lymphocytes in relation to autoimmunity. *Lancet* 2:135.

25. Cooper, M. D., Peterson, R. D. A., and Good, R. A. 1965. Delineation of the thymic and bursal lymphoid systems in the chicken. *Nature* 205:143–146.

26. Cooper, N. R., Polley, M. J., and Müller-Eberhard, M. J. 1971. Biochemical consequences of the antigen-antibody interaction, in M. Samter (ed.) *Immunological Diseases*, pp. 289–331. Boston: Little, Brown.

27. Cruchand, A. 1968. The effect of reticuloendothelial blockade on antibody production and immunologic tolerance. *Lab. Invest.* 19:15–24.

28. David, J. R. 1973. Lymphocyte mediators and cellular hypersensitivity. *N.E.J.M.* 288:143.

29. David, J. R., and Schlossman, S. 1968. The *in vitro* inhibition of peritoneal exudate cell migration by chemically defined antigens. *J. Exp. Med.* 128:1451–1459.

30. Davis, W. E., Cole, L. J., and Shaffer, W. T. 1970. Studies on synergistic thymus-bone marrow cell interactions in immunological responses. *Proc. Soc. Exp. Biol. Med.* 133:144–150.

31. Debré, P., Kapp, J. A., Dorf, M. E., and Benacerraf, B. 1975. Genetic control of specific immune suppression. II. H-2-linked dominant genetic control of immune suppression by the random copolymer L-glutamic acid D-L-Tyrosine[50] (GT). *J. Exp. Med.* 142:1447–1454.

32. De Rubertis, F. R., Zenser, T. V., Adler, W. H., et al. 1974. Role of cyclic adenosine 3′,5′-monophosphate in lymphocyte mitogenesis. *J. Immunol.* 113:151–161.

33. Dumonde, D. C., Wolstencroft, R. A., Panayi, G. S., et al. 1969. "Lymphokines": Nonantibody mediators of cellular immunity generated by lymphocyte activation. *Nature* 224:38–42.

34. Evans, R., and Alexander, P. 1971. Rendering macrophages specifically cytotoxic by a factor released from immune lymphoid cells. *Transplantation* 12:227–229.

35. Evans, R., and Alexander, P. 1972. Mechanism of immunologically specific killing of tumour cells by macrophages. *Nature* 236:168–170.

36. Feldman, M., and Basten, A. 1971. The relationship between antigenic structure and the requirement of thymus-derived cells in the immune response. *J. Exp. Med.* 134:103–119.

37. Feldman, M., and Gallily, R. 1968. Interactions in the induction of antibody formation. *Cold Spring Harbor Symp. Quant. Biol.* 32:415–421.

38. Feldman, M., and Palmer, J. 1971. The requirement for macrophages in the secondary immune response to antigens of small and large size *in vitro*. *Immunology* 21:685–699.

39. Fishman, M., and Adler, F. L. 1963. Antibody formation initiated *in vitro*.

II. Antibody synthesis in X-irradiated recipients of diffusion chambers containing nucleic acid derived from macrophages incubated with antigen. *J. Exp. Med.* 117:595–602.

40. Foley, E. J. 1953. Antigenic properties of methylcholanthrene-induced tumors in mice of the strain of origin. *Cancer Res.* 13:835–837.

41. Fox, R. A., and MacSween, J. M. 1974. The isolation of migration-inhibition factor. *Immunol. Commun.* 3:375–389.

42. Gell, P. G. H., and Benacerraf, B. 1961. The relationship between contact and delayed sensitivity: A study on the specificity of cellular immune reaction. *J. Exp. Med.* 113:571–585.

43. Gershon, R. K. 1970. T cell control of antibody production, *in* M. D. Cooper and N. L. Warner (eds.), *Contemporary Topics in Immunology*, Vol. 3. Plenum Publishing, New York. 1974.

44. Gershon, R. K. 1974., *in* M. D. Cooper and N. L. Warner (eds.), *Contemporary Topics in Immunobiology*, Vol. 3, p. 1. Plenum Press, New York.

45. Gershon, R. K., and Paul, W. E. 1971. Effect of thymus-derived lymphocytes on amount and affinity of antihapten antibody. *J. Immunol.* 106:872–874.

46. Glick, B., Chang, T. S., and Jaap, R. G. 1956. The bursa of Fabricius and antibody production. *Poult. Sci.* 35:224–229.

47. Gorer, P. A. 1958. Some reactions of H-2 antibodies "in vitro" and "in vivo." *Ann. N.Y. Acad. Sci.* 73:707–721.

48. Greaves, M. F., Torrigiani, G., and Roitt, I. 1969. Blocking of the lymphocyte receptor site for cell-mediated hypersensitivity and transplantation reactions by anti–light-chain sera. *Nature* 222:885–886.

49. Gross, L. 1943. Intradermal immunization of C3H mice against a sarcoma that originated in an animal of the same line. *Cancer Res.* 3:326–333.

50. Gudat, F. G., Harris, T. N., Harris, S., *et al.* 1970. Studies on antibody-producing cells. I. Ultrastructure of 19S and 7S antibody-producing cells. *J. Exp. Med.* 132:448–474.

51. Heber-Katz, E., and Wilson, D. B. 1976. Sheep red blood cell-specific helper activity in rat thoracic duct lymphocyte populations positively selected for reactivity to specific strong histocompatability allo-antigens. *J. Exp. Med.* 143:701–706.

52. Herzenberg, L. A. *et al.* 1976. T cell regulation of antibody responses demonstration of allotype-specific helper T cells and their specific removal by suppressor T cells. *J. Exp. Med.* 144:330–344.

53. Hutchin, P., Amos, D. B., and Prioleau, W. H., Jr. 1967. Interaction of humoral antibodies and immune lymphocytes. *Transplantation* 5:68–78.

54. Ishizuka, K., and Ishizuka, T. 1968. Induction of erythema-wheel reaction by soluble γE antibody complexes in humans. *J. Immunol.* 101:68–78.

55. Ishizuka, K., Ishizuka, T., and Campbell, D. H. 1959. Biological activity of soluble antigen-antibody complex. II. Physical properties of soluble complexes having skin-irritating activity. *J. Exp. Med.* 109:127–143.

56. Ishizuka, T., De Bernardo, R., Tomioka, H., *et al.* 1972. Identification of basophil gramlocytes at the site of histamine release. *J. Immunol.* 108:1000–1008.

57. Ishizuka, T., and Ishizuka, K. 1959. Biological activities of aggregated immunoglobulin. I. Skin reactivity and complement-fixing properties of heat-

denatured gamma globulin. *Proc. Soc. Exp. Biol. Med.* 101:845–850.

58. Jimenez, L., Bloom, B., Blume, M. R., *et al.* 1971. On the number and nature of antigen-sensitivity lymphocytes in the blood of delayed hypersensitivity human donors. *J. Exp. Med.* 133:740–751.

59. Katz, D. H., and Benacerraf, B. 1975. The function and interrelationships of T-cell receptors, Ir genes and other histocompatibility gene products. *Transplant Rev.* 22:175–195.

60. Kidd, J. G., and Tolan, H. W. 1960. The association of lymphocytes with cancer cells undergoing distinctive necrobiosis in resistant and immune hosts *Amer. J. Path.* 26:672–673.

61. Klein, G. 1966. Tumor antigens. *Ann. Rev. Microbiol.* 20:223–252.

62. Lawrence, H. S. 1949. The cellular transfer of cutaneous hypersensitivity to tuberculin in man. *Proc. Soc. Exp. Biol. Med.* 71:516–522.

63. Layton, L. L., Yamanaka, E., Lee, S., and Greene, E. W. 1962. Multiple allergies to the pollen seed antigens of *Ricinus communis. J. Allerg.* 33:234–235.

64. Levin, R. H., Landy, M., and Frie, E., III. 1964. The effect of 6-mercaptopurine on immune response in man. *N.E.J.M.* 271:16–21.

65. Liebowitz, S., and Schwartz, R. S. 1971. Malignancy as a complication of immunosuppressive therapy. *Advances in Internal Medicine* 17:95–123.

66. Lindquist, R. A. 1975. Immediate hypersensitivity, in B. A. Thomas (ed.) *Immunology,* p. 33. The Upjohn Co., Kalamazoo, Mich.

67. Litt, M. 1964. Studies in experimental eosinophilia. VI. Uptake of immune complexes by eosinophils. *J. Cell. Biol.* 23:355–361.

68. Lo Buglio, A. F., Cotran, R. S., and Jandl, J. H. 1967. Red cells coated with immunoglobulin G: Binding and sphering by mononuclear cells in man. *Science* 158:1582–1585.

69. Lohmann-Matthes, M.-L., Ziegler, F. G., and Fischer, H. 1973. Macrophage cytotoxic factor. A product of *in vitro* sensitized thymus-dependent cells. *Eur. J. Immunol.* 3:56–59.

70. McFarland, W., and Heilman, D. H. 1966. Lymphocyte foot appendage: Its role in lymphocyte function and in immunologic reactions. *Nature* 205:887–888.

71. McNeill, T. A., and Gresser, I. 1973. Inhibition of hematopoietic colony growth by interferon preparations from different sources. *Nature* 244:173–174.

72. Miller, J. F. A. P. Immunological function of the thymus. *Lancet* 2:748–749.

73. Miller, J. F. A. P., Vadas, M. A., Whitelaw, A., and Gamble, J. 1975. H-2 gene complex restricts transfer of delayed-type hypersensitivity in mice. *Proc. Natl. Acad. Sci.* 72:5095–5098.

74. Mitchell, J., and Nossal, G. J. V. 1966. Mechanism of induction of immunological tolerance. I. Localization of tolerance-inducing antigen. *Aust. J. Exp. Biol. Med.* 44:211–233.

75. Mitchison, N. A. 1971. The carrier effect in the secondary response to hapten protein conjugates. V. Use of antilymphocyte serum to deplete animals of helper cells. *Eur. J. Immunol.* 1:68–75.

76. Mohr, J. A., Killebrew, L., Mirchmore, H. G., *et al.* 1969. Transfer of delayed hypersensitivity; the role of blood transfusions in humans. *J.A.M.A.* 207:517–519.

77. Mota, I. 1964. The mechanisms of anaphylaxis. I. The production of mast cell-sensitizing antibody. *Immunology* 7:681–699.

78. Müller-Eberhard, H. J. 1961. Isolation and description of proteins related to the human complement system. *Acta Soc. Med. Upsal.* 66:152–170.

79. Nossal, G. J. V. 1966. Immunological tolerance: A new model for low zone reduction. *Ann. N.Y. Acad. Sci.* 129:822–833.

80. Nowell, P. C., Hirsch, B. E., Fox, D. H., et al. 1970. Evidence for the existence of multipotential lympho-hematopoetic stem cells in the adult rat. *J. Cell Physiol.* 75:151–158.

81. Okafor, G. O., Turner, M. W., and Hay, F. C. 1974. Localization of monocyte binding site for immunoglobulin G. *Nature* 248:228–230.

82. Oudin, J. 1974. L'Idiotype des anticorps. *Ann. Immunol. (Inst. Pasteur)* 125:309–331.

83. Ovary, Z. 1958. Immediate reactions in the skin of experimental animals provoked by antigen-antibody interaction. *Progr. Allerg.* 5:459–508.

84. Owen, R. D. 1945. Immunogenetic consequences of vascular anastomoses between bovine twins. *Science* 102:400–401.

85. Paque, R. E., Ali, M., and Dray, S. 1975. RNA extracts of lymphoid cells sensitized to DNP-oligolysines convert nonresponder lymphoid cells to responder lymphoid cells which release migration-inhibitory factor. *Cellular Immunol.* 16:261–268.

86. Paque, R. E., and Dray, S. 1970. Interspecies transfer of delayed hypersensitivity in vitro with RNA extracts. *J. Immunol.* 105:1334–1338.

87. Parish, W. E., and Coombs, R. R. A. 1968. Peripheral blood eosinophilia in guinea pigs following implantation of anephylactic and human lung. *Brit. J. Haemat.* 14:425–445.

88. Parrott, D. M. V., and De Sousa, M. A. B. 1971. Thymus-dependent and thymus-independent populations: Origin, migratory patterns and lifespan. *Clin. Exp. Immunol.* 8:663–684.

89. Paul, W. E. 1970. Functional specificity of antigen-binding receptors of lymphocytes. *Transplant. Rev.* 5:130–166.

90. Paul, W. E., and Benacerraf, B. 1977. Functional specificity of thymus-dependent lymphocytes. *Science* 195:1293–1300.

91. Paul, W. E., et al. 1968. Antigen concentration dependence of stimulation of DNA synthesis in vitro by specifically sensitized cells as an expression of the binding characteristics of cellular antibody. *J. Exp. Med.* 127:25–42.

92. Pick, E., and Turk, J. L. 1972. The biological activities of soluble lymphocyte products. *Clin. Exp. Immunol.* 10:1–23.

93. Potter, H., Rosenfeld, S., and Dressler, D. 1974. Transfer factor. *Ann. Int. Med.* 81:838–847.

94. Prehn, R. T. 1970, in M. Landy and R. T. Smith (eds.). *Immune Surveillance.* New York: Academic Press.

95. Press, J. L., Klinman, N. R., and McDevitt, H. O. 1976. Expression of Ia antigens on hapten-specific B cells. I. Delineation of B cell subpopulations. *J. Exp. Med.* 144:414–427.

96. Rich, A. R., and Lewis, M. R. 1932. The nature of allergy in tuberculosis as revealed by tissue culture studies. *Bull. Johns Hopkins Hosp.* 50:115–137.

97. Robinson, E., Ben-Hur, N., Zuckerman, H., et al. 1967. Further immunologic studies in patients with choriocarcinoma. Cancer Res. 27:1202–1204.

98. Roelants, G. E., Ryden, A., Hagg, L.-B., et al. 1974. Active synthesis of immunoglobulin receptors for antigen by T lymphocytes. Nature 247:106–108.

99. Roitt, I. M., Greaves, M. F., Torrigiani, G., et al. 1969. The cellular basis of immunological responses. A synthesis of some current views. Lancet 2:367–371.

100. Rosenthal, A. S., Lipsky, P. E., and Sheveck, E. M. 1975. Macrophage-lymphocyte interaction and antigen recognition. Fed. Proc. 34:1743–1748.

101. Rous, P. 1910. A transmissible avian neoplasm (sarcoma of the common fowl). J. Exp. Med. 12:696–705.

102. Schendel, D. J., and Bach, F. H. 1974. Genetic control of cell-mediated lympholysis in mouse. J. Exp. Med. 140:1534–1546.

103. Schoenberg, M. D., Mumak, V. R., Moore, R. D., et al. 1964. Cytoplasmic interaction between macrophages and lymphocytic cells in antibody synthesis. Science 143:964–965.

104. Schwartz, R., and Dameshek, W. 1959. Drug-induced immunologic tolerance. Nature 183:1682–1683.

105. Sela, M., and Mozes, E. 1966. Dependence of the chemical nature of antibodies on the net electrical charge of antigens. Proc. Natl. Acad. Sci. 55:445–453.

106. Shearer, G. M., Rehn, T. G., and Schmitt-Verhulst, A. 1976. Role of the murine major histocompatability complex in the specificity of "in vitro" T-cell-mediated lympholysis against chemically modified autologous lymphocytes. Transplant Rev. 29:222–248.

107. Shreffler, D. C., and David, C. S. 1975. Adv. Immunol. 20:125–196.

108. Simonesen, M. 1967. Cold Spr. Harbor Symp. Quant. Biol. 32:517–523.

109. Snell, G. D., Dausset, J., and Nathenson, S. 1976, in Histocompatability. Academic Press, New York.

110. Spirer, Z., Rudich, A., Assif, E., et al. 1974. Release of skin-reactive factor by human lymphocytes. Int. Arch. Allergy Appl. Immunol. 46:331–338.

111. Spofford, B. T., Dagnes, R. A., and Granger, G. A. 1974. Cell-mediated immunity in vitro: A highly sensitive assay for human lymphotoxin. J. Immunol. 112:2111–2116.

112. Storb, U., and Weiser, R. S. 1972. Antibodies of different immunoglobulin classes released by single cells. J. Reticuloendothel. Soc. 11:218–228.

113. Storb, U., and Weiser, R. S. 1972. Co-existence of 19S and 7S hemolysins in splenic foci. J. Reticuloendothel. Soc. 11:207–217.

114. Taylor, R. B., Duffus, W. P. H., Raff, M. C., et al. 1971. Redistribution and pinocytosis of lymphocyte surface immunoglobulin molecules induced by anti-immunoglobulin antibody. Nature 233:225–226.

115. Thomas, D. W., Roberts, W. K., and Talmage, D. W. 1975. Regulation of the immune response: Production of a soluble suppressor by immune spleen cells in vitro. J. Immunol. 144:1616–1622.

116. Thomas, L. 1959. Reaction to homologous tissue antigens in relation to hypersensitivity, in H. S. Lawrence (ed.), Cellular and Humoral Aspects of the Hypersensitivity State, p. 529. New York: Hoeber.

117. Thor, D. E., and Dray, S. 1968. The cell migration-inhibition correlate of

delayed hypersensitivity: Conversion of human nonsensitive lymph node cells with an RNA extract. *J. Immunol.* 101:469–480.

118. Tigelaar, R. E., Vaz, N. M., and Ovary, Z. 1971. Immunoglobulin receptors on mast cells. *J. Immunol.* 106:661–672.

119. Uhr, J. W., and Moller, G. 1968. Regulatory effect of antibody on the immune response. *Ann. Rev. Immunol.* 8:81–123.

120. Unanue, E. R., and Cerrothini, J. C. 1970. The immunogeneity of antigen bound to the plasma membrane of macrophages. *J. Exp. Med.* 131:711–725.

121. Ward, P. A., Remold, H. G., and David, J. R. 1970. The production of antigen-stimulated lymphocytes of a leucocytotactic factor distinct from migration-inhibitory factor. *Cell. Immunol.* 1:162–174.

122. Welsh, R. A., and Geer, J. A. 1959. Phagocytosis of mast cell granule by the eosinophilic leucocyte in the rat. *Amer. J. Path.* 35:103–111.

123. Wilson, D. B., Blyth, J. L., and Nowell, P. C. 1968. Quantitative studies on the mixed lymphocyte interaction in rats. III. Kinetics of the response. *J. Exp. Med.* 128:1157–1181.

124. Zinkernagel, R. M., and Doherty, P. C. 1976. H-2 compatability requirement for T-cell-mediated lysis of target cells infected with lymphocytic choriomeningitis virus. *J. Exp. Med.* 141:1427–1436.

CHAPTER 2

COMPARATIVE AND DEVELOPMENTAL IMMUNOLOGY

Edwin L. Cooper

Department of Anatomy
University of California
Los Angeles, California 90024

The development of the vertebrate immune system can be traced both through its ontogeny and phylogeny. With the exception of the thymus and tonsils, which develop from endoderm, organs of the immune system, including the bone marrow, spleen, and lymph nodes, develop from mesoderm. The immune system underwent major changes as animals evolved from unicellular to diploblastic to triploblastic forms with a coelomic cavity filled with leukocytes. Invertebrates grouped into these major categories respond to numerous antigens by several mechanisms, including recognition, phagocytosis, encapsulation, and specific cellular immunity. Invertebrates also produce humoral substances that inactivate infectious microorganisms. The major evolutionary pressure leading to the development of the immune system was probably to insure the body against the threat of extinction by pathogens from the external environment. The immune system also may have evolved as a safeguard against internal threats such as cancer.

Introduction

GENERAL. Understanding how the immune system developed has been greatly facilitated by an increased interest in the comparative and developmental approach to immunology (14, 19, 22, 36, 47, 48, 64). The ancestral immune cell existed among primitive invertebrates. This prototypic cell *recognizes* and *reacts* against foreign material or antigens by phagocytosis, and is conserved throughout the phylogenetic scale as macrophages, and granulocytes; mast cells are also related to the ancestral cell. The next evolutionary event occurred in coelomate invertebrates that developed diverse leukocytic types, some of which are considered to be precursors of lymphocytes and granulocytes. *Cell-mediated immune responses* (e.g., graft rejection) constitute the only known immune response of invertebrate leukocytes in which specificity and memory have been demonstrated, reactions that persist in vertebrates. Humoral substances, such as agglutinins that are structurally heterogeneous, constitute the second form of immunity in coelomate invertegrates. The third event in the evolution of immunity was the capacity for *antibody synthesis,* which first appeared among the most primitive vertebrates or cyclostome fishes. Antibody persists and has become more complicated and diverse in mammals, where five classes of antibodies or immunoglobulins are found. The principal evolutionary pressure leading to the development of immunity is considered to be protection from infectious microorganisms; according to a second view, however, the immune system evolved as an internal homeostatic mechanism, primarily against the threat of extinction by cancer.

THE ANIMAL KINGDOM AND IMMUNITY. When discussing the immune responses of different animal groups, it is often convenient to use such terms as "primitive" and "advanced," or perhaps "lower" and "higher," or "simple" and "specialized." Such terms do not imply that the immune systems of some animals are better developed than those of others; a particular animal's immune-response capacity parallels its position in the phylogenetic scale as well as its functional complexity (Fig. 1). For convenience of discussion only, those animals from protozoans through the flatworms may be considered "primitive" and the annelids, molluscs, and arthropods as "advanced." These latter three groups will also be classified as *proto-*

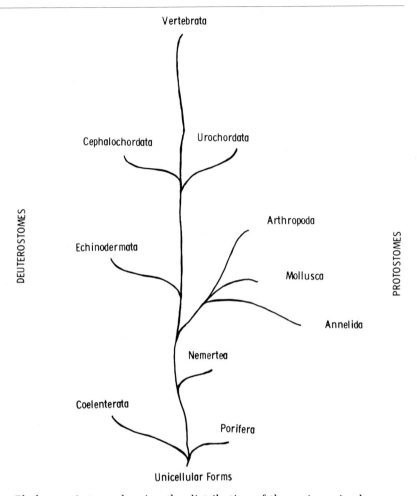

Fig. 1. Phylogenetic tree, showing the distribution of the major animal groups. The most primitive are unicellular forms. The advanced invertebrates are divided into the Protostomia and Deuterostomia. The vertebrates are believed to have evolved from the deuterostomes.

stomes, a name that is based on certain embryological developmental patterns. A second group of advanced invertebrates, the *deuterostomes,* includes the echinoderms and tunicates, the latter of which are chordates, as are vertebrates. The deuterostomes appear to have diverged from the main protostome line at a point in the phylogenetic scale after the flatworms. Regardless of their position within common taxonomic schemes, all animals have evolved immune responses built on a basic plan that functions to rid them of *non-self* material without detriment to *self.* The actual processes of immunity are academic, but that all animals have *developed* a necessary protective device, immunity, is what is crucial.

ADAPTIVE IMMUNITY. Criteria for adaptive immunity are traditionally defined on the basis of vertebrate responses, leading to the

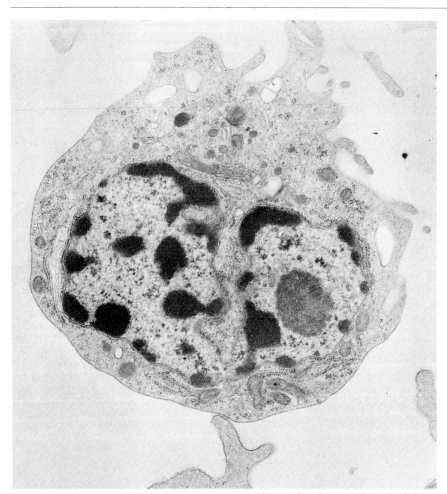

Fig. 2. Earthworm coelomocyte. (× 34,000.) This is the "basophil," which has an affinity for the basic dye of ordinary blood stains. This coelomocyte resembles the vertebrate small lymphocyte. (Courtesy of D. Scott Linthicum, Department of Pathology, University of California, San Diego, and Elizabeth Stein, Donald H. Marks, and Edwin L. Cooper, University of California, Los Angeles, California.)

erroneous assumption by classical vertebrate immunologists that invertebrates possess no form of adaptive immunity. The viewpoint taken is
that specific recognition of self and non-self, usually tested in the past
by transplanting autografts and allografts or xenografts, confirms cell-
mediated immunity as phylogenetically the earliest of specific immune
responses. Foreign grafts heal in and are vascularized, but—once recognized by the host's immune system—display visible signs of rejection. At the microscopic lovol, rejection is characterized by coelomocyte
infiltration into the grafts; most coelomocytes strongly resemble vertebrate leukocytes. Thought now focuses on the possibility that the
lymphocyte-like cells of invertebrates may represent T cell precursors
(Fig. 2).

Antibody synthesis is an attribute that seems to be peculiar to vertebrates, although invertebrates synthesize humoral substances which
may be the cell surface receptor for antigens. Unlike numerous descrip-
tions of vertebrate antibody, naturally occurring or induced, such substances in invertebrates still remain to be clearly distinguished and
defined. Progress is slow, since the conceptual and more often the technical approaches to understanding humoral synthesis in invertebrates are
still somewhat limited. A definition of adaptive immunity that encom-
passes both vertebrates and invertebrates assumes that an animal
should reach a stage at which certain characteristics of its leukocytes or
humoral substances are altered after antigen presentation.

Phylogeny

ADAPTIVE RADIATION, CONVERGENCE, AND DIVERGENCE.

Certain general concepts seek to explain the evolution of animals;
they may also serve to describe the evolution of blood cells and organs
of the immune system. A common ancestor evolved into a variety of
blood cell types by *adaptive radiation* (21). This first blood cell ancestor
probably appeared as an amoeboid wandering cell which differentiated
and specialized, becoming monocytes, granulocytes, mast cells, and
lymphocytes. Lymphocytes also developed the increased capacity to
divide, especially after contact with antigen, insuring specificity and the
more efficient recall phenomenon of *immunologic memory*, a characteristic of vertebrate immune reactions.

From structural and functional studies, lymphocyte populations are
assumed to have been derived from a common lymphocyte precursor
that diverged from the original common leukocyte ancestor. According
to some comparative immunologists, the amphibians may have represented the point where the single ancestral type split to give rise to

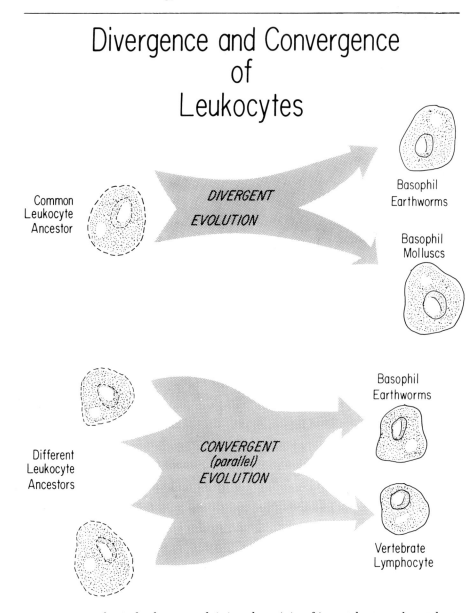

Divergence and Convergence of Leukocytes

Fig. 3. Hypothetical scheme explaining the origin of invertebrate and vertebrate leukocytes by either divergence or convergence from a leukocytic ancestor. It is probably at the level of the anuran amphibians (frogs and toads) where lymphocytes differentiated into T and B forms.

several descendant lymphocyte lines (21). These lines may have adapted by *divergent evolution* in different ways to varied organ environments (Fig. 3). Divergent evolution produced T and B lymphocytes which are, at least superficially, morphologically similar—but not functionally. The evolution of sets of similar characteristics in groups of lymphocytes of quite different evolutionary ancestry is known as *convergent evolution*. The structural and functional development of lymphocytes in mammals and lymphocyte-like cells in such animals as annelid worms may be an example of convergent evolution (7, 10, 11, 13, 15, 16, 17).

HOMOLOGY AND ANALOGY. Evolution of the immune system is intimately connected with leukocytes; and, to understand blood cell evolution, a distinction must be made between resemblances falling into two broad categories: *homology* and *analogy*. *Homology* may refer to leukocytes in different animals which share structural similarities, as a result of inheriting features from a common ancestor (Fig. 4). Homologous cells (leukocytes) or blood-cell-producing organs may resemble each other closely, for example, as do thymus lymphocytes in humans and pigs, or they may be superficially quite unlike, as in the jugular bodies of anuran amphibians and the jugular lymph nodes of humans. Jugular bodies of frogs and jugular lymph nodes of humans may resemble each other closely in their development (8, 12, 18). Whether superficially alike or unlike, homologous entities share certain basic similarities in structure referable to their common ancestor. Criteria include positional relationships to other parts of the body, similarity in vascular supply, and common ontogenetic patterns.

When cells or organs in different animals are functionally similar and have no common ancestor, this may be referred to as *analogy*. In other words, analogous cells or organs are nonhomologous but they are functionally similar (Fig. 5). Analogous entities often have little gross structural resemblance to each other, as in the case of the coelomic cavity of the earthworm, an invertebrate, and the bone marrow cavity of tetrapod vertebrates. The two entities probably have no common ancestor but, functionally, they produce and contain all types of leukocytes. Other analogous organs, such as the white body of octopus and the lymphoid aggregations of vertebrates, may have a superficial structural resemblance to each other (14). The function they share is the production of leukocytes.

CELLS OF THE IMMUNE SYSTEM. Cells of the immune system found in the circulating blood of a typical vertebrate are *granulocytes*, *lymphocytes*, and *monocytes*. All these cell types have

HOMOLOGY
OF
CELLS AND ORGANS

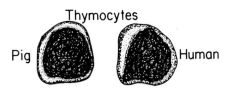

Thymocytes

Pig   Human

<u>Cells</u> that look alike
with common ancestor

or

<u>Organs</u> that look differently
with common ancestor

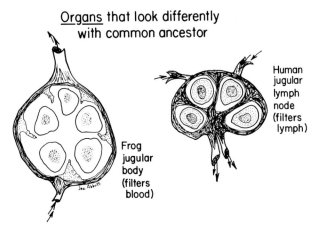

Frog
jugular
body
(filters
blood)

Human
jugular
lymph
node
(filters
lymph)

Fig. 4. Homologous cells and lymphocyte-producing organs in diverse vertebrate groups.

structural and perhaps even functional counterparts among the invertebrates (e.g., echinoderms and tunicates) and primitive vertebrates (23,
24, 26–30, 34, 37, 42–45, 50–54, 56, 59, 62, 63). The phagocytic cell,
represented by monocytes or tissue and organ macrophages, is probably
the only blood cell that has persisted since the protozoans and primitive metazoans. When food-getting and immunity became separate
functions, cells resembling granulocytes evolved. Lymphocytes evolved
when there was a still further separation among food-getting, nonspecific
immunity, and specific immunity. More progressive evolution reveals the

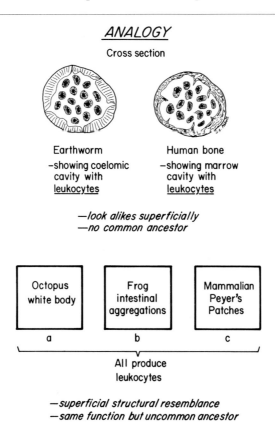

Fig. 5. Leukocytopoietic organs of an (A) octopus, (B) frog, and (C) human. The lymphocytes of the organs of the frog and human are homologous to each other. The octopus organ is similar to the vertebrate organs in function, but it has only a superficial structural resemblance to them.

existence of lymphocyte, granulocyte, and macrophage subtypes that expands what we know about the immune system.

Ontogeny and Phylogeny

THE COELOM. The ontogeny and phylogeny of the immune system derived from the origin of the third germ layer, mesoderm, and its relationship to the coelom. All organs of the vertebrate immune system come from mesoderm with the exception of the thymus, tonsils, and bursa of Fabricius (Fig. 6). The coelomic cavity of invertebrates,

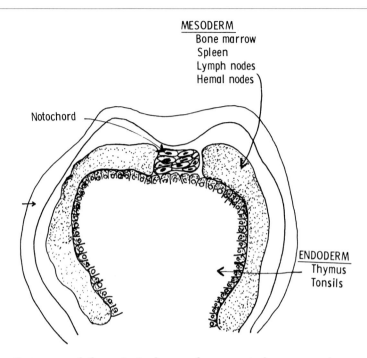

Fig. 6. Ontogeny of the principal germ layers, ectoderm, mesoderm, and endoderm. All of the cells and organs of the immune system are derived either from the mesoderm or the endoderm. (The arrow on the left indicates ectoderm.) Note the notochord, a characteristic of all chordates, including the protochordates and vertebrates.

precursor of the vertebrate peritoneal cavity, is lined by mesoderm (49). The first or primary cavity to develop in embryos is the blastocoel; the cavity of ancestral metazoans is analogous. When the gut forms, the blastocoel is reduced, usually leaving between the endoderm and the ectoderm a space, the pseudocoel. The pseudocoel results from failure of the parenchyma to completely fill the space between the body wall mesoderm and the gut wall. The pseudocoel, which is therefore derived from the blastula, is not lined by peritoneum. Acoelomate invertebrates include the flatworms (Platyhelminthes), round worms (Nemathelminthes), and ribbon worms (Nemertea). In contrast to the pseudocoel, the true coelom is the secondary cavity, which forms as an entirely new space within the mesoderm. As the coelom increases in size during development, the outer mesoderm becomes intimately associated with the body wall that is therefore lined by the parietal or somatic mesoderm; this eventually becomes the parietal peritoneum in the adult. The inner mesoderm closely invests the gut wall and other viscera so that the coelom is lined by visceral or splanchnic mesoderm known as visceral peritoneum in adults. The spleen is derived from mesoderm in this position.

THE MOUTH.   Animals such as sponges (Porifera) and hydra (Cnidaria) are metazoan invertebrates composed of only two main divisions, analogous to the two germ layers of vertebrates. When mesoderm, the third germ layer, evolved, the advanced invertebrates and coelom evolved. The so-called advanced invertebrates are also classified under two main evolutionary lines of coelomates, the Protostomia and the Deuterostomia. The protostomes include the flatworms, molluscs, annelids, and arthropods, and several minor phyla. The deuterostomes include the echinoderms, tunicates, and several minor phyla. Because the vertebrates evolved from the deuterostome line, a study of leukocytes and immunity in echinoderms and tunicates may be more meaningful if interest focuses only on vertebrates (41, 45, 50). If, on the other hand, one is to understand immunity as a biologic phenomenon, then immune mechanisms, like other physiologic processes, should be analyzed in all animal groups.

The mouth of adult protostomes is derived from the embryonic blastopore. The cleavage of the egg is usually spiral and determinate, and the mesoderm generally develops from a special blastomere, the 4d cell, which is closely associated with an endodermal stem cell. Parts of the egg are programmed to produce specific structures. Protostomes generally have a schizocoel, that is, the coelomic cavity first appears as a series of splits in the mesodermal bands. In deuterostomes, development occurs from two separate openings. The anus arises from or near the blastopore and a new mouth from a stomadaeum at a distance from the anterior border of the blastopore. Deuterostomes have a coelom known as an enterocoel, because the mesoderm forms from outpouchings of the gut. Cleavage of deuterostome eggs, in contrast to those of protostomes, is usually indeterminate and radial. Thus, specific blastomeres are not programmed to form particular parts of the body, as experimental embryologists have so adeptly proved. Experiments can actually change the destiny of blastomeres so that a whole larva will be produced from one blastomere of a two-celled or four-celled embryo (5, 61).

RECOGNITION.   Whether we are dealing with primitive animals or the more advanced protostomes and deuterostomes, the ability to distinguish between self and not-self is a universal attribute; it is not restricted to vertebrates. Indeed, this ability can be traced to the simplest protozoans. Transplantations of cell organelles in protozoans produce incompatibility reactions that are to immunity, by analogy, what primitive irritability is to the vertebrate nervous system. *Quasi-immunorecognition* is the capacity for recognition of non-self allogeneic tissue followed by incompatibility reactions; autogeneic or self-tissue never provokes incompatibility and is permanently accepted (35). Regardless of the test system, recognition is probably the most basic event in the immune response and continued analysis at all levels is crucial to understanding fundamental mechanisms. (See Fig. 7.)

RECEPTORS FOR SELF AND NON-SELF. In order for leukocytes of animals to recognize antigens, cells must possess receptors. Sloan *et al.* (1975) recently asked the important question: Do crustaceans have recognition molecules? That is, do they have receptors enabling them to recognize self so as to distinguish it from various foreign proteins and to eliminate them from the circulation (55)? Crayfish and lobsters can readily clear certain mammalian serum and albumins

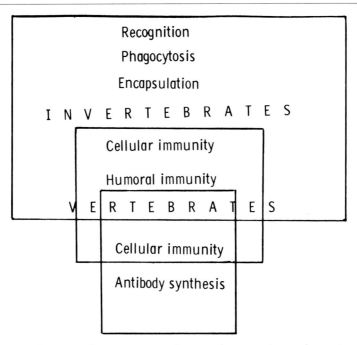

Fig. 7. Overlapping characteristics of invertebrate and vertebrate immune responses built on primordial mechanisms of recognition, phagocytosis, and encapsulation. Both animal groups share cellular and humoral immune mechanisms but antibody synthesis is purely a vertebrate attribute.

from the circulation, but the specificity of elimination is questionable. If such receptors are present, regardless of their location, whether cell-bound or -free, they may be of finite number. To test whether these receptors are saturable and wehther they possess some degree of specificity, the crayfish *Procambarus clarkii* has been injected with radioactively labeled proteins: *self* (crayfish hemocyanin) and *non-self* (bovine serum albumin [BSA] and human gamma globulin [HGG]). The response shows a marked difference in tho rate of elimination. Equilibration of self proteins occurs within 10 minutes but essentially no elimination (< 20%) after 24 hours. By contrast, non-self proteins are eliminated in significant amounts (~ 80%) within a 2-hour period. After recognition, clearance occurs, and the remaining proteins are concentrated in the gills. To understand the problem of receptors, crayfish have been injected with a mixture of labeled and unlabeled protein. In excess, the unlabeled protein always prevents the elimination of the same-labeled protein. If the excess unlabeled protein is different from the labeled protein, there is no effect on elimination:

protein A^{labeled} + protein A^{unlabeled} → defective elimination

protein A^{labeled} + protein B^{unlabeled} → no effect on elimination

In principle, this hypothesis suggests that the crayfish has naturally occurring receptors or recognition molecules for at least three groups of foreign proteins (albumins, gamma globulins, and hemocyanins). These experiments, showing clearance and blocking of binding by competitive elimination, do not precisely locate these putative receptors. Continued experimentation from various laboratories strongly supports the view that the functional analogue of vertebrate immunoglobulins is present in invertebrates.

Significance of Invertebrate Humoral Immunity: Comparison with Vertebrate Complement

POSSIBLE HOMOLOGIES. Invertebrate humoral immunity involves the presence of biologically active molecules that occur naturally or that may be induced. These molecules, by their lytic or agglutinating properties, are able to act on the antigens responsible for their induction; in this respect they resemble vertebrate antibodies. Invertebrate humoral factors do, however, lack the high degree of specificity that characterizes vertebrate antibodies. A resolution of the problem of homology rests on more detailed, primary data of molecular structure of invertebrate humoral components. The fact that hemagglutinins, bactericidins, and erythrocyte hemolysins of animals such as the spiny lobster are apparently separate entities suggests the existence of a progression from primitive to advanced among the invertebrates with respect to the presence, numbers, and kinds of separate humoral substances. Since arthropods are relatively advanced when compared with annelids and molluscs, it is possible that more primitive creatures may lack the complexity of hemolymph components that function in arthropods.

Despite important differences between invertebrate humoral substances and vertebrate antibody, both groups of molecules possess the common property of providing immune-defense mechanisms. In vertebrate animals, antigens stimulate antibody synthesis, and the resulting antibody binds to antigen-forming complexes. Under certain conditions these antigen-antibody complexes can bind to complement or to certain cells, triggering an array of inflammatory reactions. The complement system alone can be activated if the need for antigen and antibody is bypassed. Complement consists of a system of proteins that mediates a number of reactions such as cell lysis, chemotaxis, agglutination, and phagocytosis. In some invertebrates, there are hemolymph activities that resemble activities mediated by the terminal components of the vertebrate complement system. Complement-like activity represents, for now, the most striking similarity between invertebrate and vertebrate immune components (1).

HETEROGENEITY. Although there has been an emphasis on similarities of the hemagglutinins between species, and heterogeneity within species was suspected, the first information reporting different hemagglutinins (heterogeneity) within the same species was given by Hall and Rowlands, (32, 33). It is of interest that heterogeneity also exists within individuals and is most important to immunology because of its implications for antigen-binding activity. There are multiple agglutinins and possibly two independent agglutinins (LAg-1 and LAg-2). These agglutinins have been purified from hemolymph by ammonium sulfate precipitation, pevikon block electrophoresis, and gel chromatography. Each has a unique molecular size, electrophoretic mobility, and binding specificity.

The molecular weight of LAg-1 exceeds that of 19S antibody and that of LAg-2, 11S. With regard to antigen specificity, LAg-1 reacts with human and mouse erythrocytes, whereas LAg-2 reacts only with mouse erythrocytes. Both agglutinins are labile when heated at 56° for 15 minutes, require calcium ions for activity, and are inactive after treatment with trypsin or after reduction and alkylation. These agglutinins dissociate into subunits of equal size (molecular weight 55,000) in 6M urea, a characteristic which indicates that the subunits are joined by noncovalent bonds. The binding properties of these hemagglutinins have been analyzed by inhibition studies with simple saccharides, enzyme treatment of erythrocytes, absorption of agglutinins, and microagglutination preparations. LAg-2 contains an N-acetyl galactosamine (Gal NAc) site which binds to Gal NAc residues on mouse and hamster erythrocytes. LAg 1 contains an N-acetyl neuraminic acid (NANAc) site which binds to NANAc residues on human erythrocytes; LAg-1 also binds to mouse erythrocytes via the NANAc site or via a second binding site on the LAg-1 molecule.

We have accepted in the past, without much solid evidence at the molecular level, that invertebrates recognize antigens and react against them. In order for invertebrates to recognize antigens, some kind of recognition unit must be present. Recognition units or molecules or receptors should, ideally, show marked heterogeneity that represents different polymeric forms of an identical subunit or subunits. This flexibility in structure would enable the recognition unit to react with or to bind to relatively large numbers of different antigens with unique specificites. The demonstration of heterogeneity in lobster hemagglutinin is therefore profoundly important to studies of immunoevolution.

It would indeed be useful to know if such agglutinins are synthesized by cells and if these cells are in fact the ubiquitous coelomocytes. Hypothetically, the agglutinins would be found on the surface of such cells after synthesis and prior to release in the hemolymph. Although lobsters are arthropods, protostomes—and not the group (deuterostomes) from which vertebrates arose—that a measure of hemagglutinin heterogeneity exists, provides strong analogous information of much theoretical importance to understanding how immunity evolved.

IMPACT OF CELLULAR IMMUNITY IN ANNELIDS, AR-THROPODS (PROTOSTOMES), AND ECHINODERMS (DEUTERO-STOMES).

There are two broad comparative approaches to studying the evolution of immune mechanisms. Among the arthropods, which are protostomes, the greatest amount of information on immunity has focused on humoral responses. The apparent lack of specificity after executing experiments designed to show induction of humoral substances has, however, created skeptical opinions regarding invertebrate humoral immunity. Thus, any attempt to extend invertebrate humoral immune mechanisms to encompass more classical definitions of immunity are desirable. In this vein, Anderson has recently shown that insect (the cockroach, *Prodenia*) macrophages possess nonspecific receptors for several kinds of foreign material such as erythrocytes, aldehyde-treated erythrocytes, and latex beads (3). They lack Fc and C3 receptors, commonly found on mammalian macrophages and B lymphocytes. With regard to rosette formation, a characteristic of vertebrate lymphocytes, *Prodenia* macrophages form spontaneous rosettes with human and sheep erythrocytes. Rosette formation can be reversibly inhibited by cytochalasin B, but it is not affected by vinblastine or colchicine. Rosette formation by cockroach hemocytes is therefore believed to require normal microfilament function but microtubules probably do not play an important role.

It is among the annelids and echinoderms that a good deal of information exists on cell-mediated responses. Earthworms and starfishes have been grafted with autografts, allografts, and xenografts, revealing that both groups are capable of making specific immunologic distinctions between self and non-self tissue. Autografts heal and are accepted permanently; allografts and xenografts also heal in, but they are gradually destroyed by various components of the host's immune reactions. Host responses include coelomocyte migration into the transplants. In both annelids and echinoderms, short-term memory is demonstrable after regrafting previously grafted hosts (39–41, 57, 58).

This specific immunologic recall phenomenon suggests that coelomocytes do increase in number in response to a second antigenic challenge. How coelomocytes increase is a question of immense importance to immunologic theory. At least two ways can be envisioned to explain heightened coelomocyte numbers in response to a second encounter with antigen. Coelomocytes sensitive to a first antigenic encounter could be *recruited* from throughout the host or from specific *coelomocytopoietic sites*. In contrast to recruitment, coelomocytes could increase by *reproduction*; once a coelomocyte is challenged by an antigen, and assuming the presence of appropriate receptors, they would then be triggered to divide, and faster after a second challenge than during the first response. Either of the two mechanisms, recruitment or reproduction, if supported by firm evidence, would be of interest. However, specific reproduction of coelomocytes in response to antigen in invertebrates would provide evidence for elements of the *clonal selection theory* which appeared earlier in evolution than just among mammals as is generally accepted. It is highly likely that coelomocyte proliferation may indeed be the case, if the Darwinian approach to immunologic diversification is to be extended.

THE PHYLUM CHORDATA. Man, as well as many other animals, belongs to the phylum Chordata. The chordate immune system is characterized by three factors: (1) the presence of *lympho-epithelial accumulations* in the *pharyngeal region* in association with the *gill slits*; (2)

the presence of *gut-associated lymphomyeloid tissue*; *(3) the capacity to recognize and react against allogenic antigeneic components.* The phylum Chordata includes four other subphyla (26, 63, 64). The fishes, amphibians, reptiles, birds, and mammals compose the subphylum Vertebrata. These animals show *quasi-immunorecognition, cell-mediated immunity* (just as invertebrates do), and an additional characteristic, *integrated cellular and humoral immunity.* The capacity to synthesize immunoglobulins is an attribute of vertebrates only. Immunoglobulins have not been described in any of the invertebrates, nor have they been described in the two primitive chordates (also invertebrates) which comprise the second subphylum, *Urochordata.* These include the sea squirts or tunicates. The small fishlike animals (Amphioxus) belong to the third subphylum, the *Cephalochordata,* and the Hemichordata consists of the acorn worms. It will probably be accepted that homologies of various kinds exist between the lymphoid elements of the chordates. First, however, parameters such as surface characteristics of putative lymphocyte subpopulations must be defined. Only then can we draw firmer conclusions about evolutionary mechanisms.

Evolution and the Immunologic Disciplines

INTRODUCTION. The previous sections have concentrated on immunological diversification by giving glimpses of varieties of living organisms and of their various immune responses. The concept of *immunoevolution* is based on comparing structural components of immune systems of representative invertebrate and vertebrate species, including their cells, tissues, organs, and their most important and best-known products, in the case of vertebrates: antibodies. Immunoevolution is new to immunology and the concept has developed as a result of greater understanding in disciplines such as phylogeny, genetics, and embryology and such expanding subdisciplines of the parent field, immunology (e.g., immunochemistry, immunogenetics, comparative immunology, and developmental immunology).

The process of evolution means an unfolding, a gradual moving in orderly fashion from one condition to the next. One major trend in immunology has been a growing awareness of an evolution toward increased *antibody diversity* and *specificity.* Another pattern that has emerged points out the great complexity of cells and the cellular immune responses. It is assumed that both cellular and humoral immunities evolved to protect man, other vertebrates, and invertebrates from both external and internal threats to their existence. It is a popular concept now that cellular immune responses probably evolved from the invertebrates as an internal safeguard against cancer, autoimmunity, and aging, in addition to their more obvious role in preventing infections.

EVOLUTION OF GENES CODING FOR HEMOLYMPH COMPONENTS IN INVERTEBRATES.

Our present knowledge concerning the genes that coded for antibody is far less speculative than our hypotheses for how genes may have coded for invertebrate humoral substances (38). The existing similarities among the hemagglutinins suggest that they had common origins and that they may have been the first primitive receptor units that evolved and were localized on the surface of immunocytes, serving as recognition units for antigens. Speculation centers around a precursor gene that coded for a molecule of about 20,000 molecular weight; then through fusion, contiguous-gene duplication, and possible translocation, genes evolved, coding for hemolymph molecules of about 69,000 molecular weight (e.g., in the spiny lobster). Such genes could have undergone considerable mutation which ultimately produced the well-known molecules with diverse functions (e.g., hemolysins, bactericidins, and hemagglutinins) (2). As an alternative hypothesis, it has been suggested that genes coding for invertebrate hemolymph factors (e.g., hemagglutinins) was lost when vertebrates evolved. For example, a hemagglutinin occurs in the lamprey, one of the most primitive jawless fishes; its hemagglutinin differs from its immunoglobulin (46).

HUMORAL IMMUNITY AND PHYLOGENETIC CONCEPTS.

When dealing with the evolution of structure and function, we can think in terms of homology and analogy. With homology in mind, and using the classical example, we see that the vertebrate forelimb has undergone striking modifications in various animals in order to adapt to particular environmental niches. Man has arms and hands; birds have wings; whales have flippers. Despite these adaptations, the limb has remained basically the same in its morphological structure. Although the adult structures appear different from one another, they do possess, at the core, the same ancestral entities. With analogy in mind, we can see that the need for flight can be provided by wings of birds or those of bats or of butterflies (57). However, the wings of all these animals, simply by sharing the same function, are analogous, not homologous. Undoubtedly homology and analogy exist in the structures and functions of various immune systems, but these concepts have only been dealt with in reference to immunoglobulins. Despite the need to begin thinking about homology and analogy in the immune system, especially with regard to cells, the universality of immunologic responses is real, for the full array of these responses in all vertebrates has some counterpart(s) in certain ancestral invertebrate prototypic immune responses. Immunochemists have preempted the function of immunobiologists and comparative immunologists by dealing with the concept of homology as it relates to immunoglobulin structure (4). Recently, because of more precise information on invertebrate humoral substances, there has been some attempt to think of analogy, especially in trying to account for the origins of cell receptors, probably as those substances in the coelomic fluids of invertebrates (e.g., hemagglutinins).

RELATIONSHIP BETWEEN THE EVOLUTION OF IMMUNITY AND CANCER.   Neoplasia and cancer in invertebrates, fishes, amphibians, and reptiles have been the subject of two recent reviews (6, 25). A great deal of controversy once centered around the question of whether cancer really did exist in animals other than birds and mammals. The questions raised about *cancer* have been somewhat similar to those about *immunity* in more primitive creatures. Now, however, both the disciplines of *comparative oncology* and *comparative immunology* are begin-

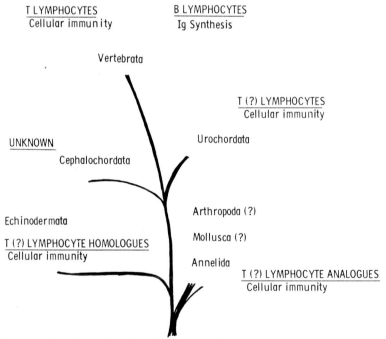

Fig. 8.   Phylum Chordata, showing the major characteristics of lymphocytes in two major subphyla: Vertebrata and Urochordata. For comparison, the protostome and deuterostome invertebrates are also shown. Extensive studies of echinoderms and annelids reveal characteristics of T cell responses, notably graft rejection.

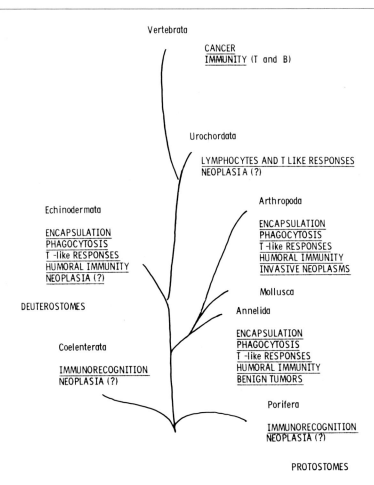

Fig. 9. Incidence of immunity and neoplasia in the animal kingdom. Although all groups have not been studied extensively, there may be a correlation between immune responsive and the capacity for cells to undergo neoplastic change.

ning to keep pace with the parent disciplines, which of course deal more with immunity and cancer in mammals. We do recognize immune mechanisms and cancer in invertebrates and primitive vertebrates. (See Fig. 8.)

The problem of immunity and neoplasia in invertebrates, just as in vertebrates, has a central core, the capacity to distinguish between self and non-self material. In essence, this describes the phenomenon of *recognition*. Exogenous infectious material introduced into invertebrates induces a state of immunity, but foreign cells from within, in the form of neoplasia, may or may not be reacted against by the immune system; this remains to be determined. Assuming a cause-and-effect relationship, animals would possess cell-mediated immunity as defense against neoplasia; thus, animals with immune systems can be expected to have neoplasia. Absence of neoplasia may be due to an effectively functioning immune system (Fig. 9). Conversely, immunologic deficiency caused by breakdown of the immune system may lead to the exposure of neoplasia. Studying both neoplasia and immunity in primitive animals such as mollusks (snails, clams) is important for understanding how both phenomena evolved (20).

It is generally accepted that some form of immunity with both specific and nonspecific components exists among the invertebrates. The mollusks and the arthropods are the only groups, however, where there are clearcut cases of known neoplastic growths with characteristics similar to those in mammals. According to Weiss, the major problem remaining to be resolved is to determine if there is a causal association between the vigor and kind of invertebrate immune reactions and their capacity to resist the abnormal growths analogous to or homologous to vertebrate neoplasia (60). It is probably safe to conclude that both neoplasia and immunity are not purely vertebrate attributes, thus accounting for the two phenomena earlier in evolution.

Final Comment

Recognition, primordial cell-mediated immunity, and vertebrate-type immune reactions represent evolutionary developments of immunity in the animal kingdom that protect organisms against infectious microorganisms. Unicellular protozoans combine food-getting and ultimate sequestration of microorganisms into one activity that occurs by chemotaxis and recognition and phagocytosis. Another mechanism for sequestering foreign material is by means of encapsulation. At this phylogenetic level, it has been presumed that self—non-self discrimination occurs by means of "proto-immunoglobulins" or other substances, which may act like receptors facilitating recognition or opsonins aiding phagocytosis. Primitive metazoans that exhibit only quasi-immuno-recognition may represent phylogenetic groups that should be examined for the existence of such cellular recognition units (35).

Another theory of importance to the evolution of recognition considers that the development of neoplasia was a strong force in the phylogeny of the entire immune system. Thus, simple recognition that encompassed combined food-getting and defense evolved into specific, primitive cellular immunity with a memory component and unknown receptors. The next step among chordates was the evolution of specific anamnestic immune responses mediated by cells with known receptors (immunoglobulins). If the dictum of Haeckel (1891) that "ontogeny recapitulates phylogeny" is still instructive, it certainly pertains to immune responsiveness (31). Indeed, the simplest manifestations of immunity are found throughout the phylogenetic sequence. Every level of metazoan complexity yields species adapted to certain environmental niches and each advancing level may possess remnants of the successive steps in the development of immunity. Each step in the immune system's ontogenesis and phylogenesis occurs in ordered fashion in both the embryologic and evolutionary development of animal species and their particular organ systems and physiologies.

REFERENCES

1. Acton, R. T., Evans, E. E., Weinheier, P. F., Cooper, E. L., Campbell, R. D., Prowse, R. H., Bizot, M., Stewart, J. E., Fuller, G. M., et al. 1972. Invertebrate Immune Mechanisms. MSS Information Corporation, New York.

2. Acton, R. T., and Weinheimer, P. F. 1974. Hemagglutinins: Primitive receptor molecules operative in invertebrate defense mechanisms, in E. L. Cooper (ed.), Contemporary Topics in Immunobiology, pp. 271–282. Plenum, New York.

3. Anderson, R. L. 1976. Expression of receptors by insect macrophages, in R. K. Wright and E. L. Cooper (eds.), Phylogeny of Thymus and Bone Marrow–Bursa Cells, North Holland, Amsterdam.

4. Atwell, J. L., and Marchalonis, J. J. 1975. Phylogenetic emergence of immunoglobulin classes distinct from IgM. J. Immunogenet. 1: 367–391.

5. Balinsky, B. I. 1970. An Introduction to Embryology. W. B. Saunders Co., Philadelphia.

6. Balls, M., and Ruben, L. N. 1976. Phylogeny of neoplasia and immune reactions to tumors, in J. J. Marchalonis (ed.), Comparative Immunology, pp. 167–208. Blackwell Scientific Publications, London.

7. Cohen, N. 1975. Phylogeny of lymphocyte structure and function. Amer. Zool. 15: 119–133.

8. Cooper, E. L. 1967. Some aspects of the histogenesis of the amphibian lymphomyeloid system and its role in immunity, in R. T. Smith, R. A. Good, and P. A. Miescher (eds.), Ontogeny of Immunity, pp. 87–102. University of Florida Press, Gainesville.

9. Cooper, E. L. 1970. Introduction to symposium on phylogeny of transplantation. Transpl. Proc. 2: 181–182.

10. Cooper, E. L. 1973. Earthworm coelomocytes: Role in understanding the evolution of cellular immunity. I. Formation of monolayers and cytotoxicity, in J. Rehácek, D. Blaskovic, W. F. Hink (eds.), Proc. III International Colloquium on Invertebrate Tissue Culture, pp. 381–404. Publishing House of the Slovak Academy of Sciences, Bratislava.

11. Cooper, E. L. 1973. Evolution of cellular immunity, in W. Braun and J. Ungar (eds.), *Non-Specific Factors Influencing Host Resistance*, pp. 11–23. S. Karger, Basel.

12. Cooper, E. L. 1973. The thymus and lymphomyeloid system in poikilo-thermic vertebrates, in A. J. S. Davies and R. L. Carter (eds.), *Contemporary Topics in Immunobiology*, pp. 13–38. Plenum, New York.

13. Cooper, E. L. 1974. Phylogeny of leukocytes: Earthworm coelomocytes in vitro and in vivo, in K. Lindahl-Kiessling and D. Osoba (eds.), *Lymphocyte Recognition and Effector Mechanisms, Proceedings of the Eighth Leukocyte Culture Conference*, pp. 155–162. Academic Press, New York.

14. Cooper, E. L. (ed.). 1975. *Invertebrate Immunology*. Contemporary Topics in Immunobiology, Volume 4, Plenum, New York.

15. Cooper, E. L. 1975. Characteristics of CMI and memory in annelids. *Adv. Exp. Med. Biol.* 64: 127–136.

16. Cooper, E. L. 1976. The earthworm coelomocyte: A mediator of cellular immunity, in R. K. Wright and E. L. Cooper (eds.), *Phylogeny of Thymus and Bone Marrow–Bursa Cells*, pp. 9–18. North Holland, Amsterdam.

17. Cooper, E. L. 1976. Cellular recognition of allografts and xenografts in invertebrates, in J. J. Marchalonis (ed.), *Comparative Immunology*, pp. 36–79. Blackwell, Oxford.

18. Cooper, E. L. 1976. Immunity mechanisms, in B. Lofts (ed.), *Physiology of the Amphibia*, pp. 163–272. Academic Press, New York.

19. Cooper, E. L. 1976. *Comparative Immunology*, Prentice-Hall, New Jersey.

20. Cooper, E. L. 1976. Immunity and neoplasia in mollusks. *Israel J. Med. Sci.* 12: 479–494.

21. Cooper, E. L. 1977. Evolution of blood cells. *Arch. Immunol.* (in press).

22. Cooper, E. L., *International Journal of Developmental and Comparative Immunology*. Pergamon Press, New York.

23. Cuenot, L. 1897. Les globules sanguins et les organes lymphoïdes des invertébrés *Arch. d'anat. Micr.* 1: 153–192.

24. Cuenot, L. 1891. Etudes sur le sang et les glands lymphatiques dans la série animale (2ᵉ Partie: Invertébrés) *Arch. Zool. Exp. Gen.* 9: 13–90.

25. Dawe, C. J., and Harshbarger, J. C. (eds.). 1969. A symposium on neoplasms and related disorders of invertebrate and lower vertebrate animals. *Natl. Cancer Inst. Monog.* 31.

26. Ermak, T. 1976. Hematogenic tissues of tunicates, in R. K. Wright and E. L. Cooper (eds.), *Phylogeny of T and B cells*, pp. 45–56. North Holland, Amsterdam.

27. Freeman, G. 1970. The reticuloendothelial system of tunicates. *J. Ret. Soc.* 7: 183–194.

28. Geddes, P. 1880. Observations sur le fluide périviscéral des oursins. *Arch. Zool.*, Ser. 8: 483–496.

29. George, W. C. 1926. The histology of the blood of *Perophora viridis* (ascidian). *J. Morphol.* 41: 31–331.

30. George, W. C. 1939. A comparative study of the blood of tunicates. *Quart. J. Microscop. Sci.* 81: 391–428.

31. Haeckel, E. 1891. Anthropogenie oder Entwickelungsgeschichte des Menschen. *Keimes- und Stammes-geschichte*. 4th rev. and enl. ed. Wilhelm Engelmann, Leipzig.

32. Hall, J. L., and Rowlands, D. T. Jr. 1974. Heterogeneity of lobster agglutinins. I. Purification and physiocochemical characterization. *Biochemistry* 13: 821–827.

33. Hall, J. L., and Rowlands, D. T. Jr. 1974. Heterogeneity of lobster agglutinins. II. Specificity of agglutinin-erythrocyte binding. *Biochemistry* 13: 828–832.

34. Hetzel, H. R. 1965. Studies on holothurian coelomocytes. II. The origin of coelomocytes and the formation of brown bodies. *Biol. Bull.* 128: 102–111.

35. Hildemann, W. H., and Reddy, A. L. 1973. Phylogeny of immune responsiveness: marine invertebrates. *Fed. Proc.* 32: 2188–2194.

36. Hildemann, W. H., and Benedict, A. A. 1975. *Immunologic Phylogeny. Advances in Experimental Medicine and Biology*. Plenum, New York.

37. Holland, N. D., Phillips, J. H., Jr., and Giese, A. C. 1965. An autoradiographic investigation of coelomocyte production in the purple sea urchin (*Strongylocentrotus purpuratus*). *Bio. Bull.* 128: 259–270.

38. Hood, L., Campbell, J. H. and Elgin, S. C. R. 1975. The organization, expression, and evolution of antibody genes and other multigene families. *Ann. Rev. Genet.* 9: 305–353.

39. Hostetter, R. K., and Cooper, E. L. 1972. Coelomocytes as effector cells in earthworm immunity. *Immunol. Commun.* 1: 155–183.

40. Hostetter, R. K., and Cooper, E. L. 1973. Cellular anamnesis in earthworms. *Cell Immunol.* 9: 384–393.

41. Hostetter, R. K., and Cooper, E. L. 1974. Earthworm coelomocyte immunity, in E. L. Cooper (ed.), *Contemporary Topics In Immunobiology*, 4, pp. 91–107. Plenum, New York.

42. Jordan, H., and Reynolds, B. D. 1933. The blood cells of the trematode, *Diplodiscus temperatus*. *J. Morphol.* 55: 119–130.

43. Jordan, H. E. 1938. Comparative hematology, in H. Downey (ed.), *Handbook of Hematology*, pp. 700–862. Hoeber Pub., New York.

44. Kindred, J. E. 1929. The leucocytes and leucocytopoietic organs of an oligochaete, *Pheretima indica* (Horst). *J. Morphol.* 47: 435–477.

45. Kollmann, M. 1908. Recherches sur les leucocytes et le tissu lymphoide des invertébrés. *Ann. Sci. Natur. Zool.*, Ser. 9, 8: 1–240.

46. Kubo, R. T., Zimmerman, B., and Grey, H. M. 1973. Phylogeny of Immunoglobulins, in M. Sela (ed.), *The Antigens*, pp. 417–477.

47. Manning, M. J., and Turner, R. J. 1976. *Comparative Immunobiology*, p. 184. Wiley, Halsted.

48. Marchalonis, J. J. 1976. *Comparative Immunology*, p. 470. Oxford, England.

49. Meglitsch, P. A. 1967. *Invertebrate Zoology*, p. 961. Oxford Univ. Press, New York.

50. Overton, J. 1966. The fine structure of blood cells in the ascidian *Perophora viridis*. *J. Morphol.* 119: 305–326.

51. Peres, J. M. 1953. Recherches sur le sang et les organes neuraux des tuniciers. *Ann. Inst. Oceanogr.*, 21: 229–359.

52. Prenant, M. 1922. Recherches sur le parenchyme des plathelminthes: Essai d'histologie comparée. *Arch. Morphol. Gen. Exp.,* 5: 1–174.

53. Roch, P. H., Valembois, P., and Du Pasquier, L. 1975. Response of earthworm leukocytes to concanavalin A and transplantation antigens, *in* W. H. Hildemann and A. A. Benedict (eds.), *Adv. Exp. Med. Biol.,* 64: 44–45. Plenum, New York.

54. Simpson, G. G. 1960. *The Meaning of Evolution. A Study of the History of Life and of Its Significance for Man,* p. 365. Yale Univ. Press, New Haven.

55. Sloan, B., Yocum, C., and Clem, L. W. 1975. Recognition of self from non-self in crustaceans. *Nature* 258: 521–523.

56. Stang-Voss, C. 1974. On the ultrastructure of invertebrate hemocytes: An interpretation of their role in comparative hematology, *in* E. L. Cooper (ed.), *Contemporary Topics in Immunobiology,* 4: 65–75. Plenum, New York.

57. Toupin, J., and Lamoureaux, G. 1976. Mitogen responsiveness of *Lumbricus terrestris* coelomocytes, *in* R. K. Wright and E. L. Cooper (eds.), *Phylogeny of Thymus and Bone Marrow Bursa-Cells,* pp. 19–25. North Holland, Amsterdam.

58. Valembois, P. 1974. Cellular aspects of graft rejection in earthworms and some other metazoa, *in* E. L. Cooper (ed.), *Contemporary Topics in Immunobiology,* 4: 121–126. Plenum, New York.

59. Vethamany, V. G., and Fung, M. 1972. The fine structure of coelomocytes of the sea urchin *Strongylocentrotus dröbachiensis.* (Müller, O. F.), *Canad. J. Zool.* 50: 77–81.

60. Weiss, D. W. 1976. Central problems in tumor immunology (Introduction and Preface). *Israel J. Med. Sci.* 12: 281–287.

61. Willier, B. H., Weiss, P. A., and Hambruger, V. 1956. *Analysis of Development,* p. 734. W. B. Saunders Co., Philadelphia.

62. Wright, R. K., and Cooper, E. L. 1975. Immunological maturation in the tunicate *Ciona intestinalis. Amer. Zool.* 15: 21–27.

63. Wright, R. K., 1976. Phylogenetic origin of the vertebrate lymphocyte and lymphoid tissue, *in* R. K. Wright and E. L. Cooper (eds.), *Phylogeny of Thymus and Bone Marrow–Bursa Cells,* North Holland, Amsterdam.

64. Wright, R. K., and Cooper, E. L. (eds.), 1976. *Phylogeny of Thymus and Bone Marrow–Bursa Cells,* p. 325. North Holland, Amsterdam.

CHAPTER 3

THE EFFECTS OF AGING ON IMMUNE FUNCTION [1]

Marguerite M. B. Kay

Geriatrics Research,
Education and Clinical Center
Veterans Administration,
Wadsworth Hospital Center
Los Angeles, California
and Department of Medicine
University of California
at Los Angeles
Los Angeles, California 90024

Normal immune functions can begin to decline shortly after an individual reaches sexual maturity. This decline is due primarily to changes in the cells although changes in the cellular milieu contribute to it. Foremost among the cellular changes are those in the stem cells as reflected in their growth properties and the availability of precursor T cells, and in the T cells, where a shift in subpopulations may be occurring. Evidence suggests that at least the shift in T cell subpopulations is secondary to the age-related structural and functional changes occurring within the thymus. Thus, the process(es) regulating involution and atrophy of the thymus could be the key to immunosenescence.

Alone, as if enduring to the end
A valiant armor of scarred hopes outworn,
He stood there in the middle of the road
Like Roland's ghost winding a silent horn.
Below him, in the town among the trees,
Where friends of other days had honored him,
A phantom salutation of the dead
Rang thinly till old Eben's eyes were dim.

—Edwin Arlington Robinson
  "Mr. Flood's Party"

I. INTRODUCTION

Aging is characterized by a declining ability of the individual to adapt to environmental stress. This decline is exemplified physiologically by an inability to maintain homeostasis. Since 1900, the 65-and-older sector has grown much faster than the rest of the population. The 75-and-older group has increased even faster. Between 1960 and 1974, 65–74-year-olds increased 23%, while over 75's increased 49%. Today, there are 22 million Americans 65 and older. This differential growth rate of age groups within the United States population is due predominantly to two factors: improved health care, such as immunizations and antibiotics, which enable individuals to live to an older age; and the decreased birth rate.

In spite of improved health care, approximately 3000 Americans aged 65 and older die per day while approximately 4000 Americans turn 65 every day. The survivors are exposed to new medicopsychosocial, economic, and biomedical crises. Medicopsychosocial problems often revolve around agonizing disabilities associated with aging, biomedically forced curtailment of normal activities, requirements for chronic medical care, and fears concerning mental deterioration. Economic and biomedical problems arise because older individuals are more susceptible to disease and therefore tend to have chronic diseases requiring more ambulatory and extended hospital medical care. It is imperative, then, that methods be found which may delay the onset or lessen the severity of the diseases associated with aging—thus prolonging the *productive* lifespan.

The immune system is perhaps the most productive field in which to conduct studies in such methods, for the following reasons:

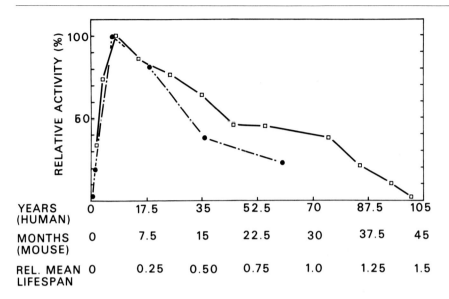

Fig. 1. Age effects on serum agglutinin titers in the human and the mouse. □, natural serum anti-A isoagglutinin titers in the human (130). ●, peak serum agglutinin response titer to sheep RBC stimulation by intact long-lived mice (80). Reprinted from *Proc. Nat. Acad. Sci.* 48: 234–238.

1.   Certain normal immune functions decline with age in humans, guinea pigs, hamsters, rats, and mice (114, 134) (Fig. 1), although the onset, magnitude, and rate of decline vary with the type of immune function and the species.

2.   The immune system is "organismal" in that it is in continual contact with most, if not all, cell, tissue, and organ systems within the body. Thus, any alteration of the immune system would be expected to affect all other systems. If one views aging as a perturbation of homeostasis, then a mobile, dynamic system such as the immune system is perhaps the ideal one in which to study such perturbations and their consequences.

3.   As immunologic vigor decreases, the incidence of infections, autoimmune and immune complex diseases, and cancer increases (41, 46, 76, 77) (Fig. 2), as in the case of immunodeficient newborns and immunosuppressed adults (34, 35, 92).

The evidence linking decreased immunologic vigor to disease includes the following: (a) the onset of decline in thymus-derived T-cell-dependent immune functions can occur as early as sexual maturity

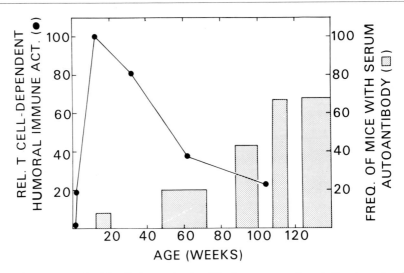

Fig. 2.   The capacity for T-cell-dependent antibody response in relation to natural antibody formation in long-lived mice. Reprinted with permission from Handbook on the Biology of Aging, C. Finch and L. Hayflick (eds.), © 1977 by Van Nostrand Reinhold Co.

when the thymus begins to involute (80), which is long before immunodeficiency diseases of the elderly are manifested; (b) immunodeficiency, wasting disease, amyloidosis, and autoimmunity in neonatally thymectomized mice and in genetically susceptible mice can be prevented, or at times even reversed, by reconstituting them with young syngeneic thymus or spleen grafts; old grafts are not effective (29, 127, 140); (c) an age-related decrease in T cell function, as determined by T-cell-dependent antibody synthesis, is associated with an increase in the frequency of antinuclear antibody in humans (108) (Fig. 3); (d) preliminary data suggest that in aging men, but not in women, autoantibodies are predictive of death from vascular causes, and that rheumatoid factor is predictive of death from cancer (77); (e) the incidence of cancer in persons with childhood immunodeficiency diseases ranges from 1 in 10 to 1 in 20, in spite of the fact that these individuals have a much shorter lifespan in which to develop cancer, whereas approximately 1 in 300 persons in the general population either has or has had cancer (34); (f) the incidence of cancer in adult-onset immunodeficiency is higher than normal and is estimated by some at 1 in every 10 affected individuals (34, 35); (g) immunosuppression both in animals and in humans increases the incidence of spontaneous tumors (e.g., the risk for an immunosuppressed transplant patient of developing reticulum cell sarcoma is 350 times that

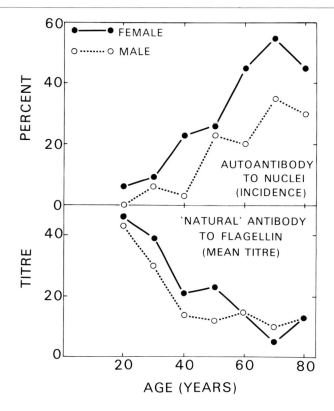

Fig. 3.   Fall in natural anti-Salmonella flagellin titer with age and rise in the incidence of antinuclear factor in humans of both sexes (108). Reprinted with permission from Rowley, Buchanan, and MacKay, Lancet 1968, Vol. 2, pg. 24.

of the normal population) (20); (h) immunosuppression enhances transplanted tumor "takes" and increases the incidence of metastases of transplanted tumors both in humans and in animals (20, 141); and (i) mortality is higher among aged humans with reduced cell-mediated immune function than among those with normal cell-mediated immune function, and death associated with cancer and cardiovascular diseases is higher among those with serum antinuclear autoantibody than among those without such antibody (76, 77, 107).

Based on these considerations, the intriguing possibility exists that a delay, reversal, or prevention of the decline in normal immune functions could delay the onset and/or minimize the severity of diseases of the elderly. However, before any attempt is made to intervene with the disease processes, it would seem that an understanding of the basic mechanism(s) responsible for the loss of immunologic vigor is not only desirable but essential. It is not surprising, therefore, that much of the research on immunosenescence has been centered on characterizing the decline and, more recently, searching for its mechanism.

In this chapter, therefore, an overview of this rapidly developing area will be presented by first discussing the age-related changes in the immune system and then by focusing attention on the mechanisms responsible for the decline in immune functions.

II. AGE-RELATED CHANGES IN IMMUNE FUNCTIONS

A. Morphology

The first hint that normal immune functions may be declining with age came from the findings of classical morphologists who showed rather convincingly both in laboratory animals and humans that the thymic lymphatic mass decreased with age as a result primarily of atrophy of the cortex, beginning at the time of sexual maturity (4, 109) (Fig. 4). Histologically, the cortex of an involuted thymus is sparsely populated

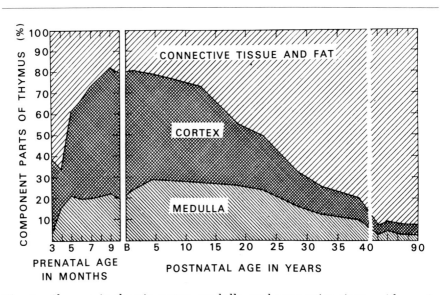

Fig. 4. Changes in thymic cortex, medulla, and connective tissue with age in humans (13). Reprinted from *American Journal of Diseases of Children*, 1932, Vol. 43: 1162–1214. © 1932, American Medical Association.

with lymphocytes, which are replaced by numerous macrophages filled with lipoid granules (62). In addition, infiltration of plasma and mast cells can be observed in the medulla as well as in the cortex (62). The proportion and number of T cells in the thymus decreases with age, as does thymus cellularity (cells per mg net weight) and thymic weight (67, 68).

The weight of the spleen of normal mice remains the same with age after adulthood (4, 67, 68). The weight of lymph nodes increases slightly with age in some strains and hybrids of mice but not in others although the total number of cells does not change significantly (67, 68). Probably more significant are the age-related histologic changes of lymphatic tissues which include diminishing germinal centers, decreased cellularity accompanied by an increase in connective tissue, and increasing numbers of plasma cells and phagocytes (23, 97, 134).

B. Cell Number

Several recent reports indicate that the number of circulating lymphocytes in humans decreases progressively during or after middle age to a level that by the sixth decade is about 70% of that of a young adult, and the decrease is due to a reduction in the absolute number of circulating T cells, while the number of B cells remains essentially the same (7, 19, 27, 68, 118). In these reports, the number of T and B cells was calculated from estimates of their concentration and proportion, based on sheep erythrocyte (E) rosettes and immunofluorescence. Others have reported that the proportion of T cells does not change with age (133, 138). In aging mice, the pattern of change in the absolute number of theta-bearing T cells varies with the strain and hybrid of strains and with the organ (67, 68). In some strains, the absolute number of T cells in the spleen and lymph nodes shows no change, while in others an increase or decrease is noted. However, changes in the number or proportion of T cells in both humans and mice are not sufficient to account for the observed decrease in immunologic functions (67, 68). Further, as will be discussed in a later section, a decrease in the number of cells bearing surface T cell markers does not necessarily mean that the number of T cells has decreased; it could mean that the number of T cells in a particular differentiation stage has decreased.

C. Cell-Mediated Immunity

There are conflicting reports in the literature concerning the effect of age on T cell functions in humans and animals (9, 40, 43, 46, 47,

89, 121). Some investigators report a decrease in delayed hypersensitivity to common skin-test antigens to which individuals have been previously sensitized (such as purified protein derivative of tuberculosis, streptokinase-streptodornase; monilia, trichophyton; and mumps), while others report no decrease except in those elderly persons with acute illness. In general, it appears that T cell functions, when assessed with an antigen to which the individuals have not been sensitized previously (such as dinitrochlorobenzene [DNCB]), decline with age. The conflicting results could be attributed to: (a) utilization of only one skin test antigen to assess T cell function, (b) selection of skin-test antigens (e.g., only a fraction of the United States population has been immunized to tuberculosis; therefore, a negative result cannot be interpreted as reflective of defective immunological memory), and (c) selection of the population samples (i.e., some studies used hospitalized patients and medical clinic populations).

A battery of common skin-test antigens should be utilized for assessing immunological memory. For assessing the ability of an individual to become sensitized to a "new" antigen, DNCB is probably the best choice, if for no other reason than to allow comparison of results between laboratories. It could, of course, be argued that any decrease in delayed hypersensitivity seen in the elderly reflects aging of the skin rather than the immune system. However, results of tumor cell rejection tests in aging mice were comparable, and since tumor cells were injected intraperitoneally in these tests, aging of the skin was not the limiting factor (43).

In vivo studies in mice indicate that T cell functions decline with age (43, 95, 125, 128). Cells from old mice have a decreased ability to mount a graft-versus-host (GVH) reaction (95, 137) even when enriched T cell populations are utilized to compensate for the possibility that old animals may have fewer T cells (137). Resistance to challenge with allogeneic tumor cells in vivo decreases dramatically with age, as does the lymphoproliferative response of draining lymph nodes to allogeneic tumor cells and the proliferative response of spleen cells to allogeneic cells (95). It is of great significance that in these studies the decline in response to phytohemagglutinin (PHA), a plant-mitogenic lectin, measured in vitro, approximated the decline in GVH and tumor cell challenge measured in vivo.

The in vitro findings show that the proliferative capacity of T cells of humans and rodents in response to plant mitogens (PHA and concanavalin A [Con A]) and allogeneic target cells declines with age (1, 32, 50, 59, 63, 67, 68, 71, 84, 95, 100, 107), and the decline is most striking in mice, regardless of their lifespan (Fig. 5). The decline in the cytotoxicity index of T cells of long-lived mice has been reported to be moderate against allogeneic tumor cells and not readily apparent against certain syngeneic tumor cells (43). The discrepancy between results of tumor cytotoxicity

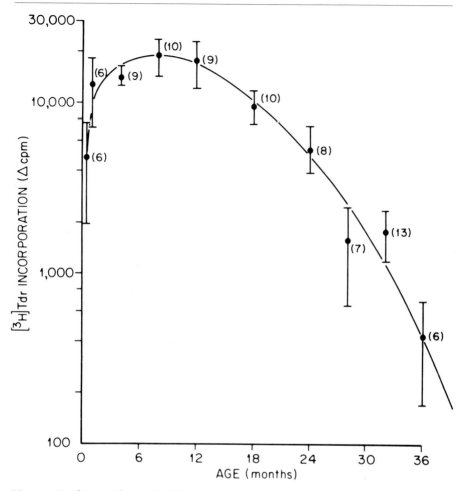

Fig. 5. Decline with age in PHA mitogenic activity of splenic T cells of long-lived mice. Reprinted from *Proc. Soc. Exp. Bio. Med.,* 1973, Vol. 144, pp. 48–53.

tests performed *in vivo* and *in vitro* may be due to inadequate culture conditions in the latter. More recently, the development of cytotoxic lymphocytes in *in vitro* mixed lymphocyte culture (MLC) reaction has been reported to decline with age (60).

There has been one report that the response to PHA in mice shows few changes with age (113). However, in this report, "middle-aged" rather than old C57Bl/6J mice were used; that is, 15–20-month-old mice were used when the mean lifespan (MLS) of the mice in that laboratory was 24 months, which is equivalent to assaying 44-to-58-year-old humans whose

MLS is 70 years. This directs attention to an important point: The age at which a mouse is "old" varies with the strain; for example, in one laboratory, the MLS of DBA/2 males is 86 weeks whereas the MLS of C57Bl/6J males is 130 weeks (71, 117). Further, the MLS of a strain can vary between laboratories depending upon the animal housing conditions; for example, C57Bl/6J which have a MLS of 130 weeks in some laboratories may have a mean lifespan of 97 weeks in others (122, 135). Thus, a 90-week-old C57Bl/6J could be considered "old" in one laboratory but "middle-aged" in another.

It should be emphasized, furthermore, that young *adult* mice (3–6 months old) rather than "young" mice ($\leq$ 2 months old) should be used as a reference point for aging studies, for the latter may be "immature" immunologically, depending on the immunologic index. Thus, using antibody response to sheep red blood cells (SRBC) as an index, it was shown that BC3F mice do not mature until 6 months of age (80). Moreover, it has been observed that the response of BC3F mice (MLS, 30 months) to PHA peaked at 8 months of age, while the response of BALB/c (MLS, 25 months) peaked by 4 months (63) in one laboratory; and in another, the PHA response of $BC3F_1$, C3H, and C57Bl/6 mice peaked between 3 and 6 months of age (67, 68). The response of CD-1 and C57Bl/6 mice to T cell mitogens (PHA and con A) is 18–33% of 8-week values for the first three weeks of life and 63% of 8-week values by 6 weeks of life; whereas the lipopolysaccharide (LPS) responses are equivalent to 8-week values as early as 7 days after birth (106). Other strains, such as C3H, do not mature until 3 months of age as determined by body weight, organ weight, number of theta-positive cells, and organ cellularity (68). A further complication encountered when using immature mice is that variability between individuals is greater than in young adults. As is evident from the above discussion, the description of mice as "old" or "young" should be based upon the survival and developmental pattern of each individual strain. This would reduce the number of conflicting reports regarding the effect of age on immune functions.

There are conflicting reports in the literature on the effect of age on the MLC reactions.[2] Some investigators reported a marked decrease in the response of cells with age (1, 61). Others reported that cells from old mice are as efficient or more so than cells from young mice both as responding and stimulating cells in the MLC reaction (137), but the same cells showed a decreased GVH index. Regarding the use of MLC index to study age effects on cell-mediated immunity, the use of X-rayed cells or hybrid cells of donors of one age group as the stimulating cells is advised over that of mitomycin-treated cells. Mitomycin may leak from the stimulating cells, and cells from old animals may be more susceptible to this drug than cells from young animals.

The helper function of T cells declines with age. This has been demonstrated in intact animals and in assays performed both *in vivo* and *in vitro* (52, 58, 102, 103). The assays employed are based on the ability of T cells to promote antibody response to "T-cell-dependent" antigens. Many of the assays have utilized foreign red blood cells as a "T-dependent" antigen. Since many of the descriptive studies have been completed, and since it is now necessary to elucidate cellular and molecular mechanisms of age-related alteration, use of antigenically undefined red blood cells as a test antigen should be discouraged because they contain many antigens, some of which are probably T-independent while others are T-dependent. Instead, defined hapten antigens, such as dinitrophenolbovine serum albumin (DNP-BSA) or the polypeptide poly-L-(Tyr, Glu)-poly-DL-Ala-poly-L-Lys(T,G-A-L) should be used for T-dependent antigen studies, and antigens such as DNP-Ficoll or pneumococcus SIII for T-independent antigen studies.

As yet, very little is known regarding the effect of age on suppressor T cell function in normal aging individuals. This is due in part to the complexities of the system. It has not been clearly demonstrated that there is a T cell which, upon stimulation, will produce only a suppressive effect. It is possible that there are subpopulations of T cells which exert both suppressive and helper effects depending upon the nature of the stimulation. Assay systems used to detect suppressor functions are often the same as those that have been used to demonstrate helper function. Depletion of a particular T cell population in order to abolish suppression often results in the abolition of helper activity. The recent development of antisera directed against allelic T cell determinants (Ly differentiation antigens) which allows identification of three T cell subsets should greatly facilitate research in the area of age effects on T cell suppressor function (17, 18). It seems that T cells expressing the Ly 1 antigen are responsible for helper- and delayed-type hypersensitivity effects, while cells expressing Ly 2,3 are responsible for suppressor effects and for cell-mediated cytolysis (17, 18). No specific function has yet been assigned to Ly 1,2,3 cells. For a complete review of suppressor cells in aging, see Reference 39.

The evidence that suppressor T cell activity declines with age was derived from studies of short-lived NZB and related mice. C-type virus infection, however, plays a major role in the pathogenesis of the disease of NZB. The causes and mechanisms of the decline in normal immune functions and of immunodeficient diseases in these animal models may be different from those occurring in long-lived mice and elderly humans. We may be observing phenotypic caricatures of old-age immune deficiency which is analogous to the phenotypic features of accelerated aging seen in progeria in humans.

D. Humoral Immunity

Normal B cell immune functions reflective of humoral immunity have been analyzed in terms of circulating levels of natural isoantibodies and heteroantibodies and in terms of antigen-induced antibody response. Circulating levels of natural antibodies have been assessed most systematically in the human, and the results show that they decline with age, starting shortly after the thymus begins to involute (33, 37, 91, 130) and after the level of serum thymosin (alleged to be a thymic hormone) begins to decline (8).

Aging rodents have been used primarily for the study of antigen-induced antibody responses, and the results show that primary, but not secondary, antibody response decreases with age (45, 70, 80, 88, 111, 112, 121, 139). They also show that the onset of decline in antibody response can occur as early as when the thymus begins to involute. This would suggest that with many types of primary antibody responses, aging is affecting the regulator T cells and not necessarily the B cells. This suspicion has been verified partially by the subsequent demonstration that the antibody response of B cells to complex antigens generally requires the help of T cells (e.g., 24), and that the antibody response to the T-independent antigens, Type III pneumococcal polysaccharide and bacterial lipopolysaccharide, does not decline appreciably with age in BALB/c and C3H mice (116) although it does in SJL/J mice. Inbred SJL/J mice have a predisposition for Hodgkin's-like reticulum cell neoplasia and may not be good models for immunodeficiency as it occurs in long-lived mice and humans.

Figure 1 relates B cell immune functions of the human and mouse to their lifespan. It can be seen that the patterns of rise and decline in B cell immune functions of the human and mouse are remarkably similar.

There have been exceptions to the "rule"; that is, reports showing no decline in primary antibody response, especially against bacterial and viral vaccines (26, 36, 70, 110, 119). Two explanations can be offered: (a) these individuals have been previously exposed to the antigen and therefore are, in fact, mounting a secondary response, and (b) the reaction is to antigens which do not require the participation of T cells; that is, they are T-independent antibody responses.

III. MECHANISMS OF THE AGE-RELATED DECLINE IN NORMAL IMMUNE FUNCTIONS

A. Cellular Milieu

The decline with age in normal immune functions may be due to changes in the cellular environment or milieu, changes in the cells of the immune system, or both. To differentiate between the influences of cells and their environment, the cell-transfer method, which assesses immunocompetent cells from young and old mice in immunologically inert old and young syngeneic recipients, respectively, was employed (2, 102, 103). The results revealed that changes both intrinsic and extrinsic to the cells affect the immune response and that about 10% of the normal age-related decline can be attributed to changes in the cellular environment, while 90% of the decline can be attributed to changes intrinsic to the old cells (102, 103).

The responsible factor(s) in the cellular environment was shown to be systemic and noncellular (103). Spleen cells from young mice were cultured with the test antigen either in the young (or old) recipient's spleen by the cell-transfer method or in the recipient's peritoneal cavity by the diffusion chamber method (44). A twofold difference in response was observed between young and old recipients at both sites, indicating that the factor(s) is systemic. The fact that the effect was observed in cells grown in cell-impermeable diffusion chambers further indicates that a noncellular factor is involved. A comparable twofold difference was also observed when bone marrow stem cells were assessed in the spleens of young and old syngeneic recipients (21), indicating that the systemic, noncellular factor(s) influences both lympho- and hematopoietic processes.

The factor(s) could be a deleterious substance of molecular or viral nature, or it could be an essential substance that is deficient in old mice. Factors of both types probably change with age, and further, several factors of each type may exist.

Unfortunately, this area of research has not progressed as rapidly as anticipated because a simple, sensitive in vitro assay to analyze mouse sera has not yet been perfected. Thus, for example, it is unclear why normal adult mouse serum is toxic for mouse immunocompetent cells grown in vitro.

B. Cellular Changes

One of the hallmarks of immunosenescence is the increase in variability of immune indices (68, 82). If more than one factor is responsible for the increase in variability, it is not surprising to find that the decline in humoral immune capacity of aging mice results from deficiencies in both the immune cells and in their milieu (2, 102, 103).

Three types of cellular changes could cause a decline in normal immune functions: (a) an absolute decrease in cell number through death caused possibly by autoimmune cells, (b) a relative decrease in cell number as a result of an increase in the number of "suppressor" cells, and

(c) a decrease in functional efficiency caused possibly by somatic mutation. One approach in resolving this problem is to first estimate the frequency of old mice with various cellular changes. This can be done by assessing the activity of reference immune cells from adult individuals in the presence of immune cells from old individuals. A response of young-old cell mixtures that was less than the sum of the responses given by pure young and pure old cells would indicate that the decreased response of old individuals was due to an increase in suppressor cells. If the response of the mixture was comparable, it would indicate that the decreased response of old individuals was caused either by a decrease in their functional efficiency or a general loss of immune cells. If the response of the mixture was higher, it would indicate that the decreased response of old individuals was caused by a selective loss of one type of immune cell that exists in excess in young individuals. The results showed that, indeed, all three types of interactions can occur (96). This supports the contention that although there may be only one underlying mechanism responsible for the loss of immunologic vigor with age, it is expressed differently between aging individuals, and this contributes to the increase with age in variability in immunologic performance.

1. STEM CELLS.   In mouse bone marrow, which contains 90% of all stem cells, the total stem cell number remains constant with age (21, 22). This indicates that stem cells can self-replicate in situ throughout the natural lifespan of the mouse, unlike stem cells passaged in vivo whose self-replicating ability can be exhausted (53, 72, 115). Further, stem cells do not lose their lympho-hematopoietic ability with age (54). On the other hand, subtle changes have been detected with age. Thus, their rate of B cell formation seems to decline with age (31), as does their ability to repair X-ray-induced DNA damage (22), and there is an absolute decrease in the number of functionally competent T cell precursors in the hematopoietic tissues of aging mice and a decrease in the proliferative capacity of some of these cells with age (132). In addition, alteration in certain kinetic parameters in spleen colony formation has been detected with age (83). Interestingly, when attempts were made to reverse these age-related kinetic parameters by enabling "old" stem cells to self-replicate in syngeneic young recipients for an extended period, it was found that kinetically they still behaved as old stem cells. However, when "young" stem cells were allowed to self-replicate in syngeneic old recipients, they behaved as old stem cells kinetically. These results indicate that the milieu of stem cells induces subtle stable changes which affect their responsiveness to differentiation-homeostatic factors.

2. MACROPHAGES.   Many of the earlier studies on the mechanism of loss in immunologic vigor with age were focused on the macrophages (5, 6, 129). It was thought that because macrophages confront antigens before the T and B cells, any defect in them could decrease immune functions without appreciable changes in the antigen-specific T and B cells. These studies showed that macrophages are not adversely affected by aging in their handling of antigens during both the induction of immune responses and phagocytosis; that is: (a) the in vitro phagocytic activity of old mice was equal to or better than that of young mice (93); (b) the activity of at least three lysosomal enzymes in macrophages increased rather than decreased with age (56); (c) the ability of antigen-laden macrophages of old mice to initiate primary and secondary antibody responses in vitro was comparable to that of young mice (93); and (d) the capacity of splenic macrophages and other adherent cells to cooperate with T and B cells in the initiation of antibody response in vitro was unaffected by age (58). Furthermore, when their antigen-processing ability was indirectly assessed by injecting young and old mice with varying doses of sheep red blood cells, it was found that the slope of regression line of the antigen dose-response curve and the minimum dose of antigen needed to generate a maximum response were significantly higher and lower, respectively, in old mice (102) (Fig. 6). Such results could be explained by assuming that the antigen-processing macrophages prevented antigen-sensitive T and B cells from responding maximally to

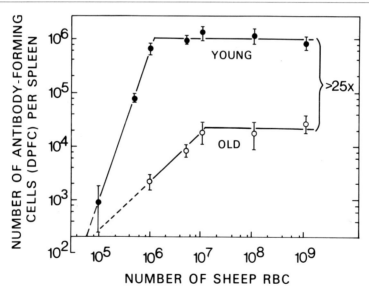

Fig. 6. Effect of antigen dose on peak antibody response of young and old mice. Vertical bars indicate 95% confidence limits (102). Reprinted by permission of The Williams & Wilkins Co., Baltimore, MD., from *Journal of Immunology,* © 1972.

limiting doses of the antigen (74), perhaps because their number or phagocytic efficiency increased with age (56). Associated with reduced antigen-processing is the failure of antigens to localize in the follicles of lymphoid tissues of antigen-stimulated old mice (73, 88). One clinical implication of these results is that the ability of individuals to detect low doses of antigens, such as syngeneic tumor antigens, can decline with age, contributing to the age-related poor immune surveillance noted against low doses of certain syngeneic tumor cells in mice (101). It also could explain why the resistance to allogeneic tumor cell challenge can decline with age by more than 100-fold in mice manifesting only a 4-fold decline in T-cell-mediated cytolytic activity against the same tumor cells (43).

3. B CELLS.   The number of B cells in the spleen and lymph nodes does not seem to change appreciably with age in long-lived mice (79), whereas it seems to increase in autoimmune-prone, relatively short-lived mice (41). In humans, studies have been limited primarily to circulating B cells, and they indicate that the number of B cells also remains relatively constant (27). Unfortunately, we do not know as yet whether the number of circulating B cells corresponds to that in the spleen and lymph nodes. In contrast to the constancy with age in the total B cell population, subpopulations of B cells may fluctuate. Support of this view comes from the observations that the number of B cells responsive to a T-cell-independent antigen decreases slightly with age in long-lived mice (102) and that the level of serum IgG and IgA tends to increase with age, while that of serum IgM tends to decrease (16, 49, 75).

Although the number of B cells remains relatively stable with age, their responsiveness to stimulation with certain T-cell-dependent antigens decreases strikingly (80, 82). When the responses of young and old mice were systematically evaluated by limiting dilution and dose-response methods, they revealed that the decline is caused by: (a) a decrease with age in the number of antigen-sensitive immunocompetent (IU) precursor units, which are made up of two or more cell types in various ratios (T_1M_1, T_2M_1, ... B_1M_1, B_2M_1, ... $T_1M_1B_1$, $T_2M_1B_3$, ... etc.) (48) and (b) a decrease in the average number of antibody-forming functional cells generated by each IU, or the immunologic burse size (IBS) (102, 103) (Fig. 3). We do not know the cause(s) for the reduction with age in both the relative number of IU and IBS. It could be due to an increase in the number of regulatory T cells which can inhibit the precursor cells making up the IU from interacting with each other, as well as inhibit the proliferation of B cells. The reason for this suspicion is that the number of Ig-bearing B cells remains constant with age (27) and the proliferative capacity of mitogen-sensitive B cells also remains unaltered with age (64, 65, 79). It could also result from an alteration in the ability of certain B cells to interact with other precursor cells making up the IU and in their ability to respond to homeostatic factors during differentiation.

4. T CELLS. Present evidence suggests that the decline in normal immune functions which accompanies aging is due primarily to changes in the T cell component of the immune system. Since involution of the thymus precedes the age-related functional decline, a "cause and effect" relationship was suspected (i.e., thymic involution results in a decreased capacity of the system to generate functional T cells). In spite of the obvious importance of establishing such a relationship on more than inferences derived from temporal events, only recently was this subjected to rigorous experimental proof. Previous experiments demonstrated that adult thymectomy accelerates the decline of immune responsiveness as evidenced by decreased hemagglutinin response to SRBC, particularly in the early response (19S) phase (87), a marked decrease in the GVH reaction, the poor general condition of the mice, and reduced antibody response to BSA (126). The effect on the latter response was less pronounced than that on the GVH. Recently, Hirokawa and Makinodan (61) transplanted thymus lobes from mice 1 day to 33 months old into young adult, T-cell-deprived recipients and assessed kinetically the emergence of T cells. They found that the ability of the thymus tissue to influence the differentiation or maturation of cells into functional T cells decreases with increasing age, and that different T cell indices exhibit differential susceptibility to thymus involution (for details, see Ref. 62).

These results indicate that thymic involution precedes and is responsible for the age-dependent decline in the ability of the immune system to generate functional T cells. What is the mechanism by which thymic involution leads to a decrease in peripheral effector cells? It appears that the primary effect of involution of the thymus is on a T-cell-differentiation pathway. Evidence suggests that a subset of T cells does not respond to stimulation, due possibly to insufficiency of hormones in the milieu and/or alterations intrinsic to the cells. The following observations support this view:

1. The proportion of lymphocytes bearing the theta antigen decreases with age, as does the amount of theta antigen on cell surfaces; yet there is no compensatory increase in B lymphocytes nor does the lymphocyte number change significantly. This suggests an increase in T cells that do not carry detectable theta receptors on their surface (15).
2. Although PHA-induced blastogenesis of cells from old mice is significantly reduced (see Fig. 4), the same cells bind ^{125}I-labeled PHA equally as well as cells from young mice (65). Because there seems to be no significant decrease in binding affinities or receptor sites for

PHA on cells of old mice, the defect cannot be in their membrane receptors.

3. The cyclic nucleotide 3′,5′-guanosine monophosphate, which has been shown to increase when T cells are stimulated by mitogens, is found in relatively low concentrations in mitogen-stimulated T cells of old mice, and it is known that the levels of cyclic nucleotides are hormone dependent (57). This suggests that the defect in T cells is intracellular and may be hormone dependent.

4. The lifespan of hypopituitary dwarf mice, which are T-cell-deficient, can be extended from 4 months to 12 months by a single intraperitoneal injection of 150×10^6 lymph node cells, but one injection of an equal number of thymocytes or 50×10^6 bone marrow cells is ineffective (30). (Lymph nodes are rich, whereas thymus and bone marrow are deficient, in *mature* T cells.)

5. Transfer of 5×10^7 to 5×10^8 thymus cells from immunologically mature congenic donors into athymic mice reconstitutes the recipient's capacity to reject allogeneic skin graft; whereas, transfer of an equal number of thymus cells from newborn mice will not (99). Presumably, the ability of thymus cell suspensions from adult mice to reconstitute graft rejections depends on the number of "competent" lymphocytes resident in the thymic medulla or from the recirculating pool which are trapped in the thymus cell suspensions.

6. Studies of "synergy" between subpopulations of lymphocytes in the MLC reaction (38, 86) suggest that lymph node "T_2" cells (amplifier cells) display a greater functional decline with age than do spleen and thymus "T_1" lymphocytes (the precursors of T_2 cells). This suggests that the mature T cells which are required for the recruitment of precursor T cells and for the MLC reaction decline with age.

7. Treatment of thymus cell suspensions with anti-TL serum and complement (which spares the more mature, TL− thymocytes which have undergone differentiation within the thymus and are about to migrate to the periphery while killing the less mature, TL+ thymocytes) does not reduce the GVH reactivity of thymocyte suspensions (131). However, the capacity of thymocytes to give superadditive GVH reactions when combined with peripheral blood leukocytes was decreased by treatment with anti-TL. These results indicate that synergy among subpopulations of T cells in GVH reactions involve the participation of "immature" T cells under the influence of mature T cells.

8. Density distribution analysis using BSA and Ficoll discontinuous gradients shows that the frequency of less-dense cells (ρ, 1.06–1.08) increases at the expense of the more-dense cells (ρ, 1.10–1.12) (79) (Fig. 7). This density shift within the lymphocyte population can also be seen in young mice shortly after they are immunized with foreign

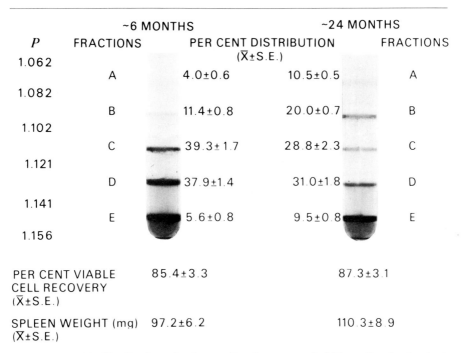

	~6 MONTHS		~24 MONTHS
P	FRACTIONS	PER CENT DISTRIBUTION ($\overline{X}$±S.E.)	FRACTIONS
1.062			
	A	4.0±0.6 10.5±0.5	A
1.082			
	B	11.4±0.8 20.0±0.7	B
1.102			
	C	39.3±1.7 28.8±2.3	C
1.121			
	D	37.9±1.4 31.0±1.8	D
1.141			
	E	5.6±0.8 9.5±0.8	E
1.156			

PER CENT VIABLE CELL RECOVERY ($\overline{X}$±S.E.)   85.4±3.3   87.3±3.1

SPLEEN WEIGHT (mg) ($\overline{X}$±S.E.)   97.2±6.2   110.3±8.9

Fig. 7. Density distribution of spleen cells of young and old long-lived mice (79). Reprinted with permission from *Federation Proceedings* 34: 153–158, 1975.

red cells or allogeneic lymphocytes and in tumor-bearing mice. In these cases, however, the spleen cell number increases, whereas in unimmunized old mice it does not. This suggests that there is a relative increase with age in immature T_1 cells at the expense of mature T_2 cells.

9.   Shortly after the thymus begins to involute and atrophy, the level of serum thymic hormone(s) decreases with age (8). It would seem reasonable to assume that this hormone(s) is necessary for terminal differentiation of T cells. This could lead to a decrease in effector cells for certain immune functions and, thus, to a deficit in T cell responsiveness.

10. The *in vitro* PHA response of T cells from old mice can be significantly increased by addition of certain chemicals (e.g., mercaptoethanol and polynucleotides) to the cultures, as can the antibody response to sheep RBC (14, 83). This supports the view that old mice are deficient in a hormone(s) that is essential for the differentiation of T cells to become responsive to a mitogen and further suggests that simple chemicals can substitute for this hormone.

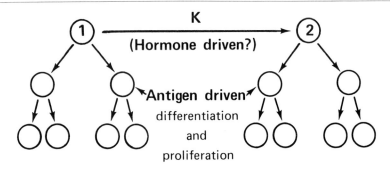

Fig. 8. Postulated model of T cell differentiation (66; for details, see text). Reprinted from *Review of Basic and Clinical Immunology*, Lange Publications, 1976, pgs. 267–8, Figure 23–7, H. H. Fudenberg, J. Caldwell, D. Stites, and J. Wells, Editors.

Figure 8 shows a possible model of T cell differentiation. In this model, T_1 (1), upon antigenic stimulation produces effector cells for certain T cell functions (such as "helper" cells for T-dependent antibody responses) and upon thymic hormone stimulation (K) produces antigen-sensitive T_2, "2," cells. Upon antigenic stimulation, T_2 produces other effector cells (such as GVH responsive cells). Each effector cell proliferates in the presence of an antigen, thus producing more effector cells. Since the level of serum thymic hormone(s) decreases with age, it would seem reasonable to assume that the effect of aging is to decrease (K). This would lead to an accumulation of T_1 cells, a decrease in T_2 cells, and, subsequently, a skewed distribution in effector T cells, which obviously can profoundly decrease immune function. There need not be only two cells in the major hormone-driven pathway, nor are there necessarily only eight effector cells.

Studies on age-related changes in T cells involved in the regulation of B cell immune responses have been minimal, due in part to lack of understanding of how these cells function. In general, a few T cells can enhance a response but many can suppress it. As discussed earlier, it is not known whether there exist two distinct subpopulations of regulator T cells, suppressor and promoter T cells, or one population of regulator T cells with the potential to promote or suppress a B cell immune response. In any event, the relative number of T cells participating in a B cell immune response decreases with age in short-lived, autoimmune-prone mice (52). This could account for the emergence of autoantibodies in the older short-lived mice. On the other hand, the relative number increases slightly in long-lived mice (102, 103). Because excessive numbers of regulator T cells tend to interfere with the B cell response to antigenic stimulation, this could account for the decline in the number of antigen-responsive IUs and IBSs. The notion that the number of regulator cells with inhibitory activities increases with age was tested by assessing the antisheep RBC response of spleen cells from young mice in the presence or absence of spleen cells from old mice (38, 83). The proliferative response of T cells from young mice to PHA and allogeneic target cells was also assessed in a similar manner. The ratio of the observed response to that which would be expected if the response of young and old cells where additive was < 1. These results indicate that spleens of old mice contain regulator cells which can interfere with the immunologic activities of spleen cells from young mice.

Finally, it should be noted that T cells may also regulate hematopoiesis (42), for it was shown that hematopoiesis of parental stem cells in heavily irradiated F·recipients can be augmented in the presence of parental T cells.

C. Thymus

All the relevant studies to date indicate that the process of involution and atrophy of the thymus is the key to the aging of the immune system. It follows, then, that the search for the cause(s) and mechanism(s) of aging of the immune system should be oriented around the thymus. The causes can be either extrinsic or intrinsic to the thymus. The most likely extrinsic cause is a possible regulatory breakdown in the hypothalamus-pineal-pituitary neuroendocrine axis in relation to thymus (10, 29). Intrinsic causes might be found at either the DNA level or the non-DNA level (for molecular theories of aging, see, for example, 123).

In regard to a neuroendocrine axis in relation to the thymus, it has been found that stress and other psychological factors can affect the immune response as measured by skin graft rejection, and primary and secondary antibody responses. Lesions in the anterior basal hypothalamus but not in the median or posterior hypothalamus can depress delayed hypersensitivity and reduce the severity of anaphylactic reactions (for review, see Ref. 120). Growth hormone and insulin have been shown to act preferentially on T-dependent immune functions, while thyroxine and sex hormones influence both T and B cell responses (for review, see Ref. 30). On the other hand, evidence is accumulating which indicates that the thymus can modulate hormone levels (12, 30). The area of thymic-neuroendocrine interactions should be an exciting and fruitful one for future aging research.

Considering intrinsic causes, three possible mechanisms of involution and atrophy can be proposed. One is clonal exhaustion (55); that is, thymus cells might have a genetically programmed clock mechanism to self-destruct and die after undergoing a fixed number of divisions, similar to the Hayflick phenomenon of human fibroblasts *in vitro*. This would require the thymus to count the cells leaving it and/or the cells to count the divisions they have undergone. Another possible mechanism is alteration of the DNA of thymus cells either randomly or through viral infection (105). The DNA-altered or mutated cells could then disrupt the self-tolerance mechanism by destroying normal cells (105). Various stable alterations of DNA can occur, including cross-linking and strand breaks (for review, see, for example, Price and Makinodan [104]). The third possible mechanism is a stable molecular alteration at the non-DNA level through subtle error-accumulating mechanisms, as proposed for those occurring at the DNA level.

At the level of the genes, evidence is mounting which indicates that genes of the H-2 system in mice and the *HLA* region in humans influence immune responsiveness and disease susceptibility (for details see 11, 85, 136).

IV. CONCLUDING REMARKS

Had we but world enough and time. . . .
—Andrew Marvell

A brief overview of the effect of age on immune function has been presented here. An attempt has been made both to summarize present knowledge and to show potential for future progress in the areas of age-related changes in immune function and mechanisms of the age-related decline.

Normal immune functions can begin to decline shortly after an individual reaches sexual maturity. Although changes in the environment of the cells are partially responsible, the decline is due primarily to changes in the cells. Foremost among the cellular changes are those in the stem cells as reflected in their growth properties and in the T cells where a shift in subpopulations may be occurring with age. The process(es) regulating involution and atropy of the thymus could be the key to immunosenescence. Future studies are expected, therefore, to focus on the area of the neuroendocrine-thymic axis.

The increasing size of the aged population is rapidly becoming the most critical socioeconomic issue on this planet and the diseases associated with loss of immunologic vigor are numerous. As our knowledge increases, it is anticipated that we will develop methods for minimizing, delaying, and preventing debilitative processes associated with aging.

This will be accomplished through the search for basic mechanisms underlying the loss of immunologic vigor and for methods to "trick" them.

LETTER TO A LITTLE SISTER
ON THE POET'S BIRTHDAY: AFFIRMATION
... fall has laced the window
with patterns we tried to create;
the wind is tossing twigs against the glass
impatient to be on its way.
... we're off to haunt the night
and search out that pilgrims' church
that stands somewhere east of ever ...

—M. M. B. Kay

NOTES

1. This is Publication No. 2 from the Geriatrics Research, Education and Clinical Center, VA Wadsworth Hospital Center, Los Angeles, California 90073.

2. Statements published in the literature notwithstanding, the MLC probably is not a good *in vitro* model of the GVH. The cell-mediated lymphocytotoxicity (CML) assay is preferred. The reasons are as follows. The MLC, at best, measures the ability of lymphocytes to recognize foreign antigens and to undergo blastogenesis. It does not directly measure the generation of effector or killer cells. Moreover, all of the cells undergoing blastogenesis in the MLC need not be cells that effect target cell killing. In this regard, the MLC index can be low even if the reacting cells have previously been "primed," or for any reason are strongly reactive to major histocompatibility differences because effector lymphocytes can be generated and, perhaps, even destroy the target before the addition of tritiated thymidine at the customary time of 48–56 hours after culture. Finally, it was found that in human renal transplant recipients a positive CML correlates well with, and often immediately precedes, an acute graft rejection episode as determined clinically; whereas the MLC is often negative immediately before and during such an episode.

REFERENCES

1. Adler, W., Takiguchi, T., and Smith, R. T. 1971. Effect of age upon primary alloantigen recognition by mouse spleen cells. *J. Immunol.* 107: 1357–1362.

2. Albright, J. F., and Makinodan, T. 1966. Growth and senescence of antibody-forming cells. *J. Cell Physiol.* 67: (Suppl. 1), 185.

3. Alexopoulos, C. and Babitis, P. 1976. Age dependence of T lymphocytes. *Lancet* 1: 426.

4. Andrew, W. 1952. *Cellular Changes with Age.* Charles C. Thomas, Springfield, Ill.

5. Aoki, T., Teller, M. N., and Robitaille, M. L. 1965. Aging and cancerigenesis. II. Effect of age on phagocytic activity of the reticuloendothelial system and on tumor growth. *J. Natl. Cancer Inst.* 34: 255–264.

6. Aoki, T. and Teller, M. N. 1966. Aging and cancerigenesis. III. Effect of age on isoantibody formation. *Cancer Res.* 26: 1648–1652.

7. Augener, W., Cohnen, G., Reuter, A., and Brittinger, G. 1974. Decrease of T lymphocytes during aging. *Lancet* 1: 1164.

8. Bach, J-F., Dardenne, M. and Salomon, J. C. 1973. Studies on thymus products. IV. Absence of serum "thymic activity" in adult NZB and (NZB × NZW) F_1 mice. *Clin. Exp. Immunol.* 14: 247–256.

9. Baer, H. and Bowser, R. T. 1963. Antibody production and development of contact skin sensitivity in guinea pigs of various ages. *Science* 140: 1211–1212.

10. Bearn, J. G. 1968. The thymus and the pituitary adrenal axis in anencephaly. *Brit. J. Exp. Path.* 49: 136–144.

11. Benacerraf, B., and McDevitt, O. H. 1972. Histocompatibility-linked immune response genes. *Science* 175: 273.

12. Besedovsky, H., and Sorkin, E. 1975. Changes in blood hormone levels during the immune response. *Proc. Soc. Exp. Biol. Med.* 150: 466–470.

13. Boyd, E. 1932. The weight of the thymus gland in health and in disease. *Amer. J. Dis. Child.* 43: 1162–1214.

14. Braun, W., Yajima, Y., and Ishizuka, M. 1970. Synthetic polynucleotides as restorers of normal antibody forming capacities in aged mice. *J. Reticuloendothel. Soc.* 7: 418–424.

15. Brennan, P. C., and Jaroslow, B. N. 1975. Age-associated decline in theta antigen on spleen thymus-derived lymphocytes of B6C F_1 mice. *Cell. Immunol.* 15: 51–56.

16. Buckley, C. G., Buckley, E. G., and Dorsey, F. C. 1974. Longitudinal changes in serum immunoglobulin levels in older humans. *Fed. Proc.* 33: 2036–2039.

17. Cantor, H., and Boyse, E. A. 1975. Functional subclasses of T lymphocytes bearing different Ly antigens. I. The generation of functionally distinct T-cell subclasses is a differentiative process independent of antigen. *J. Exp. Med.* 141: 1376–1389.

18. Cantor, H., and Boyse, E. A. 1975. Functional subclasses of T lymphocytes bearing different Ly antigens. II. Cooperation between subclasses of Ly+ cells in the generation of killer activity. *J. Exp. Med.* 141: 1390–1399.

19. Carosella, E. D., Monchanko, K., and Braun, M. 1974. Rosette-forming T cells in human peripheral blood at different ages. *Cell. Immunol.* 12: 323–325.

20. Cerilli, J., and Hatten, D. 1974. Immunosuppression and oncogenesis. *Amer. J. Clin. Pathol.* 62: 218–223.

21. Chen, M. G. 1971. Age-related changes in hematopoietic stem cell populations of a long-lived hybrid mouse. *J. Cell Physiol.* 78: 225–232.

22. Chen, M. G. 1974. Impaired Elkind recovery in hematopoietic colony-forming cells of aged mice. *Proc. Soc. Exp. Biol. Med.* 145: 1181–1186.

23. Chino, F., Makinodan, T., Lever, W. H., and Peterson, W. J. 1971. The immune system of mice reared in clean and dirty conventional laboratory farms. I. Life expectancy and pathology of mice with long life spans. *J. Gerontol.* 26: 497–507.

24. Claman, H. N., and Chaperon, E. A. 1969. Immunologic complementation between thymus and marrow cells. *Transplant. Rev.* 1: 92–113.

25. Coggle, J. E., and Proukakais, C. 1970. The effect of age on the bone marrow cellularity of the mouse. *Gerontologia* 16: 25–29.

26. Davenport, F. M., Hennessy, A. V., and Francis, T., Jr. 1953. Epidemiologic and immunologic significance of age distribution of antibody to antigenic variants of influenza virus. *J. Exp. Med.* 98: 641–656.

27. Diaz-Jouanen, E., Williams, R. C., Jr., and Strickland, R. G. 1974. Age-related changes in 'I' and B cells. *Lancet* 1: 688–689.

28. Everitt, A. V. 1973. The hypothalmic-pituitary control of ageing and age-related pathology. *Exp. Gerontol.* 8: 265.

29. Fabris, N., Pierpaoli, W., and Sorkin, E. 1972. Lymphocytes, hormones and ageing. *Nature (Lond.)* 240: 557–559.

30. Fabris, N., and Piantanell, L. 1977. Contributions of hypopituitary dwarf and athymic nude mice to the study of the relationships among thymus, hormones, and aging, *in* D. Harrison (ed.), *Genetic Effects on Aging*. National Foundation March of Dimes (in press).

31. Farrar, J. J., Loughman, B. E., and Nordin, A. A. 1974. Lymphopoietic potential of bone marrow cells from aged mice: Comparison of the cellular constitutents of bone marrow from young and aged mice. *J. Immunol.* 112: 1244–1249.

32. Fernandez, L. A., MacSween, J. M., and Langley, G. R. 1976. Lymphocyte responses to phytohaemagglutinin: Age-related effects. *Immunology* 31: 583–587.

33. Friedberger, E., Bock, G., and Fürstenheim. 1929. Zur Normalantikörper-kurve des Menschen durche die Verschiedenen Lebensalter und Ihre Bedeutung für die Erklärung der hautteste (Schick, Dick). *Z. Immunitätforsch.* 64:294–319.

34. Fudenberg, H. H. 1971. Genetically determined immune deficiency as the predisposing cause of "autoimmunity" and lymphoid neoplasia. *Amer. J. Med.* 51: 295–298.

35. Fudenberg, H. H., Good, R. A., Goodman, H. C., Hitzig, W., Kundel, H. G., Roitt, I. M., Rosen, F. S., Rowe, D. S., Selligmann, M., and Soothill, J. R. 1971. Primary immunodeficiencies. *Bull. Wld. Hlth. Org.* 45: 125–142.

36. Fulk, R. V., Fedson, D. S., Huber, M. A., Fitzpatrick, J. R., and Kasel, J. A. 1970. Antibody responses in serum and nasal secretions according to age of recipient and method of administration of A2/Hong Kong/68 inactivated influenza virus vaccine. *J. Immunol.* 104: 8–13.

37. Furuhata, T., and Eguchi, M. 1955. The change of the agglutinin titer with age. *Proc. Jap. Acad.* 31: 555–557.

38. Gerbase-DeLima, M., Meredith, P., and Walford, R. 1975. Age-related changes, including synergy and suppression, in the mixed lymphocyte reaction in long-lived mice. *Fed. Proc.* 34: 159–161.

39. Gershon, R. K., and Metzler, C. M. 1977. Suppressor cells in aging, *in* T. Makinodan and E. Yunis (ed.), *Immunity and Aging*. Plenum Press, New York (in press).

40. Giannini, D., and Sloan, R. S. 1957. A tuberculin survey of 1,285 adults with special reference to the elderly. *Lancet* 1: 525.

41. Good, R. A., and Yunis, E. J. 1974. Association of autoimmunity, immunodeficiency and aging in man, rabbits and mice. *Fed. Proc.* 33: 2040–2050.

42. Goodman, J. W., and Shinpock, S. G. 1968. Influence of thymus cells on

erythropoiesis of parental marrow in irradiated hybrid mice. *Proc. Soc. Exp. Bio. Med.* 129: 417.

43. Goodman, S. A., and Makinodan, T. 1975. Effect of age on cell-mediated immunity in long-lived mice. *Clin. Exp. Immunol.* 19: 533–542.

44. Goodman, S. A., Chen, M. G., and Makinodan, T. 1972. An improved primary response from mouse spleen cells cultured *in vivo* in diffusion chambers. *J. Immunol.* 108: 1387–1399.

45. Goullet, P., and Kaufmann, H. 1965. Ageing and antibody production in the rats. *Experimentia* 21: 46–47.

46. Gross, L. 1965. Immunologic defect in aged population and its relation to cancer. *Cancer* 18: 201–204.

47. Grossman, J., Baum, J., Fusner, J., and Condemi, J. 1975. The effect of aging and acute illness on delayed hypersensitivity. *J. Allergy Clin. Immunol.* 55: 268–275.

48. Groves, D. L., Lever, W. E., and Makinodan, T. 1970. A model for the interaction of cell types in the generation of hemolytic plaque-forming cells. *J. Immunol.* 104: 148–165.

49. Haferkamp, O., Schlettwein-Gsell, D., Schwick, H. G., and Storiko, K. 1966. Serum protein in an aging population with particular reference to evaluation of immune globulins and antibodies. *Gerontologia* 12: 30–38.

50. Hallgren, H. M., Buckley, E. C., III, Gilbertsen, V. A., and Yunis, E. J. 1973. Lymphocyte phytohemagglutinin responsiveness, immunoglobulins and autoantibodies in aging humans. *J. Immunol.* 111: 1101–1107.

51. Halsall, M. H., and Perkins, E. H. 1974. The restoration of phytohemmagglutinin responsiveness of spleen cells from aging mice. *Fed. Proc.* 33: 736.

52. Hardin, J. A., Chuseo, T. M., and Steinberg, A. D. 1973. Suppressor cells in the graft vs host reaction. *J. Immunol.* 111: 650–651.

53. Harrison, D. E. 1975. Normal function of transplanted marrow cell lines from aged mice. *J. Gerontol.* 30: 279–285.

54. Harrison, D. E., and Doubleday, J. W. 1975. Normal function of immunologic stem cells from aged mice. *J. Immunol.* 114: 1314–1317.

55. Hayflick, L. 1965. The limited *in vitro* lifetime of human diploid cell strains. *Exp. Cell Res.* 37: 614–636.

56. Heidrick, M. L. 1972. Age-related changes in hydrolase activity of peritoneal macrophages. *Gerontologist* 12: 28.

57. Heidrick, M. L. 1973. Imbalanced cycle-AMP and cyclic-GMP levels in concanavalin-A stimulated spleen cells from aged mice. *J. Cell Biol.* 57: 139a.

58. Heidrick, M. L., and Makinodan, T. 1973. Presence of impairment of humoral immunity in nonadherent spleen cells of old mice. *J. Immunol.* 111: 1502–1506.

59. Heine, K. M. 1971. Die Reaktionsfähigkeit der Lymphozyten im Alter. *Folia Haematol.* 96: 29–33.

60. Hirano, T., and Nordin, A. 1976. Age-associated decline in the *in vitro* development of cytotoxic lymphocytes in NZB mice. *J. Immunol.* 117: 1093–1098.

61. Hirokawa, K., and Makinodan, T. 1975. Thymic involution: Effect on T cell differentiation. *J. Immunol.* 114: 1659–1664.

62. Hirokawa, K. 1977. Thymus and aging, *in* T. Makinodan and E. Yunis

(eds.), *Immunity and Aging*. Plenum Press, New York (in press).

63. Hori, Y., Perkins, E. H., and Halsall, M. K. 1973. Decline in phytohemagglutinin responsiveness of spleen cells from aging mice. *Proc. Soc. Exp. Bio. Med.* 144: 48–53.

64. Hung, C-Y., Perkins, E. H., and Yang, W-K. 1975a. Age-related refractoriness of PHA-induced lymphocyte transformation. I. Comparable sensitivity of spleen cells from young and old mice to culture conditions. *Mech. Ageing Develop.* 4: 29–39.

65. Hung, C-Y., Perkins, E. H., and Yang, W-K. 1975b. Age-related refractoriness of PHA-induced lymphocyte transformation. II. ^{125}I-PHA binding to spleen cells from young and old mice. *Mech. Ageing Develop.* 4: 103–112.

66. Kay, M. M. B. 1976. Aging and the decline of immune responsiveness, in H. H. Fudenberg, J. Caldwell, D. Stites, and J. Wells (eds.), *Review of Basic and Clinical Immunology*, p. 267–268. Lange Medical Publications, Los Altos, Calif.

67. Kay, M. M. B. 1977. Immunological aging patterns: Effect of parainfluenza type I virus infection on aging mice of 8 strains and hybrids, in D. Harrison (ed.), *Genetic Effects on Aging*. The National Foundation March of Dimes (in press).

68. Kay, M. M. B., Denton, T., Union, N., Mendoza, J., and Lajiness, M. 1977. Age-related changes in the immune system of 8 medium and long-lived strains and hybrids I: Weight, cellular and functional assays. *Mech. Ageing Develop.* (in press).

69. Kishimoto, S., Tsuyuguchi, I., and Yamamura, Y. 1969. Immune responses in aged mice. *Clin. Exp. Immunol.* 5: 525–530.

70. Kishimoto, S., Takahama, T., and Mizumachi, H. 1976. In vitro immune response to the 2,4,6-trinitrophenyl determinant in age C57Bl/6J mice: Changes in the humoral response to avidity for the TNP determinant and responsiveness to LPS effect with aging. *J. Immunol.* 116: 294–300.

71. Konen, T. G., Smith, G. S., and Walford, R. L. 1973. Decline in mixed lymphocyte reactivity of spleen cells from aged mice of a long-lived strain. *J. Immunol.* 110: 1216–1221.

72. Lajtha, L. J. and Schofield, R. 1971. Regulation of stem cell renewal and differentiation: possible significance in aging. *Adv. Gerontol. Res.* 3: 131–146.

73. Legge, J. S., and Austin, C. M. 1968. Antigen localization and the immune response as a function of age. *Aust. J. Exp. Biol. Med. Sci.* 46: 361–365.

74. Lloyd, R. S., and Triger, D. R. 1975. Studies on hepatic uptake of antigen. III. Studies of liver macrophage function in normal rats and following carbon tetrachloride administration. *Immunology* 29: 253–263.

75. Lyngbye, J., and Kroll, J. 1971. Quantitative immunoelectrophoresis of proteins in serum from normal population: Season-, age-, and sex-related variations. *Clin. Chem.* 17: 495–500.

76. Mackay, I. R. 1972. Ageing and immunological function in man. *Gerontologia* 18: 285–304.

77. Mackay, I. R., Whittingham, S. F., and Mathews, J. D. 1977. The immunoepidemiology of aging, in T. Makinodan and E. Yunis (eds.), *Immunity and Aging*. Plenum Press, New York (in press).

78. Makinodan, T. 1976. Immunobiology of aging. *J. Amer. Soc. Geriat.* 24: 249–252.

79. Makinodan, T., and Adler, W. 1975. The effects of aging on the differentiation and proliferation potentials of cells of the immune system. Fed Proc. 34: 153–158.

80. Makinodan, T., and Peterson, W. J. 1962. Relative antibody-forming capacity of spleen cells as function of age. Proc. Nat. Acad. Sci. (Wash.) 48: 234–238.

81. Makinodan, T., and Peterson, W. J. 1964. Growth and senescence of the primary antibody-forming potential of the spleen. J. Immunol. 93: 886.

82. Makinodan, T., Chino, F., Lever, W. E., and Brewen, B. S. 1971. The immune systems of mice reared in clean and dirty conventional laboratory farms. II. Primary antibody-forming activity of young and old mice with long life-spans. J. Gerontol. 26: 508–514.

83. Makinodan, T., Deitchman, J. W., Stoltzner, G. H., Kay, M. M., and Hirokawa, K. 1975. Restoration of the declining normal immune functions of aging mice. Proc. 10th Internat. Congr. Gerontol. 2: 23.

84. Mathies, M., Lipps, L., Smith, G. S., and Walford, R. L. 1973. Age related decline in response to phytohemagglutinin and pokeweed mitogen by spleen cells from hamsters and a long-lived mouse strain. J. Gerontol. 28: 425–430.

85. Meredith, P. and Walford, R. L. 1977. Effect of age on the response to T and B cell mitogens in mice congenic at the H-2 locus. Immunogenetics (in press).

86. Meredith, P., Tittor, W., Gerbase-DeLima, M., and Walford, R. 1975. Age-related changes in the cellular immune response of lymph node and thymus cells in long-lived mice. Cell. Immunol. 18: 324–330.

87. Metcalf, D. 1965. Delayed effect of thymectomy in adult life on immunological competence. Nature (Lond.) 208: 1336.

88. Metcalf, D., Moulds, R., and Pike, B. 1966. Influence of the spleen and thymus on immune responses in ageing mice. Clin. Exp. Immunol. 2: 109–120.

89. Novick, A., Novick, I., and Potoker, S. 1972. Tuberculin skin testing in a chronically sick aged population. J. Amer. Geriat. Soc. 20: 455–458.

90. Pantelouris, E. M. 1972. Thymic involution and ageing: a hypothesis. Exp. Gerontol. 7: 73–81.

91. Paul, J. R., and Bunnell, W. W. 1932. The presence of heterophile and antibodies in infectious mononucleosis. Amer. J. Med. Sci. 183: 90–104.

92. Penn, I., and Starzl, T. E. 1972. Malignant tumors arising de novo in immunosuppressed organ transplant recipients. Transplantation. 14: 407–417.

93. Perkins, E. H. 1971. Phagocytic activity of aged mice. J. Reticuloendothel. Soc. 9: 642.

94. Perkins, E. H., and Makinodan, T. 1971. Nature of humoral immunologic deficiencies of the aged, in: Proc. 1st Rocky Mt. Symp. on Aging, p. 80–103, Colorado State University, Fort Collins, Colorado.

95. Perkins, E. H., and Cacheiro, L. H. A multiple-parameter comparison of immunocompetence and tumor resistance in aged Balb/c mice. Mech. Ageing Develop. (in press).

96. Peter, C. P. 1971. Synergism between spleen cells of immunologically active young and inactive aged mice. Fed. Proc. 30: 526.

97. Peter, C. P. 1973. Possible immune origin of age-related pathological changes in long-lived mice. J. Gerontol. 28: 265–275.

98. Peterson, W., and Makinodan, T. 1972. Autoimmunity in aged mice. Occurence of autoagglutinating factors in the blood of aged mice with medium and long life spans. *Clin. Exp. Immunol.* 12: 273–290.

99. Pierpaoli, W. 1975. Inability of thymus cells from newborn donors to restore transplantation immunity in athymic mice. *Immunology* 29: 465–468.

100. Pisciotta, A. V., Westring, D. W., Deprey, C., and Walsh, B. 1967. Mitogenic effect of phytohaemagglutinin at different ages. *Nature (Lond.)* 215: 193–194.

101. Prehn, R. T. 1971. Evaluation of the evidence for immune surveillance, in R. T. Smith and M. Landy (eds.), *Immune Surveillance*, pp. 451–462, Academic Press, New York.

102. Price, G. B., and Makinodan, T. 1972a. Immunologic deficiencies in senescence. I. Characterization of intrinsic deficiencies. *J. Immunol.* 108: 403–412.

103. Price, G. B., and Makinodan, T. 1972b. Immunologic deficiencies in senescence. II. Characterization of extrinsic deficiencies. *J. Immunol.* 108: 413–417.

104. Price, G. B., and Makinodan, T. 1973. Aging: Alterations of DNA-protein information. *Gerontologia* 19: 58–70.

105. Proffitt, M. R., Hirsch, M. S., and Black, P. H. 1972. Murine leukemia: A virus-induced autoimmune disease? *Science* 182: 821–823.

106. Rabinowitz, S. G. 1975. Comparative mitogenic responses of T cells and B cells in spleens of mice of varying age. *Immunological Commun.* 4: 63–79.

107. Roberts-Thomson, I., Whittingham, S., Youngchaiyud, U., and Mackay, I. R. 1974. Ageing, immune response, and mortality. *Lancet* 2: 368–370.

108. Rowley, M. J., Buchanan, H., and Mackay, I. R. 1968. Reciprocal change with age in antibody to extrinsic and intrinsic antigens. *Lancet* 2: 24.

109. Santisteban, G. A. 1960. The growth and involution of lymphatic tissue and its interrelationships to aging and to the growth of the adrenal glands and sex organs in CBA mice. *Anat. Rec.* 136: 117–126.

110. Sabin, A. B. 1947. Antibody response of people of different ages to two doses of uncentrifuged Japanese B encephalitis vaccine. *Proc. Soc. Exp. Biol. Med.* 65: 127–130.

111. Segre, D. and Segre, M. 1976. Humoral immunity in aged mice. I. Age-related decline in the secondary response to DNP of spleen cells propagated in diffusion chambers. *J. Immunol.* 116: 731–734.

112. Segre, D., and Segre, M. 1976. Humoral immunity in aged mice. II. Increased suppressor T cell activity in immunologically deficient old mice. *J. Immunol.* 116: 735–738.

113. Shigemoto, S., Kishimoto, S., and Yamamura. 1975. Change of cell-mediated cytotoxicity with aging. *J. Immunol.* 115: 307–309.

114. Sigel, M. and Good, R. A. 1972. *Tolerance, Autoimmunity and Aging*, Charles C. Thomas, Springfield, Ill.

115. Siminovitch, L., Till, J. E., and McCulloch, E. A. 1964. Decline in colony-forming ability of marrow cells subjected to serial transplantation into irradiated mice. *J. Cell. Physiol.* 64: 23–31.

116. Smith, A. 1976. The effects of age on the immune response to Type III pneumococcal polysaccharide (SIII) and bacterial lipopolysaccharide (LPS) in

Balb/c, SJL/J, and C3H mice. *J. Immunol.* 116: 469–474.

117. Smith, G. S., and Walford, R. L. 1977. Influence of the H-2 and H-1 histocompatibility systems upon lifespan and spontaneous cancer incidence in congenic mice, in D. Harrison (ed.), *Genetic Effects on Aging.* National Foundation, March of Dimes (in press).

118. Smith, M. A., Evans, J., and Steel, C. M. 1974. Age-related variation in proportion of circulating T cells. *Lancet* 1: 922–924.

119. Solomonova, K., and Vizeb, St. 1973. Immunological reactivity of senescent and old people actively immunized with tetanus toxoid. *Z. Immunitätsforsch.* 146: 81–90.

120. Stein, M., Schiavi, R. C., and Camerino, M. 1976. Influence of brain and behavior on the immune system. *Science* 191: 435–440.

121. Stjernswärd, J. 1966. Age dependent tumor-host barrier and effect of carcinogens initiated immune depression of rejection of isografted methyl cholanthrene induced sarcoma cells. *J. Natl. Cancer Inst.* 37: 505–512.

122. Storer, J. B. 1966. Longevity and gross pathology at death in 22 inbred mouse strains. *J. Gerontol.* 21: 404.

123. Strehler, B., Hirsch, G., Gusseck, D., Johnson, R., and Bick, M. 1971. Codon-restriction theory of aging and development. *J. Theor. Biol.* 33: 429–474.

124. Stutman, O. 1974. Cell mediated immunity and aging. *Fed. Proc.* 33: 2028–2032.

125. Stutman, O., Yunis, E. J., and Good, R. A. 1968. Deficient immunologic functions of NZB mice. *Proc. Soc. Exp. Biol. Med.* 127: 1204–1207.

126. Taylor, R. B. 1965. Decay of immunological responsiveness after thymectomy in adult life. *Nature (Lond.)* 208: 1334–1335.

127. Teague, P. O., and Friou, G. J. 1964. Inhibition of autoimmunity in A/J mice by transfer of isogenic thymic or spleen cells from young animals. *Arthr. Rheum.* 8: 474.

128. Teague, P. O., Yunis, E. J., Rodey, G., Fish, A. J., Stutman, O., and Good, R. A. 1970. Autoimmune phenomena and renal disease of mice. Role of thymectomy, aging, and involution of immunologic capacity. *Lab. Invest.* 22: 121–130.

129. Teller, M. N. 1972. Age changes and immune resistance to cancer. *Adv. Gerontol. Res.* 4: 25–43.

130. Thomsen, O., and Kettel, K. 1929. Die stärke der menschlichen Isoagglutinine und entsprechenden Blutkörperchenrezeptoren in verschiedenen Lebensaltern. *Z. Immunitätsforsch.* 63: 67–93.

131. Tigelaar, R. E., Gershon, R. K., and Asofsky, R. 1975. Graft-versus-host reactivity of mouse thymocytes: Effect of in vitro treatment with anti-TL serum. *Cell. Immunol.* 19: 58–64.

132. Tyan, M. L. 1977. Age-related decrease in mouse T-cell progenitors. *J. Immunol.* (in press).

133. Waldorf, D. S., Willkens, R. F., and Decker, J. L. 1968. Impaired delayed hypersensitivity in an aging population. Association with antinuclear reactivity and rheumatoid factor. *J. Amer. Med. Assoc.* 203: 831–834.

134. Walford, R. L. 1974. The immunologic theory of aging: current status. *Fed. Proc.* 33: 2020–2027.

135. Walford, R. L. 1976. When is a mouse "old"? *J. Immunol.* 117: 352–353.

136. Walford, R. L. 1976. Human B cell alloantigenic systems: their medical and biological significance, in Proceeding of the International Congress of HLA System, Elsevier, North Holland (in press).

137. Walters, C. S., and Claman, H. N. 1975. Age related changes in cell mediated immunity of Balb/c mouse. *J. Immunol.* 115: 1438–1443.

138. Weksler, M. E., and Hütterroth, T. H. 1974. Impaired lymphocyte function in aged humans. *J. Clin. Invest.* 53: 99–104.

139. Wigzell, H., and Stjernswärd, J. 1966. Age-dependent rise and fall of immunological reactivity in the CBA mouse. *J. Natl. Cancer Inst.* 37: 513 517.

140. Yunis, E. J., Hilgard, H., Sjodin, K., Martinez, C., and Good, R. A. 1964. Immunological reconstitution of thymectomized mice by injections of isolated thymocytes. *Nature (Lond.)* 201: 784–786.

141. Zukowski, G., Killen, D., and Ginn, E. 1970. Transplanted carcinoma in an immunosuppressed patient. *Transplantation* 9: 71–74.

CHAPTER 4

GENETIC CONTROL OF TUMOR IMMUNITY

Geoffrey Haughton and
Alan C. Whitmore

Department of Bacteriology
and Immunology
School of Medicine
The University of North Carolina
Chapel Hill, North Carolina 27514

Genetic factors influence tumor immunity at two distinct levels. On the one hand, they determine whether or not a given oncogenic insult will cause neoplastic transformation of normal cells and they may regulate the nature of tumor-associated neoantigens on the surface of the transformed cells. On the other hand, genetic factors influence the nature and intensity of the immune response mounted by the host against tumor-associated neoantigens.

There is neither *a priori* reason to believe, nor evidence to suggest, that the genetic mechanisms controlling immune responses to tumor antigens are any different from those controlling responses to other antigens. For this reason, it seems appropriate to start with a brief review of the general knowledge of genetic factors influencing immune responses and of the nature of immune responses to tumor-associated antigens, before considering those genetic factors peculiar to cancer.

A. INTRODUCTION

1. Genetic Control of the Immune Response

Despite the vast array of antigens against which each individual can produce specific antibodies, it is now clear that this array is not limitless and does differ among individuals. It is firmly established in a number of systems that the ability to produce specific idiotypes—serologic characteristics of monoclonal antibodies directed against particular antigens, and determined by configuration at the antigen-combining site—is under the control of polymorphic genes. These genes are linked to heavy-chain allotypes and are inherited in simple Mendelian fashion (204). It seems likely that a substantial amount of DNA is involved with idiotypic inheritance, since many examples have been described (27, 45, 98, 138, 176) and cross-overs between idiotypic and allotypic heavy-chain markers are not infrequent (46, 161).

On the basis of this polymorphism, even though it may be modified by selection following somatic mutation of hypervariable residues (38), or by insertion of episomal material (33), it is unreasonable to suppose that all individuals can respond equally to all tumor-associated antigens. This theoretically derived prediction receives support from several experimental studies. Some strains of mice are able to mount an immune response to antigens associated with murine leukemia viruses and thereby resist leukemogenesis; others are not (see below) and are thus susceptible. On the other hand, ability to mount a weak response to antigens of virus-induced murine mammary carcinoma is associated with a higher probability of developing the disease; in this case, the responsiveness can cause immune-stimulation of the neoplasm (128, 149, 210).

In addition to those genes referred to above, which limit the ability of an animal to produce antibody of a given specificity and which are genetically linked to immunoglobulin constant-region allotypic markers, are two other sets of genes influencing immune responses. The one, linked to the major histocompatibility complex, comprises a group of genes, seemingly antigen-specific and controlling the ability of particular subsets of T cells to act as helper, killer, or suppressor cells (20). Such T cells may act (respectively) as essential collaborators in antibody production by B cells, as direct cytotoxic cells (39), or specifically to suppress either of these functions (57). The mechanisms by which these influences are exerted are not well understood, but a substantial amount of the genome seems, once again, to be involved (105). Along the same lines of argument as advanced above, these polymorphic genes must surely cause divergence between individuals in their ability to mount immune responses to tumor-associated antigens.

The third set of genes influencing the immune response to antigens are scattered throughout the genome, linked neither to immunoglobulin allotype nor to the major histocompatibility complex and seem, generally, not to be antigen-specific (23). These genes control such features as the efficiency of antigen degradation by macrophages (91, 205), the ease with which the switch is made from production of IgM to IgG (25), and the general level of antigen responsiveness (24). Thus, genes in this category may also influence the individual intensity of antitumor immune responses.

The foregoing is intended only as a conceptual review; more detailed reviews on each of the components have recently been published (20, 24, 204).

2. Tumor Immunity

a. TUMOR-ASSOCIATED ANTIGENS (TAA). A wide range of tumors, arising in experimental, wild and domestic animals and in humans, have been shown to bear tumor-associated cell-surface antigens (32, 58, 66, 68, 82, 126, 182, 183). Many such antigens are immunogenic for syngeneic hosts and can evoke a graft-rejection response (12, 50, 153). In many cases, it has been shown that the primary tumor host is capable of mounting both cellular and humoral immune responses against TAA. Some persons would argue that immunogenic TAAs are found only on induced tumors and that spontaneous tumors are nonantigenic (78, 152). Such a distinction, however, is probably spurious. The definition of spontaneous tumors becomes more and more restrictive as additional environmental oncogens and endogenous oncogenes are recognized.

The pattern of cross-reactivity between TAAs of different individual tumors varies with the type of tumors studied, and to some extent, with the methods used to detect the antigens. In general, tumors induced in experimental animals by physical or chemical agents and detected by immunization/transplantation tests in syngeneic animals appear to be individually specific (12, 32, 50, 153). Immunization against one tumor will not protect against challenge with another, even though the second tumor was induced by the same chemical and in the same individual animal as the first. Some reports indicate that the same pattern of individual specific antigenicity is revealed by the *in vitro* microcytotoxicity test (13, 78). Others, however, have reported that a wider range of, albeit weaker, cross-reactivity is detectable by *in vitro* methods (75, 160, 191). On the other hand, tumors induced in experimental animals by a given oncogenic virus, regardless of histologic type or species of origin, all carry similar cross-reactive TAA detectable by immunization/transplantation tests and by a variety of *in vitro* methods (70, 71, 72, 178). It has also been reported that such virally induced tumors also bear relatively weaker individually specific antigens which can be detected both *in vivo* and *in vitro* (87, 127, 196).

The pattern of cross-reactivity seen between different human tumors, where studies are necessarily confined to *in vitro* methods, differs from both of those described above. It is generally agreed that the specificity of cellular immunity against TAA reflects the organ/histologic type of tumor being studied (74, 77, 82). For instance, there is cross-reactivity between the cellular response against all melanomas but not between the response against melanoma and that against adenocarcinoma of the breast. There are suggestions that the humoral response against TAA may be more widely cross-reactive.

b. CELL-MEDIATED IMMUNITY.   There is no doubt that lymphocytes are important in graft rejection; whether the graft be normal tissue or experimentally induced tumor (76, 106). However, the biological significance of cell-mediated immunity in spontaneous animal and human tumors is not well established. Some would argue that a weak immune response is necessary for oncogenesis in these systems (150, 151). Others have reported an apparent positive correlation between antitumor cell-mediated immunity (CMI) and clinical course of disease in human patients (86). It has recently been found that breast cancer patients sequentially evaluated before and/or after treatment are divisible into those with a strong and those with a weak antitumor CMI. Although the line of division between a strong or a weak response is somewhat indistinct at present, recurrent breast cancer has occurred only in those with a clearly weak response (Avis, personal communication).

c. SERUM-BLOCKING FACTOR (SBF). The serum of experimental animals or of human patients bearing actively growing tumors frequently contains a component termed serum blocking factor or SBF (16, 73, 81, 85). SBF is able, specifically, to subvert the antitumor cytotoxic potential of the host's own circulating lymphocytes. The specificity and cross-reactivity of SBF precisely mirrors that of antitumor cellular immunity.

SBF can be eluted from the surface of cells derived from actively growing tumors, is usually demonstrable in the circulation of the hosts of such tumors (181), disappears rapidly from the circulation following surgical removal of the tumor (80, 86) and is not found in the serum of experimental animals whose tumors are undergoing spontaneous regression (73). Its reappearance in the circulation following removal of the primary tumor frequently signals the imminent appearance of metastatic lesions (86). Presently available evidence is compatible with the idea that the activity of SBF depends upon the presence of antigen released from the tumor cells and present either as free antigen or complexed with antibody (14, 15, 16, 29, 180). The possibility that certain special types of antitumor antibody might inhibit either the induction or the expression of tumor immunity is by no means excluded. In fact, Nelson et al. (129) have recently detected an antibody in the supernatant of mouse spleen cells sensitized against syngeneic methylcholanthrene-induced sarcoma which can block cell-mediated immunity against cultured cells of the same tumor. More studies are certainly needed to define the significance and nature of substances having the activity of serum-blocking factor.

d. HUMORAL IMMUNITY. The following consideration is confined to antigens known to be immunogenic for the primary tumor host or at least for animals syngeneic with it. It thus excludes several important TAAs detectable only with antisera produced by cross-species immunization.

Complement- and lymphocyte-dependent cytotoxic antibodies (CDA and LDA, respectively), as well as precipitating antibody, reactive with a variety of animal and human tumors, have been reported (13, 63, 79, 207). Such antibodies may be directed against virally specified antigens, against phase-specific antigens, or against tumor-associated antigens of unknown etiology. The ease with which CDA, for instance, can be detected depends not only upon the quantity and quality of the antibody, but also upon details of the technique used for its detection, the source of complement used, and the concentration of the reactive antigen at the surface of the target cell. The significance of such antibodies in the primary tumor host has not been established, although examples of enhanced tumor growth, regression of tumors, and clearance of SBF from the circulation have all been reported following passive transfer to tumor-bearing hosts (19, 83). The pattern of specificity and of cross-reactivity seen with antitumor antibodies may, as one would expect, be somewhat different from that of cellular immunity.

Antitumor antibodies certainly do occur in some animals that do not bear and have not borne detectable tumors (68): for instance, in mice infected as adults with Moloney lymphoma virus (182). Similarly, antitumor antibodies have been reported present in the circulation of some healthy humans (84). The source of antigens inducing such humoral antibodies is not clear, although in some cases, a response against antigens on noncancerous hyperplasias seems to be involved (6, 9, 10, 11, 67).

B. IMMUNOGENETICS OF TUMORS

1. Immune Responses to Antigens of RNA Virus-Induced Leukemias

The genetics of tumor-specific immune responses of experimental animals have been most extensively studied in the mouse. The oncogene hypothesis of Huebner and Todaro (94) has provided the conceptual framework for this research. This hypothesis, briefly stated, is: (1) The cells of many, perhaps all, vertebrates contain information for producing C-type RNA viruses. (2) The viral information (virogene), including that portion responsible for transforming a normal cell into a tumor cell (oncogene), is most commonly transmitted from animal to progeny animal and from cell to progeny cell in a covert form. (3) Carcinogens, irradiation, and the normal aging process all favor the partial or complete activation of these genes (193). The evidence that supports this hypothesis includes the finding of oncogenic RNA viruses in a variety of spontaneous or radiation-induced lymphoreticular neoplasms (53, 60, 62, 74, 117, 168), the partial expression of C-type virus genomes in a wide variety of normal tissue and life stages (65, 93), the presence of unexpressed—but activatable—virus in every cell of cell lines derived from high-leukemia (120, 164) and low-leukemia (2) inbred mouse strains, and the proven oncogenicity of virus chemically activated from virus-negative cell lines from high- and low-leukemia mouse strains (61, 183).

It is therefore of prime importance to determine what host regulatory mechanisms exist to control the expression of these apparently ubiquitous oncogenes and what genetic variation in the efficacy of these mechanisms exists. It is of interest to the cancer immunologist which of these mechanisms has an immunological basis.

Aoki, Boyse, and Old have extensively studied the cell surface antigens of murine leukemia virus-induced tumors. One of these antigens, GCSA (for Gross cell surface antigen), is found on normal lymphoid tissue and spontaneous leukemias from high-leukemia mouse strains such as AKR and C58. GCSA is not found on normal tissues of low leukemia strains such as C57BL/6 (B6) but is present on leukemias of such strains induced by Gross passage A leukemia virus (134). Aoki et al. (7) have found that older B6 mice occasionally have antibody to GCSA in their serum, detected by immunofluorescence on a GCSA+ test cell, but that AKR mice never have detectable antibody. The production of anti-GCSA is dominant—(B6 × AKR)F$_1$ mice also produced antibody. Segregating populations were produced and tested for production of anti-GCSA antibody. C57BL/6 is H-2^b and AKR is H-2^k. In the (B6 × AKR) × AKR backcross (BC) generation H-2^{kb} segregants produced anti-GCSA but the H-2^{kk} segregants did not. This pattern was also observed in the (B6 × AKR)F2 generation: H-2^{bb} and H-2^{kb} segregants produced anti-GCSA as often as did the B6 parental strain but H-2^{kk} segregants never did.

Frank Lilly has found that in (B6 × AKR) × AKR BC populations, H-2^{kb} mice have a lower incidence of leukemia and those leukemias that do occur have a longer latent period than in the H-2^{kk} segregants (118). The H-2-linked gene affecting susceptibility to spontaneous AKR leukemia and leukemia induced in low-leukemia strains by neonatal injection of Gross passage A virus has been named Rgv-1. The findings of Aoki et al. (7) indicate that one of the ways in which Rgv-1 may exert its effect is by the immune response to GCSA.

Lilly et al. (119) have recently reported an analysis of the influence of H-2 type and infectious MLV titer in young adult mice, (detected by the tail bone assay of Rowe [162]) on the ultimate incidence of leukemia in mice of a (BALB/c × ARK) × AKR backcross generation. Inbred AKR mice (H-2^k) have a very high incidence of spontaneous leukemia (95% by 11 months) and 100% of the AKR mice have high titers of MLV in the bones of the tail (10^3 to 10^5 plaque-forming units per 0.4 ml of 2% extract of tail tissue). BALB/c mice (H-2^d) have a low incidence of leukemia and are virus negative when tested at 6 weeks of age (163). The F$_1$ hybrid between these two strains has a low incidence of leukemia (4%), but 83% are virus positive (average titer = $10^{1.7}$) at 6 weeks. This lower titer in the F$_1$s probably reflects the dominant inhibitory effect of the Fv-1^b allele contributed by the BALB/c parent. Fv-1 is the major genetic locus affecting resistance to exogenous murine leukemia viruses, both in vivo (145) and in vitro (145), and acts at some stage in the virus replication cycle after penetration and uncoating (44). Lilly et al. (108) found that the presence of MLV at 6 weeks had a highly significant effect on ultimate leukemia incidence in 335 (BALB/c × AKR) × AKR backcross mice. Fifty-five percent of the virus-positive subjects (titers greater than $10^{0.3}$) succumbed to leukemia, whereas only 9% of the virus negative mice became leukemic. H-2 also has a significant effect on leukemia incidence: 43% among H-2^{kk} segregants versus 24% among H-2^{kd} segregants. This H-2 effect on leukemia incidence was most significant in those mice with intermediate virus titers (from 10$^{1.0}$ to 10$^{2.9}$). H-2 type has a small effect on early occurrence of virus but this was not statistically significant. Whatever the mechanism of this H-2-associated effect on tumor incidence, one can assume that it does not significantly influence the detection of virus in young adult mice and that this effect is minimal in mice with a very high or very low titer of infectious MLV.

Strand et al. (187) have studied a series of H-2 congenic strains on the C57BL/10Sn (B10) background for the expression of viral proteins p30 and gp 69/71 in spleen extracts using a sensitive radioimmunoassay. They found that the levels of both proteins was low in B10 and H-2^{a,d} and H-2^d congenics (B10.A, B10.D2 and B10.A(2R), respectively) and the p30:gp69/71 ratio was much less than that found in purified virus preparations. In the H-2^k congenic strain (B10.BR), however, much higher levels of both proteins were found and the ratio of p30 to gp69/71 approached that found in purified virus. This B10.BR subline does, in fact, have high concentrations of infectious virus in its tissues. They were not inclined to interpret these results as a direct influence of genes in the H-2 complex on virus expression because not all sublines of B10.BR express infectious virus. The possibility that the Albert Einstein substrain of B10.BR differs from B10 at an unlinked (or H-2-linked) contaminating virus-inducing locus has not been excluded.

In 1972 Hanna et al. (64) reported that adult mice of certain low-leukemia strains had antibodies in their serum and in kidney eluates which neutralized infectious virus from AKR leukemia cells. This phenomenon was named autogenous immunity to endogenous RNA tumor virus and two general methods for its detection have been described: Neutralizing activity is tested by reacting infectious virus with mouse serum and then inoculating the virus on to rat XC cells to test for reduction of plaque-forming virus particles. Murine leukemia virus pseudotypes of Kirsten murine sarcoma virus may also be used to test for reduction of focus-forming capacity on mouse embryo cell cultures. Antibodies directed against virus envelope antigens may also be detected by reacting mouse serum with ^{3}H-labeled virus particles and precipitating the complexes formed with goat or rabbit antimouse immunoglobulin serum. This is the radioimmune precipitation (RIP) assay (97). These methods do not necessarily detect the same serum activities.

Ihle et al. (97) have demonstrated that low-leukemia (C57BL/6 × C3H/Anf)F1 and BALB/c mice have high titers of antivirus antibody (RIP assay) by 12 weeks of age and that this titer increases until about 1 1/2 years of age. The titer of antivirus antibody in high leukemia AKR mouse serum is very low and stays low throughout life. They have experimentally excluded the possibility that AKR serum contains a substance that inhibits the reaction of antivirus antibodies with virus. Antibodies reactive in the RIP assay of autogenous immunity to endogenous RNA tumor viruses are found in both the 19S and 7S fractions of mouse gamma globulins, but only 19S (IgM) immunoglobulins have neutralizing activity (115). Polyacrylamide gel electrophoresis of immunoprecipitates of (B6 × C3H)F1 serum and disrupted radioactively labeled AKR virus particles reveals that IgM reacts with glycoproteins with molecular weights of approximately 68,000 and 43,000 daltons and a protein of 17,000 daltons. The IgG fraction reacts only with the 17,000-dalton protein (95). These findings are in agreement with other studies indicating that both p15 and gp 69/71 (nomenclature of August et al. [8]) are located at the virion surface but only anti-gp 69/71 antibodies have neutralizing activity (96, 184).

Nowinski and Kaehler (130) have also found natural antibodies to MLV active in the RIP assay in a large number of mouse strains, including AKR and C58.

Aaronson and Stephenson (1) have also found the widespread occurrence of a serum factor which neutralized the focus-forming ability of KiMSV(MLV) pseudotypes. This activity was found in all strains tested except NIH/Swiss, including some high- (AKR) and low-leukemia strains and was assumed to be antibody. They found that this serum factor had no activity against mouse-tropic murine leukemia viruses but was highly active against xenotropic viruses (those MLVs which replicate effectively only in cells of species other than the mouse).

Levy et al. (116) have attempted to reconcile some of the differences between studies using neutralization assays and those using RIP assays by using both methods to study the effect of various immunochemical treatments on the activity of (B6 × C3H)F1 serum against both xenotropic and ecotropic (mouse-tropic, e.g., AKR MLV) viruses. The RIP titer resides mainly in the 19s IgM fraction and is directed against both xeno- and ecotropic viruses. The neutralizing activity of mouse serum however, does not co-purify with gamma-globulins and is not affected by treatment with rabbit antimouse immunoglobulin which removes RIP-active immunoglobulins. Preliminary studies attempting to characterize this neutralizing factor indicate that it is a protein with a molecular weight of less than 30,000 daltons. Fischinger et al. (48) have reported that the xenotropic virus-neutralizing activity of normal serum cannot be absorbed by purified ecotropic mouse viruses but that normal and virus-transformed mouse and cat embryo cell lines could remove this activity. This factor may not, therefore, be virus-specific.

It has been shown that natural antibody to MLV proteins occurs in both high- and low-leukemia strains (130) and that this antibody lacks biological (neutralizing) activity against mouse-tropic MLVs (115). The non-antibody serum factor with virus-neutralizing activity is directed at xenotropic MLVs which have not yet been shown to be oncogenic in mice. The early conjecture that autogenous immunity to endogenous RNA tumor viruses may play a significant role in the genetics of spontaneous murine leukemia now seems somewhat sanguine.

2. H-2 Association of Ability to Reject Transplanted Murine Tumors

During extensive studies of the induction of transplantation immunity to Friend, Moloney, and Rauscher virus-induced leukemias, McCoy et al. (125) noticed that X-irradiated syngeneic leukemias readily induced significant resistance to transplantation of C57BL/6 leukemias induced by any of these viruses. It was difficult to induce resistance in BALB/c mice, however. They found that both BALB/c and B6 leukemias induced transplantation immunity to syngeneic leukemias in B6 mice but that neither syngeneic nor allogeneic immunization was very effective in immunizing BALB/c mice. Both B6 and BALB/c tumors are therefore apparently antigenic and the difference lies in the two strains' ability to respond to the FMR transplantation antigen(s).

Sato et al. (166) have also reported genetic polymorphism among mouse strains in their ability to reject a radiation-induced BALB/c leukemia bearing the transplantation antigen X.1. F_1 hybrids between X.1 responder strains and BALB/c were not killed by the subcutaneous inoculation of 10^5 X.1$^+$ RL$\male$1 leukemia cells and BALB/c mice and F1 hybrids of BALB/c and X.1 non-responder strains did not survive the inoculation of 10^4 RL$\male$1 cells. Strains of mice carrying H-2^b (C57BL/6, C57BL/10 and AKR/H-2^b) are responders and H-2^d, H-2^k, and H-2^a (BALB/c, B10.D2, AKR, C3H/An, and A) are nonresponders. The fact that the two congenic pairs—B10-B10.D2 and AKR-AKR/H-2^b—differed in their response to X.1 suggested that an H-2-linked gene determined the ability to successfully reject RL$\male$1. To test this hypothesis, Sato et al. produced a BALB/c × (BALB/c × B6) BC generation and challenged each mouse with RL$\male$1. Fifty-eight of 68 (85.3%) of H-2^d/H-2^d homozygotes were susceptible and only 18 of 70 (25.7%) of H-2^d/H-2^b heterozygotes were susceptible. Response to X.1 is therefore controlled by a gene linked to H-2. The response of two strains carrying recombinant H-2 chromosomes, HTG and HTI, suggests that the relevant gene is in the left portion (H-2K end) of H-2 or centromeric to H-2.

Williams et al. (206) have also investigated the influence of the H-2 region on resistance to syngeneic transplanted tumors. They determined the survival time of C57BL/10 mice injected with 5×10^3 B10 methylcholanthrene-induced fibrosarcoma cells and compared this to survival of F_1 hybrids of B10 and various H-2 congenic strains. B10 × B10.BR F1 (H-2^b/H-2^k), B10 × B10.M F1 (H-2^b/H-2^f) and B10 × B10.WB F1 (H-2^b/H-2^{ja}) mice all survived longer than B10 mice and a significant percentage of long term survivors were observed. B10 × B10.D2 F1s (H-2^b/H-2^d) did not survive longer than B10 inbred mice. Recombinant congenic strains were also tested for the ability to confer transplantation resistance to the B10 fibrosarcoma upon F_1 hybrids and B10.A(5R) prolonged survival, B10.A(18R) had not effect and B10.A(2R) decreased survival time. In analogous experiments, F_1 hybrids between DBA/2 and some of the strains mentioned above were challenged with the syngeneic DBA/2 mastocytoma P815. H-2^b, H-2^s, H-2^a, and B10.A(2R), (4R), and (18R) strains all conferred longer survival times on DBA/2 F_1 hybrids, while B10.A(5R) and H-2^k did not prolong survival. Williams et al. did not report backcross studies which would confirm H-2 linkage of genes controlling resistance to histocompatible tumors but the apparent tumor-specificity of this resistance (for example: B10.BR conferred resistance to the B10 fibrosarcoma on B10 × B10.BR hybrids but did not affect survival of DBA/2 × B10.BR F1s injected with P815) indicates a possible immunological mechanism. The recombinant strains used did not permit unambiguous mapping of response to either tumor to a region within the H-2 complex.

3. Effects of H-2 on Expression of Virus-Induced Antigens

Two recent reports indicate that genes linked to the H-2 complex may influence important aspects of tumor biology at the cellular level, not just at the level of the immune response. Freedman and Lilly (57) have established tissue culture lines from tumors induced by Friend leukemia virus in the congenic strains BALB/c (H-2^d) and BALB.B (H-2^b). The BALB/c tumor cell line HFL/d, when inoculated into BALB/c recipients, readily produced a transplantable tumor. In contrast, the BALB.B tumor cell line HFL/b produced tumors in BALB.B mice that often regressed. HFL/b would reliably produce transplantable tumors only in recipients rendered anemic by repeated bleedings. Both cell lines were examined for the production of infectious FLV: The HFL/d line produced infectious virus until the thirteenth in vitro passage after which no virus could be detected in culture supernatant fluid by a number of methods. HFL/d lines did retain the defective spleen locus-forming virus (SFFV) genome, as this activity could be rescued by superinfection with "helper" murine leukemia viruses such as the endogenous BALB/c MLV. HFL/b lines, on the other, produced complete, infectious FLV through 1 year *in vitro* and 121 passages.

It is obvious that the transplantability of a tumor cell line may be influenced by the expression of cell surface antigens and that some of these antigens may be associated with the budding of virus particles from the cell surface. Freedman *et al.* (52) have therefore extended their studies of HFL/d and HFL/b to investigate their complement of virion antigen and virus-induced cell surface antigen. Transplantation resistance could be induced in both BALB/c and BALB.B mice against syngeneic tumor cell lines although this was much easier in BALB.B. Less than 10^8 HFL/b cells never produced tumors in BALB.B and 10^8 HFL/b cells produced tumors which all subsequently regressed. These mice showed strong transplantation immunity and all were able to reject large subcutaneous syngeneic tumor grafts. Smaller numbers of HFL/d cells were required to produce resistance in BALB/c recipients. BALB/c mice inoculated with 10^6 HFL/d cells all developed palpable tumors which killed 7 of 38 recipients (19%). The regressors were challenged with 10^6 HFL/d cells, which grew in all recipients and then regressed. It is not clear whether this difference in the ease of induction of transplantation resistance represents a difference in the expression of tumor-associated transplantation antigen or a difference in the ability of the host to respond to such antigen (or both).

Mice hyperimmunized with syngeneic Friend virus-induced leukemias produce cytotoxic antibodies which recognize a virus-induced cell surface antigen common to leukemias induced by Friend, Moloney, and Rauscher MLVs (the FMR antigen) (131, 133). FMR antigen could not be detected by direct cytotoxicity on primary BALB/c FLV-infected spleen cells or on HFL/d tumor cells. Primary BALB/c spleen tumor cells could absorb this antibody from FMR test serum but HFL/d cells could not. In contrast, FMR antigen was demonstrable on HFL/b cells by direct cytotoxicity and absorption.

Hyperimmune anti-FLV leukemia serum also detects a virus envelope antigen (VEA), and this antibody can be assayed by neutralization of infectious virus. Both HFL/d and HFL/b bear VEA on their cell surfaces, as demonstrated by absorption of neutralizing antibody. It is not surprising that HFL/b cells bear VEA since they produce infectious virus and its presence on HFL/d cells confirms the observations of Billelo *et al.* (22) that VEA can be expressed in the absence of virus production. One intriguing observation was that HFL/d lost almost all ability to induce transplantation resistance at about the 125th *in vitro* passage, concurrent with the loss of detectable cell surface VEA.

4. Relationships Between Tumor Antigens and Normal Histocompatibility Antigens

H-2 RESTRICTION OF CYTOTOXICITY. A number of recent studies have shown that cytotoxic T lymphocytes and target cells bearing the sensitizing antigen(s) must share serologically detectable products of the major histocompatibility complex (MHC) in order to interact effectively to give maximal cytotoxicity. This histocompatibility requirement has been demonstrated in the mouse system for target cells bearing antigens induced by lymphocytic choriomeningitis virus (213), vaccinia virus (107), ectromelia virus (54), trinitrophenyl-modified normal lymphocyte antigens (175), and minor (non-H-2) histocompatibility antigens (21). Because of the generality of these observations it should not be surprizing to find that interactions between cytotoxic T cells and tumor cells bearing tumor-specific surface antigens are similarly restricted.

Wainberg et al. (203) have studied cellular immunity directed against antigens of Rous sarcoma virus-induced tumors in an outbred population of chickens. They found that the adherence of ^{51}Cr-labeled lymphocytes from tumor-bearing chickens to Rous tumor cell monolayers was significantly higher when the target cells were autochthonous in origin rather than allogeneic. The release of isotope from ^{51}Cr-labeled Rous target cells in a standard cytotoxicity assay was also higher with autochthonous than with allogeneic combinations.

Chesebro and Wehrly (36) have studied the development of cell-mediated immunity during recovery from Friend leukemia virus-induced splenomegaly in mice. One incidental observation made during these studies was that H-2^{aa} attacker cells were unable to lyse H-2^{bb} tumor cells that were lysed by H-2^{bb}- or H-2^{ab}-immune T cells. H-2^{aa} T cells were able, however, to lyse target tumor cells induced in B10.A(4R) × A.BY F1 mice. B10.A(4R) bears a recombinant H-2 haplotype with the H-2K and Ir-IA regions of H-2^a and the Ir-1B, Ir-C, S, and H-2D regions of H-2^b. Partial H-2 identity seems to be required for cytotoxic interaction. Blank et al. (26) have confirmed these findings using FLV-induced tumor cell lines induced in BALB.B (H-2^b) and BALB.K (H-2^k) congenic mice and H-2^{bk} F1 hybrids. Peritoneal exudate cells (PEC) from BALB.B mice immunized with H-2^b tumor cells were able to lyse H-2^b and H-2^{bk} targets but not H-2^k. The killing observed in this system is abolished by treatment with anti-Thy.1 and complement and is therefore T cell mediated.

Gomard et al. (59) have studied the target specificity of cytotoxic T lymphocytes (CTL) produced by the injection of adult mice with Moloney murine sarcoma virus and assayed by ^{51}Cr release from Moloney MLV-induced leukemia target cells. In agreement with the previously cited studies, they found that H-2^b (C57BL/6 and BALB.B) CTL lysed H-2^b but not H-2^d targets, H-2^d (BALB/c and B10.D2) CTL lysed H-2^d but not H-2^b targets, and H-2^{db} F1 CTL lysed both H-2^b and H-2^d target cells. They also showed that F1 CTL produced by immunization with H-2^b tumor cells were specific for H-2^b targets and that immunization with H-2^d tumor cells produced CTL specific for H-2^d targets.

Trinchieri et al. (194) have found that cytotoxic mouse spleen cells generated against syngeneic SV40-transformed mouse cells are specific for target cells syngeneic with the immunizing cells.

Two general mechanisms for this MHC-controlled restriction of cytotoxicity have been proposed (41): (a) In addition to the immunologically specific interaction between effector cell receptor and target cell antigen, effector and target cell must also interact through the products of the MHC located at the cell surface, perhaps through an MHC-coded receptor for "self" antigens. (b) The "non-self" antigen recognized as foreign by the cytotoxic cell is an altered normal histocompatibility antigen or a complex of normal and virus-induced antigens. The resulting "non-self" determinant would then be different for each outbred individual or inbred strain in which that antigen is induced. The findings of Gomard et al. (59) that cytotoxic T lymphocytes produced in H-2^{bd} heterozygotes by immunization with H-2^b Moloney sarcomas were unable to lyse H-2^d tumor cells, even though they shared MHC determinants, argue against the first possibility. Two recent studies indicate that cytotoxic T lymphocytes can specifically lyse virus-infected or chemically modified allogeneic cells. Zinkernagel (212) produced radiation chimeras by injecting bone marrow cells from C3H mice into lethally irradiated C3H × DBA/2 F$_1$ hybrids. The lymphocytes of such mice are of C3H origin and are specifically tolerant of DBA/2 antigens. When these mice are infected with lymphocytic choriomeningitis virus, T cells isolated from their spleens will kill LCM virus-infected H-2^k or H-2^d target cells but not virus-infected H-2^b cells or normal H-2^d cells. Von Boehmer and Haas (200) produced radiation chimeras by injecting DBA/2 bone marrow cells into lethally irradiated CBA × DBA/2 F$_1$ hybrids and immunized them with TNP-modified CBA spleen cells. The resulting cytotoxic T lymphocytes would specifically kill TNP-CBA spleen cells and not normal CBA cells or TNP-modified DBA/2 spleen cells. It is apparent, therefore, that in these two experimental systems H-2 identity is not a prerequisite for efficient cytotoxic interaction.

A wide variety of experimental studies show that the relationship between tumor-associated surface antigens (TASA) and normal histocompatibility antigens is more intimate and complex than just the similarity of the methods used for their detection.

Two laboratories have shown that the tumor-associated transplantation antigens of chemically induced tumors cross-react with normal histocompatibility antigens carried by mice of certain other strains.

Martin et al. (121) have studied the transplantation antigen(s) of a lung tumor (No. 85) induced in C3Hf mice by injection of a pregnant female with 1-ethyl-1-nitrosourea. This tumor grows very poorly in normal C3Hf adults but will grow in sublethally irradiated C3Hf mice, unirradiated C3H (which transmits murine mammary tumor virus strain S [MMTV S] via the milk), and unirradiated C3Hf × A F₁ hybrids. C3Hf mice immunized with tumor 85 before irradiation will reject subsequent challenges with the tumor. Not all F₁ hybrids with C3Hf strain mice will accept tumor 85: C3Hf × DBA/2 and C3Hf × C57BL/6 F₁ hybrids are resistant to tumor transplantation and although some tumors will grow briefly in C3Hf × NIH/Swiss F₁s, most ultimately regress. Martin et al. then performed an experiment to test the hypothesis that tumor 85 expresses a rejection antigen recognized as foreign by C3Hf mice but not by C3H or C3Hf × A F₁s because they possess a normal antigen or antigens which cross-react with the tumor 85 antigen. Groups of C3Hf mice were immunized with normal lung tissue from strains A, C3H, C57BL/6 or DBA/2, sublethally irradiated and injected with 10⁵ tumor 85 cells. Progressive tumor growth occurred in C3Hf mice immunized with DBA/2 and B6 lung, as in unimmunized, irradiated C3Hf mice. In contrast, severely impaired tumor growth was observed in C3Hf mice immunized with A, C3H lung, or lung tumor 85 cells, or in nonirradiated C3Hf mice.

Strain C3Hf was derived from strain C3H in 1945 by foster-nursing a C3H litter on an MTV-free C57BL/6 mother (122) and does not transmit MTV-S, although it does contain a gamete-transmitted, avirulent form, MTV-L (147). Strain C3H and strain C3Hf are no longer histocompatible (122). Martin et al. think it unlikely that the antigen in question is related to MTV because DBA/2 mice also transmit MTV (and normal DBA/2 lung does not immunize against tumor 85) and C3Hf × A F₁ mice foster-nursed on C57BL/6 mothers are as susceptible to tumor 85 as non-fostered C3Hf × A F₁s. It has not been demonstrated, however, that mammary tumors induced in the highly susceptible C3Hf strain by foster-nursing on C3H mothers do not bear the lung tumor TATA and will not immunize C3Hf recipients against challenge with tumor 85.

Martin et al. (121, 122) have used the microcytotoxicity assay (MC) to confirm that the lymph node cells of C3Hf mice immunized with lung tumor 85 or LNCs from tumor-bearing (A × C3Hf) F₁ mice will reduce the survival of tumor 85 cells and normal strain A or C3H lung cells (but not C3Hf or C57BL/6 lung cells) during 30 to 40 hours of co-cultivation. Lymphoid cells of C3Hf mice immunized with normal A or C3H lung tissue will also reduce the survival of tumor 85 cells in vitro.

In summary, the results of Martin et al. (121, 122) indicate that at least one lung tumor induced in a C3Hf mouse by transplacental chemical carcinogenesis bears an antigen or antigens, detectable by both *in vivo* transplantation methods and the *in vitro* microcytotoxicity assay, which cross-reacts with normal alloantigens found on lung tissue of strain A and C3H, but not C57BL/6 or C3Hf, mice.

Analogous findings have been reported by Invernizzi and Parmiani (99) for a sarcoma (ST-5) induced in a BALB/c mouse by methylcholanthrene. They found that immunization of BALB/c mice with C3Hf or C57BL/6 normal tissue allografts provided highly significant protection against the growth of ST-5 tumor cells. No protection was observed after immunization with W/Fu rat skin or sheep red blood cells. This cross reactivity is apparently tumor-specific, as allo-immunization with C3Hf or B6 tissues provided no protection against another MC-induced BALB/c tumor—B2. The TATAs of tumor ST-5 are apparently complex. The immunogenicity of a tumor may be assessed by determining to what degree immunization (by injection of tumor followed by excision after a short period of growth) protects against subsequent tumor challenge compared with a group of unimmunized controls. Invernizzi and Parmiani (99) found that ST-5 was immunogenic in BALB/c recipients and in (C3Hf × BALB/c) F_1 hybrids but did not provide significant protection for (BALB/c × B6) F_1 hybrids. They suggest that this could be explained by hypothesizing that ST-5 bears two distinct TATAs, both of which are found on normal B6 (and BALB/c × B6 F_1) tissues but only one of which is found on C3Hf (and C3Hf × BALB/c F_1) tissues.

Parmiani and Invernizzi (137) have extended these observations to 2 other MC-induced BALB/c sarcomas and have shown that immunization with DBA/2 skin provides significant protection against growth of tumor ST2. Immunization with C3Hf skin provided slight but significant protection (prolonged latent period) and B6 or AKR tissues did not protect. Protection against another sarcoma—TZ15—was only provided by AKR tissues and not the C3Hf, B6, or DBA/2 tissues. The specificity of this antitumor immunity was confirmed by mixing LNCs from alloimmune mice with tumor cells, incubation *in vitro* for 2 hours at 37C and injection into syngeneic recipients (the Winn test). Parmiani and Invernizzi also immunized BALB/c mice with tumors ST2 and TZ15 and compared the mean survival time of allogeneic skin grafts on these mice *versus* unimmunized controls. The survival of C3Hf, B6, DBA/2, and AKR skin was shortened on ST2-immune mice while only C3Hf and AKR skin survival was shortened on TZ15-immune mice. Immunization with tumor gave antiskin immunity with broader specificity than normal tissue-induced tumor immunity.

In immunogenicity tests tumor ST2 was immunogenic in all strains and F_1 hybrids tested except (C3HF × BALB/c) F_1 and TZ15 was immunogenic in all hybrids, including (BALB/c × AKR)F$_1$. Parmiani and Invernizzi interpret these results to indicate antigenic complexity analogous to that observed for tumor ST-5 (99). ST2 bears at least 2 TATAs, all of which are present on C3Hf normal tissue and only some are present on DBA/2 normal tissue. AKR normal tissue bears an antigen also present on tumor TZ15, but that tumor bears at least one other antigen not found on AKR tissue.

The studies of Martin et al. (121, 122) and of Parmiani and Invernizzi (99, 137) on transplantation antigens of chemically induced mouse tumors may be considered analogous to the findings that certain cell-surface antigens of MMTV-induced tumors (35) and the TL antigen of spontaneous and radiation-induced leukemias (30, 132) are also found in other strains as normal alloantigens. Bodmer (28) has proposed a genetic model for complex (polymorphic) loci under which these observations are readily explained. Bodmer suggested that the histocompatibility phenotype of a mammal may not simply be the direct expression of all alleles present, but the result of control genes which normally select one of a number of closely linked genes for expression. These closely linked genes are homologous and presumably arose by gene duplication. The expression of "alloantigens" on tumor cells observed by Martin et al. (121) and Invernizzi and Parmiani (99, 137) would then represent a breakdown in the normal control function resulting in the expression of normally silent genes.

Studies by Schrader et al. (159) indicate that H-2 antigens and virus-induced or tumor-associated cell surface antigens are physically closely associated on the surface of mouse tumor cells. When the H-2^b antigens of C57BL/6 tumor EL4 were capped in vitro by incubation with anti-H-2^b serum at 4C followed by incubation with fluorescein-conjugated goat antimouse immunoglobulin at 37C and fixed with formaldehyde to prevent further capping, viral antigens (detected with rabbit anti-Rauscher leukemia virus followed by tetramethyl rhodamine-conjugated goat antirabbit immunoglobulin) were found in caps with H-2 antigens. Patching of H-2 antigens in the presence of sodium azide, an inhibitor of capping, also induced co-patching of viral antigens (169).

Schrader and Edelman (170) have also shown that H-2 antigens participate in the lysis of syngeneic tumor cells by cytotoxic T lymphocytes. Lysis of H-2^b EL4 target cells by immune C57BL/6 T cells and lysis of H-2^d P388 target cells by immune BALB/c and DBA/2 T cells were specifically inhibited by anti-H-2^b and anti-H-2^d sera, respectively. Two lines of evidence indicate that the H-2 antigens of the cytotoxic cells are not involved in this inhibition: (1) the lysis of allogeneic cells is not inhibited by antiserum to the H-2 antigens of the effector cells, even at effector:target cell ratios as low as 0.4 to 1; and (2) the lysis of H-2^b EL4 cells by (C57BL/6

× DBA/2)F1 hybrid cytotoxic cells was inhibited by antiserum to H-2^b antigens found on both target and effector cells but not by antiserum to H-2^d antigens found only on effector cells.

Similar studies have also been reported by Germain et al. (56) who found that the lysis of P815 or SL2 tumor cells by syngeneic immune DBA/2 lymphocytes was inhibited by anti-H-2^d sera while anti-H-2^k sera failed to inhibit the lysis of SL2 cells by cytotoxic (C3H × DBA/2)F1 hybrid lymphocytes.

Further evidence for the close biological relationship between normal and tumor-associated cell surface antigens comes from a number of studies which show an inverse relationship between the quantity of normal H-2 antigens and TASAs expressed on tumor cell surfaces (31, 37, 69, 192, 195).

5. Immunosuppression, Congenital Immunodeficiencies, and Cancer in Mice and Humans

A. IMMUNOSUPPRESSION. Strong evidence has accumulated that immunosuppression of rodents leads to increased susceptibility to oncogenesis by papovaviruses and adenoviruses. Vandeputte et al. (198) first demonstrated that neonatal thymectomy of rats increased the incidence of tumors in animals infected at birth with polyoma virus, and that it prolonged the period of postnatal susceptibility to oncogenesis. Allison and Taylor (5) reported similar findings using SV40 in rats but could find no evidence of increased susceptibility to chemical carcinogenesis following neonatal thymectomy. Tumor incidence resulting from infection of adult mice with polyoma or adenovirus 12 was increased from zero to almost 100% by treatment of the mice with ALS (3, 4). It has been reported that ALS treatment does not influence the titer of antiviral antibody generated and that immune lymphoid cells, but not immune serum, could reduce the tumor incidence in immunodepressed animals (110, 111, 196). This finding has been quoted in support of the contention that the influential immune response being eliminated is that against the tumor cells rather than that against the virus (100). However, this may not be so, since all that has been demonstrated is that the influential immune response is cellular rather than humoral, without direct evidence regarding the specificity of the response.

The effect of immunosuppression on tumor induction by RNA tumor viruses is, in general, to increase susceptibility. ALS treatment increases the number of spleen foci induced by Friend leukemia virus (190) and increases the incidence of leukemias induced by Moloney (112), Rauscher

(90) and Gross (201) leukemia viruses in mice. Law (112) also found that neonatal thymectomy drastically reduced the incidence of Moloney leukemias, and East and Harvey (43) observed that the late lymphocytic leukemia induced by the MuLV component of Harvey-strain murine sarcoma virus was completely eliminated by neonatal thymectomy. These last two observations are probably due to a complete lack of target cells rather than an effect of immunosuppression. The incidence of sarcoma induced by Moloney-strain murine sarcoma virus has been shown to increase under immunosuppression by cortisone (167), cyclophosphamide (47), ALS (113), neonatal thymectomy (114), and in mice homozygous for the mutation nude (189). The frequency of regression of these tumors is also reduced by these treatments. East and Harvey (143) have also found that sarcoma incidence and early erythroblastic splenomegaly induced by the Harvey strain of murine sarcoma are increased by neonatal thymectomy.

It is possible that the immune responses that are being suppressed in these experiments with viruses of the murine leukemia-sarcoma complex are directed against virus and not cell surface antigens. Resistance to Moloney sarcoma induction can be transferred by immune serum (47, 144); the increased susceptibility of ALS-treated mice to Friend spleen focus formation is accompanied by a profound increase in virus multiplication (190) and nonproducer tumor cells transformed by defective murine sarcoma viruses are neither immunogenic nor immunosensitive (185).

In contrast to the other RNA tumor virus systems described above, it has been found that neonatal thymectomy of C3H/Bi females infected with MTV decreases the incidence of mammary tumors by about 50% (123). It is noteworthy that this is a system in which the primary host appears to be unresponsive to the major TATA of his tumor.

Embryonic bursectomy of chickens has no effect on the incidence of Rous sarcoma virus-induced tumors (124, 156) or Marek's disease (139), indicating that feedback inhibition of cellular immunity by humoral antibody is unimportant in facilitating tumor development. Neonatal thymectomy, however, increases the incidence of both virus-induced neoplasms (157, 174).

In contrast to the dramatic effects of immunosuppression on tumor induction by DNA viruses, similar treatment of rodents has little or no effect on chemical carcinogenesis or on the appearance of spontaneous tumors. Balner and Dersjant (17) reported that neonatal thymectomy did not influence oncogenesis by 3-methylcholanthrene (MCA), and this was confirmed by Allison and Taylor (5). There were conflicting reports concerning the influence of ALS on tumor induction by MCA. Balner and Dersjant (18), Cerilli and Treat (34), and Rabbat and Jeejeebhoy (155) all reported a modest increase in tumor incidence and abbreviation of the latent period, following ALS treatment; whereas Fisher *et al.* (49) reported that there was no effect. In view of this discrepancy, the question was reexamined in this laboratory.

Since the effect of ALS was clearly not great, we took the following precautions. A single large batch of ALS prepared in a pony by immunization with mouse thymocytes was used. This serum was highly potent. Following four doses of 0.06 ml given during the first week, single weekly doses of 0.06 ml were sufficient to maintain a prolonged state of immunosuppression as demonstrated by the inability of the mice to reject an H-2-incompatible, MCA-induced tumor. We used a dose of MCA which was intermediate between those used by previous workers. In three separate experiments we tested 408 mice representing 10 different inbred strains and could not see any effect of ALS treatment on tumor incidence, latency, incidence of metastasis or antigenicity of the tumors induced. The third experiment compared two groups of 50 B10.D2 (old) mice matched for age and sex with littermates randomized between the two groups. The cumulative tumor incidence and death curves of the ALS-treated and control groups were superimposed. We thus concluded that the immune response which can be suppressed with ALS, while effective in preventing growth of allogeneic transplanted tumors, is largely ineffectual in preventing the appearance of primary neoplasms induced by injection in mice of 250 or 500 μg of MCA (202).

The complementary conclusion, that the immune response which could be suppressed with ALS was not responsible for preventing the development of spontaneous tumors in CBA mice, was reached by Simpson and Nehlsen (177). They treated a large group of mice with ALS for the duration of their lifespan and maintained a continuous state of immunosuppression. The treatment group did not show any higher incidence of spontaneous tumors than the untreated control group. This experiment included an unintended internal control in that one sample of ALS was inadvertently contaminated with polyoma virus. Most of the animals injected with this preparation succumbed to polyoma viral oncogenesis (Nehlsen, personal communication).

Thus although experimental oncogenesis by DNA viruses is strongly influenced by cellular immune responsiveness, there is little evidence from experimental animals that chemical or "spontaneous" oncogenesis is similarly affected. Data obtained from chronically immunosuppressed patients (mainly kidney transplant recipients) are, at least superficially, discordant with those derived from experimental animals. The rate of tumor development in this group of patients is much greater (10–20 times) than in the general population in a comparable age range (42, 140, 141). However, the spectrum of tumors seen in these patients is very different from that which occurs in the general population. Approximately 40% of the tumors are of mesenchymal origin, with the great majority of these being malignant lymphomas. Of the remaining 60%, fully two-thirds are skin cancers or carcinoma of the cervix or the lip. Schwartz has pointed out that these are "precisely those in which oncogenic viruses are suspected as etiologic agents" (172) and has suggested that "immunity against an infectious oncogenic virus may be a more relevant question than surveillance against a barely immunogenic malignant cell" (173). It has also been postulated that the high incidence of malignant lymphomas in these patients results from chronic antigenic stimulation by the graft itself, combined with immunosuppression adequate to eliminate a feedback regulatory mechanism limiting lymphocytic proliferation (109, 171).

B. CONGENITAL IMMUNODEFICIENCY.   As with the studies of deliberate immunosuppression, there is discordance between the data derived from observations of immunodeficiency in humans and in experimental animals. Kersey et al. (100) reported 118 cases of human malignancy associated with various forms of primary immunodeficiency disease. Although the data do not permit calculation of precise incidence rates, they are clearly higher than in the general population. As with the tumors in immunosuppressed patients, the great majority (75%) are lymphoreticular tumors or leukemias, possibly resulting from the chronic antigenic stimulation associated with these patients' extreme susceptibility to infection.

Mice homozygous for the mutation *nude* are hairless, have no thymus (136), and the thymus-dependent areas of their peripheral lymphoid organs (spleen, lymph nodes and Peyer's patches) are almost without lymphocytes (40). About 5% of the cells in lymph nodes of *nu/nu* mice are killed by treatment with anti-Thy.1 serum plus complement while approximately 50% of the lymph node cells of normal controls are sensitive to anti-Thy.1 treatment (158). Wortis et al. (209) have shown that *nu/nu* bone marrow cells can effectively repopulate the thymuses of lethally irradiated normal mice but normal fetal liver cells cannot restore the thymuses of nude mice and thymic rudiments from nude mice are not populated with host lymphocytes when grafted into normal recipients. Nude mice therefore have normal thymocyte precursors, but their thymus epithelium is defective and fails to induce the differentiation of thymocytes into mature T cells (209).

Because of this defect in thymocyte differentiation, immunological phenomena mediated by or requiring the participation of T lymphocytes are severely reduced or do not occur at all in *nude* mice. These phenomena include rejection of transplanted allogeneic (142, 208) and xenogeneic (148) tissue, in vivo PHA responsiveness (208), and antibody responses to thymus dependent antigens (104, 154).

If one of the functions of the immune system is to eliminate nascent clones of neoplastic cells, then one might expect nude mice to develop more tumors after experimental treatment with carcinogens than their normal littermates.

Stutman (188) has shown that nu/nu mice were no more susceptible to tumor induction by 3-methylcholanthrene than their normal littermates and that the observed tumors in both groups had similar latent periods. Vandeputte et al. (199) have shown that nude mice are highly susceptible to oncogenesis by polyoma virus. All nude mice infected with 3×10^7 PFU of polyoma virus at 3 to 6 weeks of age developed tumors while none of their normal littermates were susceptible. Stutman has also studied the susceptibility of the nude mouse to another oncogenic virus—the Moloney murine sarcoma virus (189). All the mice in Stutman's experiments developed sarcomas but most of the tumors in normal mice regressed (100% to 87%, depending on the strain) whereas none of the tumors in nu/nu homozygotes regressed. Another interesting observation was that most of the tumors that appeared in normal mice had regressed before the appearance of tumors in the nude mice. In summary, the mutation nude apparently has no effect on induction of tumors by methylcholanthrene, but it profoundly affects polyoma virus oncogenesis and the regression of Moloney MSV-induced tumors.

If surveillance against neoplastic cells is one of the functions of the immune system, one might also expect nude mice to show a higher incidence of spontaneous tumors than their normal littermates. Experimental tests of this expectation are complicated by the fact that nude mice are highly susceptible to infection and their lifespan in conventional colonies is extremely short. Since most spontaneous tumors arise late in life, the observation periods for nude and control mice must be carefully matched. Rygaard and Povlsen (165) observed 7,900 nude mice (of various genetic backgrounds) for an average of 3 months, and 900 nudes for 7 months under specific pathogen-free conditions, and 2,000 nudes for 4 months under conventional conditions and observed no malignancies. Spontaneous tumor incidence in normal mice of otherwise similar genetic constitution during the same period was not specified. Outzen et al. (135) have maintained nude mice in germ-free conditions by delivering into sterile isolators by Caesarean section and foster nursing on germ-free mothers. If sterility is maintained, germ-free nude mice have a life expectancy of greater than 20 months. Outzen et al. found no difference between germ-free nude and conventional normal mice in the cumulative percentage of spontaneous tumors appearing versus age, but a very high proportion of the tumors which appeared in nude mice were lymphoreticular tumors including lymphocytic lymphomas and leukemias, highly anaplastic leukemias, a granulocytic leukemia, and a plasmacytoma. This observation compares with the extremely high incidence of lymphoreticular tumors in humans with immunodeficiency diseases (55) and transplant patients undergoing immunosuppression (140).

It is tempting to attribute this difference between human and experimontal animal data to the germ-free environment in which the athymic mice are kept, and to suggest that their relative susceptibility to some forms of viral oncogenesis is due to lack of response to the virus rather than to tumor cell surface antigen.

6. Genetic Variation in Killer (K) Cell Activity

In 1975, Kiessling et al. (102) observed that the spleen cells of unimmunized young adult mice of certain strains were specifically cytotoxic for syngeneic Moloney virus-induced leukemias. The cells responsible for this in vitro cytotoxicity are found mainly in the spleen, where they increase in activity from birth to about 3 months of age and decrease thereafter (101). Kiessling et al. (101) have also shown that the effector cell mediating this natural cytotoxicity is found in nude mice and is present in those spleen cells left after treatment with carbonyl iron to remove phagocytic cells, anti-Thy.1 plus complement to remove T lymphocytes, and passage through antimouse IgG columns to remove B lymphocytes.

A number of other laboratories have also reported the existence of cytotoxic cells in the spleens of unimmunized young adult mice. Sendo et al. (173) have described natural cytotoxicity for the BALB/c radiation-induced leukemia RL♂1. They found that the effector cell in their system was nonadherent and was enriched in the effluent of nylon-wool columns (which removes Ig-bearing cells). Sendo et al. (173) also found that the age-specific variation in natural killer cell activity correlated well with the age-specific variation in susceptibility to transplantation of syngeneic or semisyngeneic RL♂1 tumor cells. A high percentage of B6 and C58 mice show killer cell activity when tested at 2 months (when (B6 × BALB/c)F1 and (C58 × BALB/c)F$_1$ mice are resistant to transplantation with RL♂1 cells) but this natural cytotoxicity can not be demonstrated in mice greater than 4 months old, when F$_1$ hybrid mice are more susceptible to RL♂1 challenge (173). Zarling et al. (211) have found natural cytotoxicity to K36 spontaneous AKR leukemia cells in non-phagocytic spleen cells of some strains. Herberman et al. (89) used the Rauscher leukemia virus-induced C57BL/6 leukemia RBL-5 to demonstrate natural cytotoxic cells with a strain distribution very similar to that observed by Kiessling et al. (102). Herberman et al. (88) found that the natural killer cell in their system, the N-cell, was found in high concentrations in the spleens of nude mice, was not affected by anti-Thy.1 plus complement, was not adherent or phagocytic and did not have cell surface receptors for immunoglobulin or antigen-antibody complexes. The strain distribution of natural killer cell activities found against a number of different target cells is listed in Table 1.

A number of genetic studies indicate that the occurrence of K cell activity is under the control of more than one gene and is correlated with the ability to reject transplanted, semisyngeneic leukemias. Petranyi et al. (143) found that the cytolytic activities of spleen cells from F1 hybrids between low-activity strain A mice and high-activity strains C57BL, C57L, CBA, and C3H strains were all as high as the high-activity parental strains. Natural K cell activity is therefore completely dominant. When 77 (A × C58BL) × A backcross mice were tested for anti-YAC-1 cytolytic activity, the individual cytolytic activities were broadly distributed over the ranges of activities observed in A and A × C57BL F1 parental mice. Significant association was found with H-2 type and the B (black) coat color gene but not with C (albino). They concluded that K cell activity is under polygenic control.

Kiessling et al. (103) compared the strain distribution of in vitro K cell activity with the ability of (A × test strain) F_1 hybrids to reject small numbers (10^3 to 10^5) of YAC-1 injected subcutaneously. F_1 hybrids with high-activity strains (C57BL/6, C57L, C3H, CBA, and DBA/2) were all significantly more resistant to YAC-1 challenge than hybrids with low-activity strains (A.SW, A.CA, and A.BY). Petranyi et al. (144) expanded these studies to investigate tumor susceptibility and K cell activity in a number of (A × high-activity strain) × A BC generations. They tested a larger series of (A × C57BL) × A BC mice and again observed a significant association of K cell activity with H-2 type but failed to confirm the previously reported association with the B coat color gene (143). A slight but significant association of K cell activity with C (albino) was observed in this series. Seventy-two (A × C57BL) × A BC mice were splenectomized and the spleens tested for cytolytic activity and the BC mice were each challenged with 5 × 10^3 YAC cells. H-2^{ab} mice were significantly less susceptible to tumor growth than H-2^{aa} individuals, but no association with coat color was observed. Petranyi et al. (144) also found that tumor susceptibility, measured by average tumor diameter and percent tumor incidence, was greater in mice with low cytolytic activity (0–50% corrected lysis) than in mice with high (greater than 50% corrected lysis) cytolytic activity. No association of cytolytic activity or in vivo tumor susceptibility with the Ig-1 allotype locus, C5 complement structural

Table 1.   Strain distribution of natural cytotoxicity in spleens of young adult mice.

Target Cell (Origin)	Strains		References
	With Natural Cytotoxicity	Without Natural Cytotoxicity	
YAC-1 (Moloney virus-induced A/Sn leukemia)	CBA BALB/c C57BL C3H	A/Sn A.CA A.SW	Kiessling et al. 1975 (102) Petranyi et al. 1975 (143)
K36 (Spontaneous AKR leukemia)	C57BL/6 C57BL/10 C57L RF	AKR C58 B10.BR PL	Zarling et al. 1975 (211)
RBL-5 (Rauscher virus-induced leukemia)	C57BL/6 BALB/c C3H/HeN CBA	A/Jax	Herberman et al. 1975 (89) Herberman et al. 1975 (88)
RL 1 (Radiation-induced BALB/c leukemia)	C57BL/6 C58 male C3H/He	AKR BALB/c DBA/2 female C3H/He	Sendo et al. 1975 (173)

gene, sex, or the enzyme markers *ip-1, Gpi-1, Mod-1, Gpd-1,* or *Es-1* was observed.

REFERENCES

1. Aaronson, S. A., and Stephenson, J. R. 1974. Widespread natural occurrence of high titers of neutralizing antibodies to a specific class of endogenous mouse type-C virus. *Proc. Natl. Acad. Sci.* 71: 1957–1961.

2. Aaronson, S. A., Todaro, G. J., and Scolnick, E. M. 1971. Induction of murine C-type viruses from clonal lines of virus-free BALB/3T3 cells. *Science* 174: 157–159.

3. Allison, A. C., Berman, L. D., and Levey, R. H. 1976. Increased tumor induction by adenovirus type 12 in thymectomized mice and mice treated with anti-lymphocyte serum. *Nature* 215: 185–187.

4. Allison, A. C. and Law, L. W. 1968. Effects of antilymphocyte serum on virus oncogenesis. *Proc. Soc. Exp. Biol. Med.* 127: 207–212.

5. Allison, A. C. and Taylor, R. B. 1967. Observations on thymectomy and carcinogenesis. Cancer Res. 27: 703–707.

6. Ankerst, J., Steele, G., and Sjögren, H. O. 1974. Cross-reacting tumor associated antigen(s) of adenovirus type 9-induced fibroadenomas and a chemically induced mammary carcinoma in rats. Cancer Res. 34: 1794–1800.

7. Aoki, T., Boyse, E. A. and Old, L. J. 1966. Occurrence of natural antibody to the G (Gross) leukemia antigen in mice. Cancer Res. 26: 1415–1419.

8. August, J. T., Bolognesi, D. P., Fleissner, E., Gilden, R. V., and Nowinski, R. C. 1974. A proposed nomenclature for the virion proteins of oncogenic RNA viruses. Virology 60: 595–601.

9. Avis, F., Avis, I., Cole, A. T., Fried, F., and Haughton, G. 1975. Antigenic cross reactivity between benign prostatic hyperplasia and adenocarcinoma of prostate. Urology 5: 122–130.

10. Avis, F., Avis, I., Newsome, J. F., and Haughton, G. 1976. Antigenic cross-reactivity between adenocarcinoma of the breast and fibrocystic disease of the breast. J. Natl. Cancer Inst. 56: 17–25.

11. Avis, F., Mosonov, I., and Haughton, G. 1974. Antigenic cross-reactivity between benign and malignant neoplasms of the human breast. J. Natl. Cancer Inst. 52: 1041–1049.

12. Baldwin, R. W. 1975. Immunity to methylcholanthrene-induced tumours in inbred rats following atrophy and regression of the implanted tumors. Brit. J. Cancer 9: 652–657.

13. Baldwin, R. W., and Embleton, M. J. 1971. Demonstration by colony inhibition measurements of cellular and humoral immune reactions to tumor-specific antigens associated with aminoazo-dye-induced rat hepatomas. Int. J. Cancer 7: 17–25.

14. Baldwin, R. W., Embleton, M. J., and Robins, R. A. 1973. Cellular and humoral immunity to rat hepatoma-specific antigens correlated with tumor status. Int. J. Cancer 11: 1–10.

15. Baldwin, R. W., Price, M. R., and Robins, R. A. 1972. Blocking of lymphocyte-mediated cytotoxicity for rat hepatoma cells by tumor-specific antigen-antibody complexes. Nature New Biol. 238: 185–187.

16. Baldwin, R. W., Price, M. R., and Robins, R. A. 1973. Inhibition of hepatoma-immune lymph-node cell cytotoxicity by tumor-bearer serum, and solubilized hepatoma antigen. Int. J. Cancer 11: 527–535.

17. Balner, H., and Dersjant, H. 1966. Neonatal thymectomy and tumor induction with methylcholanthrene in mice. J. Natl. Cancer Inst. 36: 513–521.

18. Balner, H., and Dersjant, H. 1969. Increased oncogenic effect of methylcholanthrene after treatment with antilymphocyte serum. Nature 224: 376–738.

19. Bansal, S. C., and Sjögren, H. O. 1972. Counteration of the blocking of cell-mediated tumor immunity by inoculation of unblocking sera and splenectomy: Immunotheraputic effects on primary polyoma tumors in rats. Int. J. Cancer 9: 490–509.

20. Benacerraf, B., and Katz, D. H. 1975. The histocompatibility-linked immune response genes. Adv. Cancer Res. 21: 121–173.

21. Bevan, M. J. 1975. Interaction antigens detected by cytotoxic T cells with the major histocompatibility complex as modifier. Nature 256: 419–421.

22. Bilello, J. A., Strand, M., and August, J. T. 1974. Murine sarcoma virus gene expression: Transformants which express viral envelope glycoprotein in the absence of the major internal protein and infectious particles. *Proc. Natl. Acad. Sci.* 71: 3234–3238.

23. Biozzi, G., Asofsky, R., Lieberman, R., Stiffel, C., Mouton, D., and Benacerraf, B. 1970. Serum concentrations and allotypes of immunoglobulins in two lines of mice genetically selected for "high" or "low" antibody synthesis. *J. Exp. Med.* 132: 752–764.

24. Biozzi, G., Stiffel, C., Mouton, D., and Bouthilllier, Y. 1975. Selection of lines of mice with high and low antibody responses to complex immunogenes, in: B. Benacerraf (ed.), *Immunogenetics and Immunodeficiency*, pp. 179–227. University Park, Baltimore.

25. Biozzi, G., Stiffel, C., Mouton, D., Bouthillier, Y., and Decreusefond, C. 1974. La régulation génétique de la synthèse des immunoglobulines au cours de la réponse immunologique. *Ann. Immunol. (Inst. Pasteur)* 125C: 107–142.

26. Blank, R. J., Freedman, H. A., and Lilly, F. 1976. T-lymphocyte response to Friend virus-induced tumour cell lines in mice of strains congenic at H-2. *Nature* 260: 250–252.

27. Blomberg, B., Geckeler, W. R., and Weigert, M. 1972. Genetics of the antibody response to dextran in mice. *Science* 177: 178–180.

28. Bodmer, W. F. 1973. A new genetic model for allelism at histocompatibility and other complex loci: Polymorphism for control of gene expression. *Transpl. Proc.* 5: 1471–1475.

29. Bowen, J. G., Robins, R. A., and Baldwin, R. W. 1975. Serum factors modifying cell mediated immunity to rat hepatoma D23 correlated with tumor growth. *Int. J. Cancer* 15: 640–650.

30. Boyse, E. A., and Old, L. J. 1969. Some aspects of normal and abnormal cell surface genetics. *Ann. Rev. Genet.* 3: 269–290.

31. Boyse, E. A., Stockert, E., and Old, L. J. 1968. Isoantigens of the H-2 and Tla loci of the mouse. Interactions affecting their representation on thymocytes. *J. Exp. Med.* 128: 85–95.

32. Brannen, G. E., Adams, J. S., and Santos, G. W. 1974. Tumor-specific immunity in 3-methylcholanthren-induced murine fibrosarcomas. I. *In vivo* demonstration of immunity with three preparations of soluble antigens. *J. Natl. Cancer Inst.* 53: 165–175.

33. Capra, J. D., and Kindt, T. J. 1975. Antibody diversity: Can more than one gene encode each variable region? *Immunogenetics* 1: 417–427.

34. Cerilli, G. J., and Treat, R. C. 1969. The effect of antilymphocyte serum on the induction and growth of tumor in the adult mouse. *Transplantation* 8: 774–782.

35. Chang, S., Nowinski, R. C., Nishioka, K., and Irie, R. F. 1972. Immunological studies on mouse mammary tumors. VI. Further characterization of a mouse mammary antigen and its distribution in lymphatic cells of allogeneic mice. *Int. J. Cancer* 9: 409–416.

36. Chesebro, B., and Wehrly, 1976. Studies on the role of the host immune response in recovery from Friend virus leukemia. II. Cell-mediated immunity. *J. Exp. Med.* 143: 85–99.

37. Cikes, M., Friberg, S., Jr., and Klein, G. 1973. Progressive loss of H-2 antigens with concomitant increase of cell-surface antigen(s) determined by Moloney leukemia virus in cultured murine lymphomas. *J. Natl. Cancer Inst.* 50: 347–362.

38. Cohn, M. 1971. The take-home lesson-1971. *Ann. N.Y. Acad. Sci.* 190: 529–584.

39. Davies, S., Shearer, G. M., Mozes, E., and Sela, M. 1975. Genetic control of the murine cell-mediated immune response *in vivo*. II. H-2 linked responsiveness to the synthetic polypeptide poly (tyr, glu)-poly (DL-ala)--poly(lys). *J. Immunol.* 115: 1530–1532.

40. De Sousa, M. A. B., Parrott, D. M. V., and Pantelouris, E. M. 1969. The lymphoid tissues in mice with congenital aplasia of the thymus. *Clin. Exp. Immunol.* 4: 637–644.

41. Doherty, P. C., and Zinkernagel, R. M. 1975. A biological role for the major histocompatibility antigens. *Lancet* i: 1406–1409.

42. Doll, R., Payne, P., and Waterhouse, J. 1966. *Cancer Incidence on Five Continents. A Technical Report (UICC)*. Springer-Verlag, New York.

43. East, J., and Harvey, J. J. 1968. The differential action of neonatal thymectomy in mice infected with murine sarcoma virus-Harvey (MSV-H). *Int. J. Cancer* 3: 614–627.

44. Eckner, R. J. 1973. Helper-dependent properties of Friend spleen locus forming virus: Effect of the Fv-1 gene on the late stages in virus synthesis. *J. Virol.* 12: 523–533.

45. Eichmann, K., and Kindt, T. J. 1971. The inheritance of individual antigenic specificities of rabbit antibodies to streptococcal carbohybrates. *J. Exp. Med.* 134: 532–552.

46. Eichmann, K., Tung, A. S., and Nisonoff, A. 1974. Linkage and rearrangement of genes encoding mouse immunoglobulin heavy chains. *Nature* 250: 509–511.

47. Fefer, A. 1969. Immunotherapy and chemotherapy of Moloney sarcoma virus-induced tumors in mice. *Cancer Res.* 29: 2177–2183.

48. Fischinger, P. J., Ihle, J. N., Bolognesi, D. P., and Schafer, W. 1976. Inactivation of murine xenotropic oncornavirus by normal mouse sera is not immunoglobulin-mediated. *Virology* 71: 346–351.

49. Fisher, J. C., Davis, R. C., and Mannick, J. A. 1970. The effects of immunosuppression on the induction and immunogenicity of chemically induced sarcomas. *Surgery* 68: 150–157.

50. Foley, E. J. 1953. Antigenic properties of methylcholanthrene-induced tumors in mice of the strain of origin. *Cancer Res.* 13: 835–837.

51. Freedman, H. A., and Lilly, F. 1975. Properties of cell lines derived from tumors induced by Friend virus in BALB/c and BALB/c -H-2ʙ mice. *J. Exp. Med.* 142: 212–223.

52. Freedman, H. A., Lilly, F., and Steeves, R. A. 1975. Antigenic properties of cultured tumor cell lines derived from spleens of Friend virus-infected BALB/c and BALB/c—H-2ᵇ mice. *J. Exp. Med.* 142: 1365–1376.

53. Friend, C. 1957. Cell-free transmission in adult Swiss mice of a disease having the character of a leukemia. *J. Exp. Med.* 105: 307–318.

54. Gardner, I. D., Bowern, N. A., and Blanden, R. V. 1975. Cell-mediated cytotoxicity against ectromelia virus-infected target cells. III. Role of the H-2 gene complex. *Eur. J. Immunol.* 5: 122–127.

55. Gatti, R. A., and Good, R. A. 1971. Occurrence of malignancy in immunodeficiency diseases. A literature review. *Cancer* 28: 89–98.

56. Germain, R. N., Dorf, M. E., and Benacerraf, B. 1976. Inhibition of T-cell-mediated tumor-specific lysis by alloantisera directed against the H-2 serological specificities of the tumor. *J. Exp. Med.* 142: 1023–1028.

57. Gershon, R. K., Maurer, P. II., and Merryman, C. F. 1973. A cellular basis for genetically controlled unresponsiveness in mice: Tolerance induction in T-cells. *Proc. Natl. Acad. Sci.* 70: 250–254.

58. Glaser, M., Herberman, R. B., Kirchner, H., and Djeu, J. Y. 1974. Study of the cellular immune response to Gross virus-induced lymphoma by the mixed lymphocyte-tumor interaction. *Cancer Res.* 34: 2165–2171.

59. Gomard, E., Duprez, V., Henin, Y., and Levy, J. P. 1976. H-2 region product as determinant in immune cytolysis of syngeneic tumor cells by anti-MSV T lymphocytes. *Nature* 260: 707–709.

60. Graffi, A. 1957. Chloroleukemia of mice. *Ann. N.Y. Acad. Sci.* 68: 540–558.

61. Greenberger, J. S., Stephenson, J. R., Moloney, W. C., and Aaronson, S. A. 1975. Different hematological diseases induced by type C viruses chemically actuated from embryo cells of different mouse strains. *Cancer Res.* 35: 245–252.

62. Gross, L. 1951. "Spontaneous" leukemia developing in C3H mice following inoculation, in infancy, with AK-leukemic extracts or AK-embryos. *Proc. Soc. Exp. Biol. Med.* 76: 27–32.

63. Hakala, T. R., Lange, P. H., Castro, A. E., Elliott, A. Y., and Fraley, E. E. 1974. Antibody induction of lymphocyte-mediated cytotoxicity against human transitional-cell carcinomas of the urinary tract. *New Engl. J. Med.* 291: 637–641.

64. Hanna, M. G., Tennant, R. W., Yuhas, J. M., Clapp, N. K., Batzing, B. L., and Snodgrass, M. J. 1972. Autogenous immunity to endogenous RNA tumor virus antigens in mice with a low natural incidence of lymphoma. *Cancer Res.* 32: 2226–2234.

65. Hartley, J. W., Rowe, J. W., Capps, W. I., and Heubner, R. J. 1969. Isolation of naturally occuring viruses of the murine leukemia virus group in tissue culture. *J. Virol.* 3: 126–132.

66. Haughton, G. 1965. Moloney virus-induced leukemias of mice: Measurement in vitro of specific antigen. *Science* 147: 506–507.

67. Haughton, G., Avis, F., and Mosonov, I. 1974. The immune response to lung cancer: Potential importance for diagnosis, prognosis and therapy, *in:* G. F. Murray (ed.), *Cancer of the Lung,* pp. 27–37. Stratton, New York.

68. Haughton, G., and Nash, D. R. 1969. Transplantation antigens and viral carcinogenesis. *Progr. Med. Virol.* 11: 248–306.

69. Haywood, G. R., and McKhann, C. F. 1971. Antigenic specificities on murine sarcoma cells. Reciprocal relationship between normal transplantation antigens (H-2) and tumor-specific immunogenicity. *J. Exp. Med.* 133: 1171–1187.

70. Hellström, I. 1965. Distinction between the effects of antiviral and anticellular polyoma antibodies on polyoma tumor cells. *Nature* 208: 652–653.

71. Hellström, I., Evans, C. A., and Hellström, K. E. 1969. Cellular immunity and its serum-mediated inhibition in Shope-virus-induced rabbit papillomas. *Int. J. Cancer* 4: 601–607.

72. Hellström, I., and Hellström, K. E. 1969. Studies on cellular immunity and its serum-mediated inhibition in Moloney-virus-induced mouse sarcomas. *Int. J. Cancer* 4: 587–600.

73. Hellström, I., and Hellström, K. E. 1970. Colony-inhibition studies on blocking and non-blocking serum effects on cellular immunity to Moloney sarcomas. *Int. J. Cancer* 5: 195–201.

74. Hellström, I., and Hellström, K. E. 1972. Newer concepts of cancer of the colon and rectum: Cellular immunity to human colonic carcinomas. *Dis. Col. Rect.* 15: 100–105.

75. Hellström, I., and Hellström, K. E. 1972. Murine bladder tumors as models for human immunity. *Natl. Cancer Inst. Monogr.* 35: 125–127.

76. Hellström, I., and Hellström, K. E. 1973. Some recent studies on cellular immunity to human melanomas. *Fed. Proc.* 32: 156–159.

77. Hellström, I., Hellström, K. E., Bill, A. H., Pierce, G. E., and Yang, J. P. S. 1970. Studies on cellular immunity to human neuroblastoma cells. *Int. J. Cancer* 6: 172–188.

78. Hellström, I., Hellström, K. E., and Pierce, G. E. 1968. *In vitro* studies of immune reactions against autochthonous and syngeneic mouse tumors induced by methylcholanthrene and plastic discs. *Int. J. Cancer.* 3: 467–482.

79. Hellström, I. E., Hellström, K. E., Pierce, G. E., and Bill, A. H. 1968. Demonstration of cell-bound and humoral immunity against neuroblastoma cells. *Proc. Natl. Acad. Sci.* 60: 1231–1238.

80. Hellström, I., Hellström, K. E., and Sjögren, H. O. 1970. Serum mediated inhibition of cellular immunity to methylcholanthrene-induced murine sarcomas. *Cell. Immunol.* 1: 18–30.

81. Hellström, I., Hellström, K. E., and Sjögren, H. O. 1971. Some recent information on "blocking antibodies" as studied in vitro. *Transplant. Proc.* 3: 1221–1227.

82. Hellström, I., Hellström, K. E., Sjögren, H. O., and Warner, G. A. 1971. Demonstration of cell-mediated immunity to human neoplasms of various histological types. *Int. J. Cancer* 7: 1–16.

83. Hellström, I., Hellström, K. E., Sjögren, H. O., and Warner, G. A. 1971. Serum factors in tumor-free patients cancelling the blocking of cell-mediated tumor immunity. *Int. J. Cancer* 8: 185–191.

84. Hellström, I., Pierce, G. E., and Hellström, K. E. 1969. Human tumor-specific antigens. *Surgery* 65: 984–989.

85. Hellström, I., Sjögren, H. O., Warner, G., and Hellström, K. E. 1971. Blocking of cell-mediated tumor immunity by sera from patients with growing neoplasms. *Int. J. Cancer* 7: 226–237.

86. Hellström, I., Warner, G. A., Hellström, K. E., and Sjögren, H. O. 1973. Sequential studies on cell-mediated tumor immunity and blocking serum activity in ten patients with malignant melanoma. *Int. J. Cancer* 11: 280–292.

87. Heppner, G. H., and Pierce, G. 1969. *In vitro* demonstration of tumor-

specific antigens in spontaneous mammary tumors of mice. *Int. J. Cancer* 4: 212–218.

88. Herberman, R. B., Nunn, M. E., Holden, H. T., and Lavrin, D. H. 1975. Natural cytotoxic reactivity of mouse lymphoid cells against syngeneic and allogeneic tumors. II. Characterization of effector cells. *Int. J. Cancer* 16: 230–239.

89. Herberman, R. B., Nunn, M. E., and Lavrin, D. H. 1975. Natural cytotoxic reactivity of mouse lymphoid cells against syngeneic and allogeneic tumors. I. Distribution of reactivity and specificity. *Int. J. Cancer* 16: 216–229.

90. Hirsch, M. S., and Murphy, F. A. 1968. Effects of anti-thymocyte corum on Rauscher virus infection of mice. *Nature* 218: 478–479.

91. Howard, J. G., Christie, G. H., Courtenay, B. M., and Biozzi, G. 1972. Studies on immunological paralysis. VIII. Pneumococcal polysaccharide tolerance and immunity differences between the Biozzi high and low responder lines of mice. *Eur. J. Immunol.* 2: 269–273.

92. Huang, A. S., Besmer, P., Chu, L., and Baltimore, D. 1973. Growth of pseudotypes of vesicular stomatitis virus with N-tropic murine leukemia virus coats in cells resistant to N-tropic viruses. *J. Virol.* 12: 659–662.

93. Huebner, R. J. 1967. The murine leukemia sarcoma virus complex. *Proc. Natl. Acad. Sci.* 58: 835–842.

94. Huebner, R. J., and Todaro, G. J. 1969. Oncogenes of RNA tumor viruses as determinants of cancer. *Proc. Natl. Acad. Sci.* 64: 1087–1094.

95. Ihle, J. N., Hanna, M. G., Roberson, L. E., and Kenney, F. T. 1974. Autogenous immunity to endogenous RNA tumor virus: Identification of antibody to select viral antigens. *J. Exp. Med.* 139: 1568–1581.

96. Ihle, J. N., Hanna, M. G., Schafer, W., Hunsmann, G., Bolognesi, D. P., and Huper, G. 1975. Polypeptides of mammalian oncornaviruses. III. Localization of p15 and reactivity with natural antibodies. *Virology* 63: 60–67.

97. Ihle, J. N., Yuronic, M., and Hanna, M. G. 1973. Autogenous immunity to endogenous RNA tumor virus. Radioimmune precipitation assay of mouse serum antibody levels. *J. Exp. Med.* 138: 194–208.

98. Imanishi, T., and Mäkelä, O. 1974. Inheritance of antibody specificity. I. Anti-(4-hydroxy-3-nitrophenyl) acetyl of the mouse primary response. *J. Exp. Med.* 140: 1498–1510.

99. Invernizzi, G., and Parmiani, G. 1975. Tumour-associated transplantation antigens of chemically induced sarcomata cross reacting with allogeneic histocompatibility antigens. *Nature* 254: 713–714.

100. Kersey, J. H., Spector, B. D., and Good, R. A. 1975. Primary immunodeficiency and malignancy, in D. Bergsma (ed.), *Immunodeficiency in Man and Animals, Birth Defects: Original Articles Series, Vol. XI*, p. 289–296. Sinauer, Sunderland, Mass.

101. Kiessling, R., Klein, E., Pross, H., and Wigzell, H. 1975. "Natural" killer cells in the mouse, II. Cytotoxic cells with specificity for mouse Moloney leukemia cells. Characteristics of the killer cell. *Eur. J. Immunol.* 5: 117–121.

102. Kiessling, R., Klein, E., and Wigzell, H. 1975. "Natural" killer cells in the mouse. I. Cytotoxic cells with specificity for mouse Moloney leukemia cells. Specificity and distribution according to genotype. *Eur. J. Immunol.* 5: 112–117.

103. Kiessling, R., Petranyi, G., Klein, G., and Wigzell, H. 1975. Genetic variation of in vitro cytolytic activity and in vivo rejection potential of non-immunized semi-syngeneic mice against a mouse lymphoma line. *Int. J. Cancer* 15: 933–940.

104. Kindred, B. 1971. Immunological unresponsiveness of genetically thymus-less (nude) mice. *Eur. J. Immunol.* 1: 59–61.

105. Klein, J. 1974. Genetic polymorphism of the *histocompatibility - 2* loci of the mouse. *Ann. Rev. Genetics* 8: 63–77.

106. Klein, G., Sjögren, H. O., Klein, E., and Hellström, K. E. 1960. Demonstration of resistance against methylcholanthrene-induced sarcomas in the primary autochthonous host. *Cancer Res.* 20: 1561–1572.

107. Koszinowski, U., and Thomssen, R. 1975. Target cell-dependent T cell-mediated lysis of vaccinia virus-infected cells. *Eur. J. Immunol.* 5: 245–251.

108. Krontiris, T. G., Soeiro, R., and Fields, B. N. 1973. Host restriction of Friend leukemia virus. Role of the viral outer coat. *Proc. Natl. Acad. Sci.* 71: 2549–2553.

109. Krueger, G. R. F. 1972. Chronic immunosuppression and lymphomagenesis in man and mice. *Natl. Cancer Inst. Monogr.* 35: 183–190.

110. Law, L. W. 1966. Studies of thymic function with emphasis on the role of the thymus in oncogenesis. *Cancer Res.* 26: 551–574.

111. Law, L. W. 1969. Studies of the significance of tumor antigens in induction and regression of neoplastic diseases: Presidential address. *Cancer Res.* 29: 1–21.

112. Law, L. W. 1970. Effects of antilymphocyte serum on the induction of neoplasms of lymphoreticular tissues. *Fed. Proc.* 29: 171–174.

113. Law, L. W., Ting, R. C., and Allison, A. C. 1968. Effects on antilymphocyte serum on induction of tumors and leukemia by murine sarcoma virus. *Nature* 220: 611–612.

114. Law, L. W., Ting, R. C., and Stanton, M. F. 1968. Some biologic, immunogenic, and morphologic effects in mice after infection with a murine sarcoma virus. I. Biologic and immunogenic studies. *J. Natl. Cancer Inst.* 40: 1101–1112.

115. Lee, J. C., Hanna, M. G., Ihle, J. N., and Aaronson, S. A. 1974. Autogenous immunity to endogenous RNA tumor virus: Differential reactivities of IgM and IgG to virus envelope antigens. *J. Virol.* 14: 773–781.

116. Levy, J. A., Ihle, J. N., Oleszko, O., and Barnes, R. D. 1975. Virus-specific neutralization by a soluble non-immunoglobulin factor found naturally in normal mouse serum. *Proc. Natl. Acad. Sci.* 72: 5071–5075.

117. Lieberman, M., and Kaplan, H. S. 1959. Leukemogenic activity of filtrates from radiation-induced lymphoid tumors of mice. *Science* 130: 387–388.

118. Lilly, F. 1966. The inheritance of susceptibility to the Gross leukemia virus in mice. *Genetics* 53: 529–539.

119. Lilly, F., Duran-Reynals, M. L., and Rowe, W. P. 1975. Correlation of early murine leukemia virus titer and H-2 type with spontaneous leukemia in mice of the BALB/c × AKR cross: A genetic analysis. *J. Exp. Med.* 141: 882–889.

120. Lowy, D. R., Rowe, W. P., Teich, N., and Hartley, J. W. 1971. Mouse leukemia virus: High-frequency activation in vitro by 5-iododeoxyuridine and 5-bromodeoxyuridine. *Science* 174: 155–156.

121. Martin, W. J., Esber, E., Cotton, W. G., and Rice, J. M. 1973. Derepression of alloantigens in malignancy. Evidence for tumour susceptibility alloantigens and for possible self-reactivity of lymphoid cells active in the microcytotoxicity assay. Brit. J. Cancer 28: Suppl. I, 48–61.

122. Martin, W. J., Esber, E., Cotton, W. G., and Rice, J. M. 1975. Normal tissue alloantigens and genetic control of susceptibility to tumors: Microcytotoxicity studies on resistant C3Hf and susceptible (A × C3Hf) F1 mice inoculated with transplacentally induced C3Hf lung tumor. J. Immunol. 115: 289–295.

123. Martinez, C. 1964. Effect of early thymectomy on development of mammary tumours in mice. Nature 203: 1188.

124. McArthur, W. P., Carswell, E. A., and Thorbecke, G. J. 1972. Growth of Rous sarcoma in bursectomized chickens. J. Natl. Cancer Inst. 49: 907–909.

125. McCoy, J. L., Fefer, A., and Glynn, J. P. 1967. Comparative studies on the induction of transplantation resistance in BALB/c and C57BL/6 mice in three murine leukemia systems. Cancer Res. 27: 1743–1748.

126. Mohanakumar, T., Metzgar, R. S., and Miller, D. S. 1974. Human leukemia cell antigens: Serologic characterization with xenoantisera. J. Natl. Cancer Inst. 52: 1435–1444.

127. Morton, D. L., Miller, G. F., and Wood, D. A. 1969. Demonstration of tumor-specific immunity against antigens unrelated to mammary tumor virus in spontaneous mammary carcinomas. J. Natl. Cancer Inst. 42: 289–301.

128. Mühlbock, O., and Dux, A. 1974. Histocompatibility genes (the H-2 complex) and susceptibility to mammary tumor virus in mice. J. Natl. Cancer Inst. 53: 993–996.

129. Nelson, K., Pollack, S. B., and Hellström, K. E. 1975. In vitro synthesis of tumor-specific factors with blocking and antibody-dependent cellular cytotoxicity (ADC) activities. Int. J. Cancer 16: 932–941.

130. Nowinski, R. C., and Kaehler, S. L. 1974. Antibody to leukemia virus: Widespread occurance in inbred mice. Science 185: 869–871.

131. Old, L. J., Boyse, E. A., and Lilly, F. 1963. Formation of cytotoxic antibody against leukemias induced by Friend virus. Cancer Res. 23: 1063–1068.

132. Old, L. J., Boyse, E. A., and Stockert, E. 1963. Antigenic properties of experimental leukemias. I. Serological studies in vitro with spontaneous and radiation-induced leukemias. J. Natl. Cancer Inst. 37: 977–986.

133. Old, L. J., Boyse, E. A., and Stockert, E. 1964. Typing of mouse leukaemias by serological methods. Nature 201: 777–779.

134. Old, L. J., Boyse, E. A., and Stockert, E. 1965. The G (Gross) leukemia antigen. Cancer Res. 25: 813–819.

135. Outzen, H. C., Custer, R. P., Eaton, G. J., and Prehn, R. T. 1975. Spontaneous and induced tumor incidence in germfree "nude" mice. J. Reticuloendothel. Soc. 17: 1–9.

136. Pantelouris, E. M. 1968. Absence of a thymus in a mouse mutant. Nature 217: 370–371.

137. Parmiani, G., and Invernizzi, G. 1975. Alien histocompatibility determinants on the cell surface of sarcomas induced by methylcholanthrene. I. In vivo studies. Int. J. Cancer 16: 756–767.

138. Pawlak, L. L., Mushinski, E. B., Nisonoff, A., and Potter, M. 1973. Evi-

dence for the linkage of the IgCH locus to a gene controlling the idiotypic specificity of anti-p-azophenyl-arsonate antibodies in strain A mice. *J. Exp. Med.* 137: 22–31.

139. Payne, L. N., and Rennie, M. 1970. Lack of effect of bursectomy on Marek's disease. *J. Natl. Cancer Inst.* 45: 387–397.

140. Penn, I., and Starzl, T. E. 1972. Malignant tumors arising de novo in immunosuppressed organ transplant recipients. *Transplantation* 14: 407–417.

141. Penn, I., and Starzl, T. E. 1973. Immunosuppression and cancer. *Transplant. Proc.* 5: 943–947.

142. Pennycuik, P. R. 1971. Unresponsiveness of nude mice to skin allografts. *Transplantation* 11: 417–418.

143. Petranyi, G. G., Kiessling, R., and Klein, G. 1975. Genetic control of "natural" killer lymphocytes in the mouse. *Immunogenetics.* 2: 53–61.

144. Petranyi, G. G., Kiessling, R., Povey, S., Klein, G., Herzenberg, L., and Wigzell, H. 1976. The genetic control of natural killer cell activity and its association with in vivo resistance against a Moloney lymphoma isograft. *Immunogenetics* 3: 15–28.

145. Pincus, T., Hartley, J. W., and Rowe, W. P. 1971. A major genetic locus affecting resistance to infection with murine leukemia viruses. I. Tissue culture studies of naturally occuring viruses. *J. Exp. Med.* 133: 1219–1233.

146. Pincus, T., Rowe, W. P., and Lilly, F. 1971. A major genetic locus affecting resistance to infection with murine leukemia viruses. II. Apparent identity to a major locus described for resistance to Friend leukemia virus. *J. Exp. Med.* 133: 1234–1241.

147. Pitelka, D. R., Bern, H. A., Nandi, S., and DeOme, K. B. 1964. On the significance of virus-like particles in mammary tissues of C3Hf mice. *J. Natl. Cancer Inst.* 33: 867–884.

148. Povlsen, C. O., and Rygaard, J. 1971. Heterotransplantation of human adenocarcinomas of the colon and rectum to the mouse mutant nude. A study of nine consecutive transplantations. *Acta Path. Microbiol. Scand., A* 79: 159–169.

149. Prehn, R. T. 1969. Influence of X-irradiation and the milk agent on growth of transplanted mouse mammary tumors. *J. Natl. Cancer Inst.* 43: 1215–1220.

150. Prehn, R. T. 1971. Perspectives on oncogenesis: Does immunity stimulate or inhibit neoplasia? *J. Reticuloendothelial. Soc.* 10: 1–16.

151. Prehn, R. T. 1971. Immunosurveillance, regeneration and oncogenesis. *Progr. Exp. Tumor Res.* 14: 1–24.

152. Prehn, R. T. 1976. Do tumors grow because of the immune response of the host? *Transplant. Rev.* 28: 34–42.

153. Prehn, R. T., and Main, J. M. 1957. Immunity to methylcholanthrene-induced sarcomas. *J. Natl. Cancer Inst.* 18: 769–778.

154. Pritchard, H., Riddaway, J., and Micklem, H. S. 1973. Immune responses in congenitally thymusless mice. II. Quantitative studies of serum immunoglobulins, the antibody response to sheep erythrocytes, and the effect of thymus allografting. *Clin. Exp. Immunol.* 13: 125–138.

155. Rabbat. A. G., and Jeejeebhoy, H. F. 1970. Heterologous antilymphocyte serum (ALS) hastens the appearance of methylcholanthrene-induced tumors in

mice. *Transplantation* 9: 164–166.

156. Radzichovskaja, R. 1967. Effect of bursectomy on the Rous virus tumor induction in chickens. *Nature* 213: 1259–1260.

157. Radzichovskaja, R. 1967. Effect of thymectomy on Rous virus tumor growth induced in chickens. *Proc. Soc. Exp. Biol. Med.* 126: 13–15.

158. Raft. M. C., and Wortis, H. H. 1970. Thymus dependence of θ-bearing cells in the peripheral lymphoid tissues of mice. *Immunology* 18: 931–942.

159. Rauscher, F. J. 1962. A virus-induced disease of mice characterized by erythrocytopoiesis and lymphoid leukemia. *J. Natl. Cancer Inst.* 29: 515–543.

160. Reiner, J., and Southam, C. M. 1969. Further evidence of common antigen properties in chemically induced sarcomas of mice. *Cancer Res.* 29: 1814–1820.

161. Riblet, R., Weigert, M., and Makela, O. 1975. Genetics of mouse antibodies. II. Recombination between V_H genes and allotype. *Eur. J. Immunol.* 5: 778–781.

162. Rowe, W. P. 1972. Studies of genetic transmission of murine leukemia viruses by AKR mice. I. Crosses $Fv\text{-}1^n$ strains of mice. *J. Exp. Med.* 136: 1272–1285.

163. Rowe, W. P., and Hartley, J. W. 1972. Studies of genetic transmission of murine leukemia viruses by AKR mice. II. Crosses with $Fv\text{-}1^b$ strains of mice. *J. Exp. Med.* 136: 1286–1301.

164. Rowe, W. P., Hartley, J. W., Lander, M. R., Pugh, W. E., and Teich, N. 1971. Noninfectious AKR mouse embryo cell lines in which each cell has the capacity to be activated to produce infectious murine leukemia virus. *Virology* 46: 866–876.

165. Rygaard, J., and Povlsen, C. O. 1974. The mouse mutant *nude* does not develop spontaneous tumors. An argument against immunological surveillance. *Acta Path. Microbiol. Scand.*, B 82: 99–106.

166. Sato, H., Boyse, E. A., Aoki, T., Iritani, C., and Old, L. J. 1973. Leukemia-associated transplantation antigens related to murine leukemia virus. The X.1 system: Immune response controlled by a locus linked to H-2. *J. Exp. Med.* 138: 593–606.

167. Schachat, D. A., Fefer, A., and Moloney, J. B. 1968. Effect of cortisone on oncogenesis by murine sarcoma virus (Moloney). *Cancer Res.* 28: 517–520.

168. Schoolman, H. M., Spurrier, W., Schwartz, S. O., and Szanto, P. B. 1957. Studies in leukemia. VII. The induction of leukemia in Swiss mice by means of cell-free filtrates of leukemic mouse brain. *Blood* 12: 694–700.

169. Schrader, J. W., Cunningham, B. A., and Edelman, G. M. 1975. Functional interactions of viral and histocompatibility antigens at tumor cell surfaces. *Proc. Natl. Acad. Sci. USA* 72: 5065–5070.

170. Schrader, J. W., and Edelman, G. M. 1976. Participation of the H-2 antigens of tumor cells in their lysis by syngeneic T cells. *J. Exp. Med.* 143: 601–614.

171. Schwartz, R. S. 1972. Immunoregulation, oncogenic viruses, and malignant lymphomas. *Lancet* i: 1266–1269.

172. Schwartz, R. S. 1974. Immunosuppression and neoplasia, in: L. Brent and J. Holborow (eds.), *Progress in Immunology II*, Vol. 5, pp. 229–232. North-Holland, Amsterdam.

173. Sendo, F., Aoki, T., Boyse, E. A., and Buato, C. K. 1975. Natural occur-

ence of lymphocytes showing cytotoxic activity to BALB/c radiation-induced leukemia RL♂1 cells. *J. Natl. Cancer Inst.* 55: 603–609.

174. Sharma, J. M., Witter, R. L., and Purchase, H. G. 1975. Absence of age-resistance in neonatally thymectomised chickens as evidence for cell-mediated immune surveillance in Marek's disease. *Nature* 253: 477–479.

175. Shearer, G. M., Rehn, T. G., and Garbarino, C. A. 1975. Cell-mediated lympholysis of trinitrophenyl-modified autologous lymphocytes. Effector cell specificity to modified cell surface components controlled by the H-2K and H-2D serological regions of the murine major histocompatibility complex. *J. Exp. Med.* 141: 1348–1364.

176. Sher, A., and Cohn, M. 1972. Inheritance of an idiotype associated with the immune response of inbred mice to phosphorylcholine. *Eur. J. Immunol.* 2: 319–326.

177. Simpson, E., and Nehlsen, S. L. 1971. Prolonged administration of anti-thymocyte serum in mice. II. Histopathological investigation. *Clin. Exp. Immunol.* 9: 79–98.

178. Sjögren, H. O. 1965. Transplantation methods as a tool for detection of tumor-specific antigens. *Progr. Exp. Tumor Res.* 6: 289–322.

179. Sjögren, H. O., and Borum, K. 1971. Tumor-specific immunity in the course of primary polyoma and Rous tumor development in intact and immuno-suppressed rats. *Cancer Res.* 31: 890–900.

180. Sjögren, H. O., Hellström, I., Bansal, S. C., and Hellström, K. E. 1971. Suggestive evidences that "blocking antibodies" of tumor-bearing individuals may be antigen-antibody complexes. *Proc. Natl. Acad. Sci.* 68: 1372–1375.

181. Sjögren, H. O., Hellström, I., Bansal, S. C., Warner, G. A., and Hellström, K. E. 1972. Elution of "blocking factors" from human tumors, capable of abrogating tumor-cell destruction by specifically immune lymphocytes. *Int. J. Cancer* 9: 274–283.

182. Sjögren, H. O., Hellström, I., and Klein, G. 1961. Resistance of polyoma virus immunized mice to transplantation of established polyoma tumors. *Exp. Cell Res.* 23: 204–208.

183. Sobczak, E., and de Vaux Staint Cyr, C. 1971. Study of the *in vivo* fixation of antibodies on tumors provoked in hamsters by injection of SV40-transformed cells (TVS₅ C1₂). *Int. J. Cancer* 8: 47–52.

184. Steeves, R. A., Strand, M., and August, J. T. 1974. Structural proteins of mammalian oncogenic RNA viruses: Murine leukemia virus neutralization by antisera prepared against purified envelope glycoprotein. *J. Virology* 14: 187–189.

185. Stephenson, J. R., and Aaronson, S. A. 1972. Antigenic properties of murine sarcoma virus-transformed BALB/3T3 nonproducer cells. *J. Exp. Med.* 135: 503–513.

186. Stephenson, J. R., Greenberger, J. S., and Aaronson, S. A. 1974. Oncogenicity of an endogenous C type virus chemically activated from mouse cells in culture. *J. Virology* 13: 237–240.

187. Strand, M., Lilly, F., and August, J. T. 1974. Genetic control of the expression of murine leukemia virus proteins in tissues of normal young adult mice. *Cold Spring Harbor Symp. Quant. Biol.* 39: 1117–1122.

188. Stutman, O. 1974. Tumor development after 3-methylcholanthrene in immunologically deficient athymic-nude mice. *Science* 183: 534–536.

189. Stutman, O. 1975. Delayed tumor appearance and absence of regression in nude mice infected with murine sarcoma virus. *Nature* 253: 142–144.

190. Stutman, O., and Dupuy, J. M. 1972. Resistance to Friend leukemia virus in mice: Effect of immunosuppression. *J. Natl. Cancer Inst.* 49: 1283–1293.

191. Taranger, L. A., Hellström, I., Chapman, W. H., and Hellström, K. E. 1972. In vitro demonstration of common tumor antigens in mouse and rat bladder carcinomas. *Proc. Am. Assoc. Cancer Res.* 13: 56.

192. Ting, C. C., and Herberman, R. B. 1971. Inverse relationship of polyoma tumour specific cell surface antigen to H-2 histocompatibility antigens. *Nature New Biology* 232: 118–120.

193. Todaro, G. J., and Heubner, R. J. 1972. The viral oncogene hypothesis: New evidence. *Proc. Natl. Acad. Sci.* 69: 1009–1015.

194. Trinchieri, G., Aden, D. P., and Knowles, B. B. 1976. Cell-mediated cytotoxicity to SV40-specific tumor-associated antigens. *Nature* 261: 312–314.

195. Tsakraklides, E., Smith, C., Kersey, J. H., and Good, R. A. 1974. Transplantation antigens (H-2) on virally and chemically transformed BALB/3T3 fibroblasts in culture. *J. Natl. Cancer Inst.* 52: 1499–1504.

196. Vaage, J. 1968. Nonvirus-associated antigens in virus-induced mouse mammary tumors. *Cancer Res.* 28: 2477–2483.

197. Vandeputte, M. 1969. Antilymphocyte serum and polyoma oncogenesis in rats. *Transplant. Proc.* 1: 100–105.

198. Vandeputte, M., Denys, P., Leyten, R., and De Somer, P. 1963. The oncogenic activity of the polyoma virus in thymectomized rats. *Life Sci.* 2: 475–478.

199. Vandeputte, M., Eyssen, H., Sobis, H., and de Somer, P. 1974. Induction of polyoma tumors in athymic nude mice. *Int. J. Cancer* 14: 445–450.

200. von Boehmer, H., and Haas, W. 1976. Cytotoxic T lymphocytes recognize allogeneic tolerated TNP-conjugated cells. *Nature* 261: 141–142.

201. Vredevoe, D. L., and Hayes, E. F. 1969. Effect of antilymphocytic and antithymocytic sera on the development of mouse lymphoma. *Cancer Res.* 29: 1685–1690.

202. Wagner, J. L., and Haughton, G. 1971. Immunosuppression by antilymphocyte serum and its effect on tumors induced by 3-methylcholanthrene in mice. *J. Natl. Cancer Inst.* 46: 1–10.

203. Wainberg, M. A., Markson, Y., Weiss, D. W., and Doljanski, F. 1974. Cellular immunity against Rous sarcomas of chickens. Preferential reactivity against autochthonous target cells as determined by lymphocyte adherance and cytotoxicity tests in vitro. *Proc. Natl. Acad. Sci., U.S.A.* 71: 3565–3569.

204. Wiegert, M., Potter, M., and Sachs, D. 1975. Genetics of the immunoglobulin variable region. *Immunogenetics* 1: 511–523.

205. Wiener, E., and Bandieri, A. 1974. Differences in antigen handling by peritoneal macrophages from the Biozzi high and low responder lines of mice. *Eur. J. Immunol.* 4: 457–463.

206. Williams, R. M., Dorf, M. E., and Benacerraf, B. 1975. H-2-linked genetic control of resistance to histocompatible tumors. *Cancer Res.* 35: 1586–1590.

207. Wood, W. C., and Morton, D. L. 1970. Microcytotoxicity test: Detection in sarcoma patients of antibody cytotoxic to human sarcoma cells. *Science* 170: 1318–1320.

208. Wortis, H. H. 1971. Immunological responses of "nude" mice. *Clin. Exp. Immunol.* 8: 305–317.

209. Wortis, H. H., Nehlsen, S., and Owen, J. J. 1971. Abnormal development of the thymus in "nude" mice. *J. Exp. Med.* 134: 681–692.

210. Yunis, E. J., Martinez, C., Smith, J., Stutman, O., and Good, R. A. 1969. Spontaneous mammary adenocarcinoma in mice: Influence of thymectomy and reconstitution with thymus grafts or spleen cells. *Cancer Res.* 29: 174–178.

211. Zarling, J. M., Nowinski, R. C., and Bach, F. H. 1975. Lysis of leukemia cells by spleen cells of normal mice. *Proc. Natl. Acad. Sci. U.S.A.* 72: 2780–2784.

212. Zinkernagel, R. M. 1976. Virus-specific T-cell-mediated cytotoxicity across the H-2 barrier to virus-altered alloantigens. *Nature* 261: 139–141.

213. Zinkernagel, R. M., and Doherty, P. C. 1974. Restriction of *in vitro* T cell-mediated cytotoxicity in lymphocytic choriomeningitis within a syngeneic or semiallogeneic system. *Nature* 248: 701–702.

CHAPTER 5

EFFECTS OF THE LYMPHOID TISSUE MICRO-ENVIRONMENT ON IMMUNITY

T. L. Feldbush,
A. van der Hoven, and
D. Lafrenz

Departments of
Microbiology and Urology
College of Medicine
University of Iowa and
the Veterans Administration Hospital
Iowa City, Iowa 52240

The ordered migration of lymphocytes through the reticuloendothelial system contributes significantly to the microenvironment of the immune system. This chapter focuses on the controversies in this area, such as: (1) the recirculating characteristics of antigen-experienced and antigen-inexperienced lymphocytes, (2) the influence of antigen and adjuvant on the homing patterns of cells and how this relates to lymphocyte triggering, and (3) the stimulatory and inhibitory effects of growing tumors on lymphocyte trapping and how this may effect both prognosis and treatment.

I. INTRODUCTION

Not too long ago, lymphocytes were considered to be cells which occurred in patches throughout the body as well as in discrete nodes and in the blood, and were felt by many cytologists to have something to do with immune responses. Within the last two decades, the term lymphocyte has been shown to encompass a large heterologous population of nomadic cells which pass freely from the vasculature into the fixed recticulum and then back into the vasculature. Beginning with the classic experiments of Gowans (42, 43), we have come to realize that many lymphocytes are capable of leaving the lymph nodes by way of the efferent lymphatics, traveling to the blood and then passing back into the nodes through high-walled endothelial venules. As evidenced in a recent review by Ford (26), a large amount of experimental evidence now exists concerning the migratory patterns of T and B cells, their transit time through the spleen and lymph nodes and the role of lymphocyte recirculation in establishing the proper microenvironmental conditions which are so important to the integrity of the immune system.

The present review is not intended to be a comprehensive survey of this classic literature but will deal instead with some of the more recent controversies regarding lymphocyte recirculation, such as: (1) the recirculating characteristics of lymphocyte subpopulations, (2) the effect of antigen and adjuvant on the recirculating pattern of cells, and (3) the influence of a growing tumor on the specific and nonspecific trapping of lymphocytes in the draining lymphoid tissue.

II. METHODS USED FOR STUDYING RECIRCULATION

An important functional distinction should first be made between circulating and recirculating lymphocytes. The detection of a lymphocyte in the thoracic duct lymph (TDL) or the peripheral blood does not provide sufficient evidence to classify a cell as recirculating. Only if one can show that a cell is capable of repetitive passage from the blood to the lymph is it appropriate to conclude that the cell is capable of recirculation. For example, Strober (112) has shown that TDL can be used to reconstitute the primary immune response in irradiated rats to horse spleen ferritin (HSF), presumptive evidence for the recirculation of HSF virgin B cells. However, Strober (113) further showed that the HSF-specific virgin B cell could not be recovered from the TDL of an irradiated intermediate host cannulated 24 hours after the injection 5×10^8 thoracic duct cells from a normal donor. Thus, by definition, the HSF-specific virgin B cells are circulating but are not capable of recirculation.

All studies of lymphocyte migration utilize some means of marking the cells, one of the most common methods employing radioactive isotopes. Labeling lymphocytes in vitro or in vivo is relatively easy and the ability to detect these cells both macroscopically and microscopically in the lymphoid tissues has been reasonably well delineated. Problems associated with the labeled cells, however, must be kept in mind since these could influence the interpretation of results. For example, ^{51}Cr-sodium chromate does not label lymphocytes uniformly (67) and in some cases the ^{51}Cr label is not excreted from the body following death of the lymphocyte (105) but instead appears to be ingested by phagocytes. Labeling lymphocytes with ^{3}H-thymidine in vitro appears to mark only large cells (77) while labelling in vivo for various periods of time can preferentially label short or long-lived lymphocytes (19). Labelling in vitro with ^{3}H-uridine in the rat labels T lymphocytes 10 to 15 times more intensely than B lymphocytes (66). However, Gutman and Weissman (53) have not shown a differential uptake of uridine by mouse T and B cells.

Functional markers have also been used successfully to follow the migration of lymphocytes, but in these experiments the major aim is the differential migration of lymphocyte subpopulations rather than the whole lymphocyte population. For example, Strober and Dilley (118) and Strober (114) have examined the ability of virgin and memory B cells to recirculate and found that the memory cells are quite capable of recirculating from blood to lymph while the virgin cells are not. Sprent and Miller (108, 109) have studied T cells activated to H-2 determinants (T.TDL) and have shown that while the precursor cells are readily recirculating, only a very small proportion of the T.TDL will recirculate. Furthermore, some of the T.TDL may leave the circulation, undergo division and then rejoin the recirculating pool. Koster et al. (73, 74) and McGregor et al. (80) have reported that the lymphocytes which mediate immunity to L. monocytogenes do not recirculate but are capable of circulation since they can readily accumulate in the peritoneum.

III. ROUTE AND KINETICS OF RECIRCULATION

There is no question that both B and T lymphocytes recirculate (26), although, as discussed below, there is still a great deal of controversy regarding the recirculation of T and B lymphocyte subpopulations. Thymic derived lymphocytes comprise approximately 80–85 percent of the mouse TDL population (104), 65–80 percent of the rat TDL population (90), and 60–75 percent of the human peripheral blood lymphocyte pool (100). Most, if not all, of these cells are recirculating, migrating into the lymph nodes (26), spleen (26), bone marrow (68, 99, 94), tonsils (72), appendix (65), Peyer's patches (125), and probably the bronchial associated lymphoid tissue. An average of 15 hours is required for the unstimulated T cell to migrate through the lymph nodes (28, 45) and 5 hours for passage through the spleen (23).

B cell recirculation has been most successfully studied by using purified populations of cells. In rats, Howard (66) and Nieuwenhuis and Ford (86) prepared B cell enriched fractions by collecting TDL from rats which were thymectomized, lethally irradiated, and reconstituted with bone marrow obtained from donors chronically drained of thoracic duct cells to remove the T cells from the marrow. Nieuwenhuis and Ford (86) also used complement receptor-bearing TDL from normal animals while Sprent (104) employed nude mice. Upon intravenous injection into normal recipients, the B cells localized predominantly in the spleen and lymph nodes (104) with the remaining 10–20 percent recoverable from the thoracic duct for at least 48 hours after injection (66). These recirculating B cells are long lived, being labeled in vivo with ^{3}H-thymidine only after 7 days of continuous infusions, as opposed to the short-lived nonrecirculating B cells described by Strober (114, 115). Thus it seems quite likely that at least a given subpopulation of B cells is able to recirculate.

The kinetics of B cell recirculation is quite different from that of the T cell, with the B cells demonstrating a slower transit time. Following intravenous injection of labeled B cells, approximately 23–30 hours (24) or more (66) are needed for the cells to pass through the lymph nodes while, as stated above, T cells require 15 hours. Similarly, in the spleen the transit time of B cells may be at least four times as long as the 5–6-hour transit time of T cells (86). These observations appear to explain the finding that during chronic drainage of the thoracic duct the ratio of B to T cells in the lymph increases with time so that by 4 days 40–50 percent of the TDL are B cells (104).

In the lymph nodes (Fig. 1), labeled T and B cells enter from the blood within 10 minutes after intravenous injection by passing through the postcapillary venules (PCV) (28, 41, 52, 67, 86). The cells then disperse progressively throughout the deep cortex with subsequent partitioning of the T and B cells occurring after a few hours. The B cells seem to accumulate in the paracortical areas with a tendency to converge in the primary follicles and germinal centers (86). This pattern persists for up to 48 hours with the B cells eventually returning to the medulla and leaving via the efferent lymphatic ducts. The T cells, on the other hand, move directly

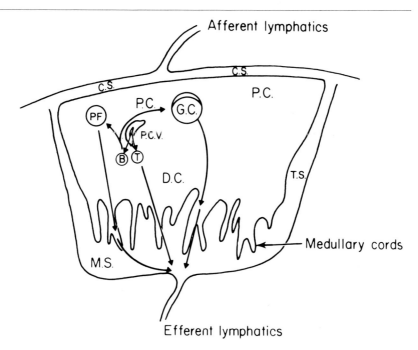

Fig. 1. *Recirculation through the lymph nodes.* The proposed routes followed by both B and T cells through the lymph node are shown by the arrows and discussed in the text. Abbreviations used: *T*, thymus-derived lymphocyte; *B*, thymus-independent lymphocyte; *PCV*, post-capillary venule; *GC*, germinal centre; *PF*, primary follicle; *PC*, paracortical area; *DC*, deep or diffuse cortex; *CS*, circular sinus; *MS*, medullary sinus; *TS*, trabecular sinus.

from the deep cortex to the medullary region and then out through the efferent lymphatics (26).

Rat lymphocytes enter the splenic white pulp, localizing initially in the marginal zone and later on in the outer region of the periarteriolar lymphoid sheath (PALS) (23, 24, 41, 47). The rate of lymphocyte flow into the white pulp appears to be related to their concentration in the blood (23, 24). As depicted in Figure 2, both the T cells and B cells cross the marginal zone (26, 52) with the T cells migrating through the outer zone of the PALS and then returning to the red pulp via marginal zone bridging channels (82). The B cells also migrate through the outer region of the PALS but never penetrate the central zone, localizing instead in the lymphocyte corona surrounding the germinal centers (86). This B cell concentration in the lymphocyte corona seems to reach a peak within 24 hours of their initial entrance into the spleen.

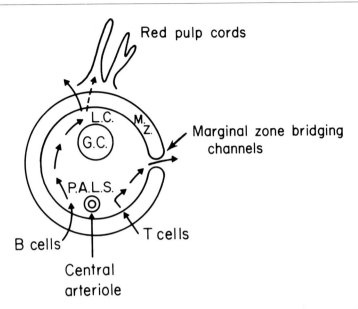

Fig. 2. *Recirculation through the spleen.* The proposed routes followed by both B and T cells through the spleen are shown by the arrows and discussed in the text. Abbreviations used: *T*, thymus-derived lymphocyte; *B*, thymus-independent lymphocyte; *MZ*, marginal zones; *PALS*, periarteriolar lymphoid sheath; *GC*, germinal centre; *LC*, lymphocyte corona surrounding the germinal center.

The factors which control the selective migration of T and B cells through the PCV and the different areas of the lymph node and spleen are not well understood. Some evidence has accumulated which points to a specific interaction between lymphocyte surface receptors and the PCV which allows the cells to attach and subsequently penetrate into the node (35, 38, 127–131). Alteration of lymphocyte homing by surface modifications using such agents as glycosidase (35), trypsin (127, 128), and neuraminidase (129) have all led to decreased numbers in both the spleen and lymph nodes, while treatment with concanavalin A (con-A) (38) and X-irradiation (11) led to decreased lymph node homing and increased spleen homing. All of these studies, however, suffer from the same criticism: that these manipulations may have caused gross alterations of the cell surface which had little to do with sites that regulate migration (26). Indeed every report shows increased homing to the liver, which is usually associated with cell death. Furthermore, the migration of different lymphocyte subpopulations may not be controlled by the same factor(s).

In a recent study, Freitas and deSousa (31) treated lymph node cells with concanavalin A and phytohemagglutinin and studied their migration to the spleen, lymph node, and liver in normal and splenectomized mice. In these animals they found a decreased localization in the lymph nodes and increased localization in the spleen by 24 hours post injection, but by 72 hours, the cells relocalized normally. Their apparent *in vivo* recovery and a lack of increased liver homing attested to the viability of the treated population. In splenectomized mice, no decrease in liver homing could be seen. This observation, together with their inability to produce a modified homing pattern with chymotrypsinized con-A (a modified form of con-A which still binds to sugar receptors but does not agglutinate cells), led the authors to speculate that cell surface carbohydrates were not responsible for the altered lymphocyte migration. Instead, this resulted from a biochemical alteration of the membrane which produced an enhanced retention of the cells in the natural body filters, such as the lungs and spleen.

In our laboratory we have also been able to produce altered lymphocyte homing without cell death and we have data to suggest that different factors may influence the homing patterns of different lymphocyte subpopulations (Crouse, Feldbush, and Evans, unpublished observation). In our initial experiments, rat lymph node cells were labeled *in vitro* with ^{51}Cr and then subjected to various levels of X-irradiation before intravenous injection into syngenic recipients. As shown in Table 1, irradia-

Table 1.   Organ distribution of Cr-labeled and X-irradiated LBN lymph node cells.[a]

Tissue Sampled	Exposure (R)			
	0	100	300	800
Spleen	14.6 ± 0.2[b]	20.8 ± 0.8	22.4 ± 0.8	24.4 ± 0.7
Lymph node	18.8 ± 1.2	16.1 ± 1.5	11.8 ± 0.4	11.0 ± 0.2
Liver	19.0 ± 0.5	20.7 ± 1.2	22.7 ± 0.3	22.5 ± 0.5
Lungs	2.3 ± 0.1	0.9 ± 0.1	0.7 ± 0.0	0.6 ± 0.1
Small intestine	2.7 ± 0.2	1.9 ± 0.2	2.0 ± 0.1	1.8 ± 0.1
Peripheral blood	2.1 ± 0.2	1.0 ± 0.1	0.8 ± 0.1	0.9 ± 0.0
Bone marrow	3.6 ± 0.2	5.5 ± 0.3	9.5 ± 0.1	9.3 ± 0.4

a. These results are expressed as the mean percentage of the injected activity recovered in the various organs and tissues at 22–24 hours post-irradiation and injection into syngeneic unirradiated LBN hosts.
b. ± Standard error of the mean.

tion resulted in a dose-dependent shift in lymphocyte homing increasing in the spleen and bone marrow and decreasing in the lymph nodes, lungs, small intestinal and peripheral blood. At the same time, only a slight increase in liver homing was observed, negating gross cell damage as an explanation for our results. These findings are similar to those seen in mice following in vitro treatment of lymphocytes with irradiation (11) or con-A (31). The effect of in vitro irradiation on a lymphocyte subpopulation was tested using the functional marker of the memory cells. Lymph node cell suspensions from dinitrophenylated bovine gamma globulin (DNP-BGG) immunized rats were prepared, irradiated with 200 R and injected intravenously into unirradiated intermediate hosts and irradiated syngeneic adoptive controls. The adoptive control animals were then

Table 2.   Secondary anti-DNP antibody response in LBN rats receiving serially transferred control or irradiated LN cells.

Group[a]	Days After Challenge		
	7	11	14
A Intermediate controls Control LN cells	2.635 ± 0.195[b]	3.289 ± 0.120	3.051 ± 0.104
B Intermediate controls 200 R LN cells	1.035 ± 0.201	2.990 ± 0.421	2.907 ± 0.384
C Final hosts Control LN cells	0.015 ± 0.003	0.053 ± 0.013	0.063 ± 0.018
D Final hosts Control Spl cells	0.012 ± 0.033	0.053 ± 0.011	0.062 ± 0.017
E Final hosts 200 R LN cells	0.006 ± 0.001	0.018 ± 0.003	0.017 ± 0.001
F Final hosts 200 R Spl cells	0.011 ± 0.003	0.027 ± 0.006	0.017 ± 0.005

a. Intermediate controls received normal or irradiated lymph node cells from immune donors and final hosts received lymph node cells or spleen cells from intermediate hosts after allowing 24 hours for cell homing.

b. Mean antigen-binding-capacity (ABC) ± 1 standard error of the mean.

challenged with DNP-BGG and the effect of the irradiation on the ability of the memory cells to differentiate into antibody forming cells was determined. The influence of the irradiation on the homing of the memory cells was studied by recovering both spleen cells and lymph node cells from the intermediate host and injecting them into irradiated adoptive recipients which were then challenged. The results of a typical experiment are shown in Table 2. Antibody responses were measured by the Farr technique (20) and are reported as the μg of DNP bound per milliliter of whole serum. By comparing groups A and B it is apparent that the irradiation of memory cells delays, but does not destroy their ability to respond. This would seem to confirm the lack of increased liver homing in Table 1. In groups C through F it is obvious that 200 R irradiation drastically reduces (73% reduction) the homing of memory cells to both the spleen and the lymph node. Thus, from these data, it would appear that irradiation affects memory cell homing differently than it affects the homing of ^{51}Cr-labeled cells. More experimentation is needed on the nature of lymphocyte surface receptors and their influence on lymphocyte recirculation, especially utilizing functional markers.

IV. RECIRCULATION OF ANTIGEN-REACTIVE T AND B CELLS

The number of B lymphocytes which can respond to a given antigen is small. Klinman (71) has estimated the clonal frequency in a nonimmune animal to fall within the range of 1 in 6×10^4 to 1 in 4×10^7 depending upon the antigen. Therefore, it is of great selective advantage to the host if it can create the proper microenvironment in which a large number of lymphocytes pass through an area of antigen concentration. Teleologically, lymphocyte recirculation could enhance this opportunity for interaction between antigen and specific lymphocytes. However, before one accepts lymphocyte recirculation as a panacea, it is necessary to examine the assumptions upon which this theory is based. Ford (26) has outlined three theorems: 1) the recirculating pool should contain lymphocytes which are reactive to a number of antigens; 2) the cells must circulate through regions in which antigen is localized and the antigens must remain immunogenic; and 3) a selective stimulation of sessile cells as opposed to recirculating cells should not occur. A fourth requirement should also be considered, that the recirculating population represents a cross section of the various lymphocyte subpopulations.

The presence of specific antigen-reactive lymphocytes in the circulating pool and their importance to the development of immune responses have been shown in a variety of ways. Taliaferro and Taliaferro (120) and

Hall and Morris (56) showed that local irradiation of a draining lymphoid organ before antigen injection had no effect upon the magnitude of the immune response even though the levels of irradiation were higher than that required to produce immunosuppression following whole-body exposure. These results would imply that the recirculating lymphocyte pool was adequate to restore the level of immunocompetent cells in these lymphoid structures such that normal (56) or even augmented responses could occur (120). Ford and Gowans (28) examined the phenomenon more closely by use of a technique for perfusing the surgically isolated rat spleen. The lymphocyte concentration of the blood perfusing the spleen was manipulated in order to determine the effect of lymphocyte migration on the immune response. Normal and lymphocyte-depleted spleens responded normally to the antigen sheep red blood cells (SRBC) when the concentration of lymphocytes in the perfusate was normal. However, when the perfusate was depleted of cells, both normal and depleted spleens were much less responsive to SRBC stimulation. The results suggest that the magnitude of the immune response is dependent upon the concentration of lymphocytes migrating through the spleen but not on the total number of lymphocytes present. The same conclusions can be drawn from the observations of McGregor and Gowans (79) who showed that rats depleted of recirculating lymphocytes by chronic drainage from the thoracic duct were severely suppressed in their ability to mount a primary anti-SRBC response.

The presence of virgin lymphocytes specific for SRBC (46), flagellin (101, 112), DNP (119), and bovine serum albumin (111) could be shown in the thoracic duct by adoptive transfer to irradiated syngeneic recipients. On the other hand, virgin lymphocytes specific for horse spleen ferritin, diphtheria toxoid, and tetanus toxoid were shown to be nonrecirculating cells (117, 118). Memory cells specific for a variety of antigens such as ϕX174 (48), DNP-BGG (20), horse spleen ferritin (117, 118), and fowl gamma globulin (98) have been shown to be recirculating. In fact, in every experiment known to these authors, memory cells are part of the recirculating pool of lymphocytes.

The recirculating nature of lymphocytes involved in primary and secondary antibody-forming responses has also been demonstrated by specific depletion experiments. It is theorized that if the recirculating pool of lymphocytes provide the bulk of the specific immunocompetent cells involved in primary or secondary immune responses, then injection of an antigen into a donor animal before collection of the TDL should result in an accumulation of reactive cells in the draining lymphoid organs and a concomitant removal from the TDL. As predicted, specific depletions have been shown with SRBC (81, 96, 106), DNP-BGG (96), tetanus toxoid

(25), and purified protein derivative (61), and it has been shown to be a property of both B cells (96, 106) and T cells (96).

All of the above investigations have involved antibody formation, but the same type of results have also been reported for the T cells which participate in cell-mediated immune reactions. The first observation was the finding by Billingham and Brent (7) that a cell circulating in the peripheral blood of adult mice was capable of causing a graft-versus-host (GvH) reaction in newborn mice. Later, Gowans (44) showed that GvH reactive cells were also present in the TD of rats. Since these original observations, many investigators have shown that the TD contains lymphocytes which are capable of transferring allograft immunity and delayed hypersensitivity, proliferating in response to allogeneic lymphocytes or antigen in vitro, and generating specific cytotoxic cells (for review see 49). Specific depletion of T cells reactive to allogeneic antigens has also been shown. Ford and Atkins (27) injected TDL from a parental rat into an irradiated F_1 hybrid and then collected the TDL from the recipient. This procedure should allow for the specific retention of lymphocytes reactive to the F_1 hybrid in the lymphoid organs of the host while permitting T cells reactive to different Ag-B antigens to recirculate. As anticipated, for the first 12–36 hours after injection into the F_1 hybrid the TDL contained very few cells capable of inducing GvH reactions against the same type of F_1 hybrid but contained normal levels of cells reactive to a third-party host. After 36 hours, reactive cells again appeared in the TD but not in the same number as found in normal donors. In similar experiments Rowley et al. (96) and Sprent et al. (110) injected F^1 hybrid lymphocytes intravenously into parental strain mice and found that the TD contained depleted numbers of GvH reactive cells specific for the F_1 hybrid. This was due, presumably, to the recruitment of reactive T cells out of the recirculation and into the site of antigen localization.

Admittedly, the preceding review has presented only a brief survey of the literature dealing with the antigen specificity and immunocompetence of recirculating lymphocytes, but it would seem adequate to answer the theorems posed by Ford (26). Without doubt the recirculating pool does contain both T and B lymphocytes which are reactive to a variety of antigens. Based upon the antigen-specific depletion experiments, the lymphocytes do appear to migrate through regions in which antigen is localized and there does not appear to be a selective stimulation of sessile cells as opposed to recirculating cells. The fourth proposition regarding the recirculating characteristics of lymphocyte subpopulations cannot be answered as easily. As discussed below, there are still questions concerning the ability of both T and B cells to become recirculating without an antigen-driven differentiation step.

V. RECIRCULATION OF VIRGIN AND MEMORY CELLS

Based upon the evidence presented in the preceding section it would seem likely that virgin T cells (those which have not undergone an antigen-driven maturation step) are recirculating. There are, however, results which would argue that this generalization may not always be accurate. One of the earlier attempts to classify T cells into subpopulations utilized their homing and recirculating characteristics in addition to their content of the theta antigen (92). A T_1 cell population was envisaged as an immature T cell which localized in the spleen as compared to the lymph nodes, was short lived as evidenced by their rapid disappearance in adult thymectomized mice, possessed relatively large amounts of theta antigen, and did not recirculate. The T_2 population was more mature, long lived, homed predominantly to the lymph nodes and was recirculating. Raff and Cantor (92) proposed that the $T_1 \to T_2$ maturation process was antigen driven, thus implying that only antigen experienced T cells could recirculate. More recently, Cantor et al. (10) confirmed the distribution of the T_1 and T_2 cell subpopulations by tagging the cells with fluorescence-labeled anti-theta antibody and subsequently separating them on the fluorescent-activated cell sorter. The bright-staining T cells (T_1 cells possessing large amounts of theta antigen) homed predominantly to the spleen of irradiated recipients and were reduced in donor animals within 30 days of adult thymectomy. The dull T cells (T_2 with small amounts of theta antigen) were found mostly in the TD, homed to the lymph nodes, and were not affected by adult thymectomy.

Simpson and Cantor (103) and Araneo et al. (2) have studied the functional properties of the T_1 and T_2 cells, employing adult thymectomy to produce a mouse depleted in T_1 or antilymphocyte serum (ALS) to enrich for the T_1 cells. It is presumed in these experiments that ALS depletes predominantly the recirculating T cells and thus acts upon the T_2 population. Using bovine serum albumin (BSA) as the antigen, adult thymectomy had no effect upon the primary in vivo response but severely inhibited the generation of memory cells (103). These results show that the primary response is due to the T_2 cell population which has been generated from the T_1 cells by environmental antigens, while the memory cells are the result of an antigen-driven $T_1 \to T_2$ conversion. Araneo et al. (2) came to the same conclusion when they showed that ALS inhibited primary responses to SRBC but did not adversely effect the development of memory. Furthermore, they showed that ALS partially inhibited (50%) the development of sensitized T cells active in delayed hypersensitivity reactions.

From these experimental results one may question the ability of the antigen-inexperienced T cell to recirculate. This does not negate the possible existence of T cells in the recirculating pool which are able to cooperate in primary immune responses and to generate sensitized T cells, but it does argue that this cell may be the product of an antigen-driven maturation step. In the normal animals one would presume that these antigen-experienced cells exist as a product of environmental antigens but this awaits definitive proof.

Another area of controversy concerns the ability of virgin B cells to recirculate. As previously stated, TDL from non-immune donors are able to adoptively transfer the primary immune response to SRBC, flagellin, horse spleen ferritin, DNP, and bovine serum albumin (46, 101, 111, 112, 117–119). The specific depletion experiments of Miller and Mitchell (81), Ford (25), and Hay et al. (61), in which lymphocytes specifically reactive to SRBC, DNP-BGG, tetanus toxoid, and PPD could be removed from the recirculating pool by the deposition of antigen in the lymphoid tissue, also argues for the presence of virgin cells in the TD. However, alternate explanations for these results can be envisaged. For example, Strober and Dilley (117, 118) have shown that the presence of a virgin B cell in the TD does not necessarily mean that it recirculates. They found that primary precursor B cells specific for horse spleen ferritin were present in the thoracic duct of non-primed rats. However, these cells could not recirculate, as shown by their inability to recover them in the thoracic duct lymph of an intermediate host (20–100 times depletion). Thus, it may be possible to find virgin cells circulating, but this does not necessarily mean that they can recirculate.

Another possible explanation for the presence of apparent antigen specific B cells in the TD of non-primed animals would state that these are not virgin cells. As in the case of T cells, the antigen specific B cell may represent the product of an antigen driven maturation, presumably by environmental antigens. For example, Schrader and Vadas (98) have found that fowl gamma globulin specific virgin B cells were adherent to glass beads when passed through a column, but memory cells specific for the same antigen were nonadherent. DNP-specific spleen cells from nonimmune donors displayed both adherent and nonadherent properties, suggesting that the animals had been sufficiently stimulated by environmental antigens to generate memory cells to DNP. Similarly, Strober and Dilley (117, 118) have shown that the unprimed B cells responsive to ferritin are short lived as judged by the ability of large doses of ^{3}H-thymidine to destroy them while memory B cells were long lived. Like the memory cells, unprimed B cells specific for DNP were long lived.

A third alternative explanation, which may apply to the depletion experiments, would propose that T cells rather than B cells have been recruited into the antigen containing lymphoid tissue. Functionally, this would have the same effect of depleting the ability of the TDL to restore the response of irradiated animals to a specific thymus-dependent antigen.

Taken together, these results would suggest that, as yet, we cannot conclude that the recirculating pool of lymphocytes contain both virgin T and B cells for all antigens. Without doubt, lymphocyte recirculation is necessary for the development of good primary responses. However, the important cell type(s) responsible for this activity may need further characterization.

VI. EFFECTS OF ANTIGEN AND ADJUVANT ON LYMPHOCYTE RECIRCULATION

In spite of the fact that we do not yet fully understand all the factors which control lymphocyte recirculation nor the exact nature of the lymphocyte subpopulations capable of recirculating, we have been able to show that the ordered migration of lymphocytes through the reticuloendothelial system is quite important to the integrity of the immune system. The microenvironment created by the dynamic fluxes in lymphocyte migration and the effect of antigen and/or adjuvant on this environment are partially responsible for the development of immune responses. Based upon evidence gathered from a variety of sources, we know that the following events usually occur in the generation of an immune response: (1) antigen reaches the draining lymphoid tissues and there induces an accumulation of both specific antigen-reactive cells and other lymphocytes; (2) antigen interacts with at least three cell types, namely B cells, T cells, and macrophages, the former two of which are specific for the particular antigen; and (3) antibody formation develops first in the draining lymphoid tissue and later systemically due to the emigration of transitional cells and memory cells which ultimately home to distal lymph nodes. In light of these basic observations it would seem appropriate to examine more closely the specific and nonspecific effects of antigen and/or adjuvant on lymphocyte recirculation and to evaluate how this may relate to an altered microenvironment.

A. Nonspecific Effects

The introduction of antigen or adjuvant has profound effects on the dynamics of cellular traffic through the lymph node or spleen. Exposure of a lymph node to antigen, whether soluble, or particulate, results in a drastic decrease in cell output in the efferent lymph (54, 55, 57). Thus, the physical nature of the antigen is not important to this phenomenon.

This lymph node "shut-down" is followed by a period of increased efflux of the cells which exit from the stimulated node were derived from the increase in cells leaving the node is not the result of any significant contribution of cells by the afferent lymph (55), nor is it the result of cellular proliferation within the node, as only 4% of the cells released were actually produced within the node (58). This means that the majority of the cells which exit from the stimulated node were derived from the recirculating population. These findings were construed to represent a transient reduction in the rate at which lymphocytes recirculated from the blood to the lymph (57).

Antigen and/or adjuvant also have the capacity to cause cellular changes within the node, resulting in hypercellularity (122, 133). The early phase of hypercellularity is proposed to be the result of augmented cellular traffic to the stimulated node while the later phase is presumably due to cellular proliferation (121, 126). This was shown using ^{51}Cr-labeled lymphocytes which demonstrated a markedly enhanced (fourfold) homing to stimulated nodes or spleen as opposed to unstimulated lymphoid tissue (8, 17, 121, 137). The cells homing to the stimulated nodes retain their capacity to recirculate normally in an adoptive recipient (17) and those cells draining from the stimulated node show no preferential homing. This would imply that the early increased cell localization is a function of the effects of antigen and/or adjuvant on the lymphoid tissue rather than an alteration in the recirculating cell population. Furthermore, this trapping of lymphocytes was shown to be indiscriminate, in that nonantigen-reactive cells as well as reactive cells home (8) to the stimulated lymph node or spleen, and the number of labeled cells present was a linear function of the number of cells injected (137, 138). In studies using isolated perfused spleens (23, 24, 28), the rate of entry of cells into the organ was dependent upon the concentration of the cells in the perfusate, that is, cell entry follows first order kinetics.

The increased influx of cells to the stimulated spleen was at the expense of cells travelling to the lymph nodes (8, 25, 137), and increased influx to the stimulated nodes was at the expense of cells travelling to unstimulated nodes (137) with no concomitant effect on splenic localization. This enhanced flow is transient in the spleen, existing for 24–48 hours after antigen contact (8, 137) and may even be followed by restricted cell entry in 4–7 days (8, 134). Lymph nodes, also demonstrate maximal trapping for 24–48 hours after antigen injection but show a slow decline in this phenomenon over the course of the entire primary immune response (9, 133, 137).

More recent evidence also supports the concept of augmented cellular traffic rather than the hypothesis of altered rates of recirculation. The induction of a primary immune response does not alter the rate at which an equilibrium is reached between the labeled cells present in the blood and lymph (60). A more detailed study has shown that the transit time in a stimulated node was not altered by antigen in comparison to the unstimulated contralateral node. However, labeled cells present in the node at the time of antigen contact were prevented from leaving the node, although this effect is only transient (1 hour) (9). The two mechanisms of augmented cellular traffic and antigen-induced transient "shut-down" were shown to operate separately, implying control by separate mechanisms.

In summary, stimulation of a lymphoid organ results in an immediate but transient closing of the node to cellular emigration and a subsequent increased influx of cells into this organ. The shut-down would apparently function immediately to increase the probability of an antigen-reactive cell already present in the lymphoid organ to make contact with antigen, while changes in cellular dynamics would result in an increased frequency of antigen reactive cells entering the antigen stimulated nodes from the recirculating pool, that is, recruitment.

B. Mechanisms of Trapping

The mechanisms regulating lymphocyte trapping have not been elucidated. However, some evidence exists which would give the T cell the role of modulator in lymphocyte recirculation. Under normal circumstances, injection of mice with alum-precipitated BGG results in an increase in lymph node weight and subsequent lymphocyte proliferation. Addition of the adjuvant B. pertussis accelerated the lymph node weight increase and produced a heightened level of DNA synthesis. However, in T cell depleted mice only cellular hyperplasia occurs without the preceding influx of small lymphocytes from the recirculating pool (121). Zatz and Gershon (134) observed a similar T cell dependence of lymphocyte trapping in T-cell-deprived mice immunized with SRBC or KLH or undergoing GvH reactions. In these experiments, the amount of trapping was reduced but it was never completely abolished. This residual localization may have been due to a possible role for the macrophage in controlling lymphocyte migration to antigen stimulated lymphoid organs (33), or to a radiation resistant, non-antigen specific mechanism (8). It is, of course, possible that all three systems may play a role in the regulation of lymphocyte trapping.

The spleen provides a special case in that it is subject to another form of control, namely the restricted entry of cells late after administration of antigen or initiation of a GvH response. This restricted localization was demonstrated to possess immunologic specificity in that tolerance or presensitization abrogates this effect and the rate of appearance of the restricted entry was dependent upon the concentration of antigen used for induction of the primary response. A role for the T cell in modulation of this effect has also been implicated (135).

C. Specific Effects on Recirculating Populations

In addition to its effects on recirculation dynamics, antigen is also able to directly influence the composition of the recirculating population of lymphocytes. As previously described, irradiation of an isolated spleen at levels which are cytotoxic does not ablate the ability of the animal to mount a response to SRBC administered intravenously. However, the kinetics of the response show approximately a 2-day delay (102) and may even result in an enhanced response (120). On the other hand, if splenic irradiation is followed by sublethal whole-body irradiation, the response is inhibited (102). Therefore, antigen-reactive cells which are able to re-populate the spleen and contribute to the immune response are present in the recirculating population.

In experiments using isolated rat spleens, perfusion with lymphocyte-free modified blood resulted in decreased responses to SRBC (28). Cells which were released into the perfusate were subsequently shown to be able to respond to SRBC (24). This argues that for a response to occur there must be contact with antigen by incoming cells. This concept is supported by the observation that perfusion of the isolated spleen with normal blood allows for a normal response. In addition, perfusion of the spleen with lymphocyte-free blood for 5 hours allows for cells released from the spleen to reenter this organ at approximately normal levels. Exposure to antigen at this time results in a normal response. If after the 5-hour perfusion, excess cells are added with antigen, slightly augmented responses can be observed (28). The magnitude of the response is thus directly proportional to the number of cells entering the spleen at the time of antigen exposure. These experiments do not directly show antigen-specific recruitment but rather that the recirculating population does contribute to the response. In light of the previously discussed changes in recirculation dynamics, this contribution is intuitively practical and physiological.

In order to demonstrate actual retention of antigen-reactive recirculating cells in the same experimental system, the antigen-sensitized, isolated spleen was perfused with immune cells. Cells released by the spleen were unable to transfer a secondary response, although transplanted fragments of the perfused spleen were able to do so without further exposure to antigen (25). Such selection of the antigen-reactive cells from the recirculating population was also shown to be antigen-specific. Perfusion of the spleen with TDL from tetanus toxoid and swine influenza virus-immune animals plus tetanus toxoid selectively depletes those cells responsive to the corresponding antigen. The cells released into the perfusate were not impaired in their ability to adoptively transfer the response to swine influenza virus.

Selective recruitment of cells by antigen should also result in concomitant reduction of antigen-reactive cells in the recirculating population, as was shown in a series of studies. TDL from SRBC-immune donors was transferred to adoptive recipients which were then challenged with SRBC. Daily collections of TDL from the adoptive recipients were made and the cells tested for their capacity to transfer the secondary response to an adoptive recipient. It was shown that TDL was unable to transfer the response if collected 1 to 2 days after challenge. However, by the third day the capacity had returned and, using 5-day post antigen TDL, enhanced indirect PFC were obtained (110). Using memory cells to DNP-BGG and HSA, selective depletion of TDLs specific to hapten and carrier were shown (96), although here the capacity to transfer responsiveness was never totally abolished. Selective depletion of cells capable of initiating GvH reactivity from nonimmune donors was also demonstrated using this adoptive recipient protocol (96, 110).

Intuitively, it was expected that the specific recruitment of cells would result in enriched populations of antigen-specific cells within the stimulated organ. Thus, animals injected intravenously with SRBC 24 hours before the removal of their spleens were used as donors in adoptive recipients. Challenge of the recipient and assay for PFC on day 7 results in depressed responsiveness. This depression was specific to the antigen used in priming, the responsiveness to other antigens being unimpaired. Time studies demonstrated that this depression was greatest at day one and wained with time, bearing a direct relationship to the unresponsiveness observed in TDL (107). If this refractory period was due to impaired ability of antigen specific cells in the spleen to recirculate, normal function should express itself in vitro. Microculture assay of stimulated spleens one day after antigen showed rapid and elevated responses to antigen. The TDL of such animals were specifically unresponsive. Therefore, the unresponsiveness observed in the adoptive recipient is not due to the rapid generation of suppressor cells, but rather an alteration of the homing properties of reactive cells as the result of contact with antigen (106).

In summary, the presence of antigen and/or adjuvant in a lymphoid organ allows for both specific and nonspecific sequestration of antigen-reactive cells from the recirculating pool. As the result of antigen contact, reactive cells have a refractory impairment of their ability to recirculate causing them to localize at the site of antigen. This series of events allows ample opportunity for antigen-triggering of both B and T cells. As suggested by Nieuwenhuis and Ford (86), antigen interaction with both T and B cells in the spleen may occur initially in the marginal zone (Fig. 2) but more likely it takes place in the outer zone of the PALS. After the T cells are stimulated, they are retained in the PALS for at least 36 hours (26). The B cells continue to migrate through this area of sequestered T cells and thus have the additional opportunity for cellular interaction. This hypothesis is consistent with the known areas of antigen localization, the presence of macrophages, B cells and T cells and the effects of antigen on lymphocyte recirculation. Once stimulated by antigen, the B cells migrate either to the red pulp cords, where they become antibody forming cells, or possibly to the germinal centers where they become memory cells.

In the lymph nodes (Fig. 1), Nieuwenhuis and Ford (86) have suggested that T and B cell stimulation occurs in the paracortex in a manner similar to that seen in the PALS. The stimulated B cells are then diverted from their normal course of migration to the medullary cords where they become antibody-forming cells. Conversely, those B cells which are destined to become memory cells migrate into the germinal centers following antigen triggering.

D. Appearance of Antigen-Stimulated Cells in the Recirculation

Not all antigen-triggered lymphocytes remain at the site of antigen depot. In the classic experiments by Hall et al. (59), primitive undifferentiated basophilic blastlike cells appeared in efferent lymph of antigen-stimulated lymph nodes. These basophilic cells were shown to be responsible for propagating the immune response throughout the body and they depended upon an intact lymphatic pathway for their transport. This view was supported by experiments which showed that these cells were capable of initiating immune responses in other lymph nodes of the same animal and of transferring active immunity between chimeric twins.

As discussed previously, antigen-triggered effector T cells and memory cells have also been shown to leave the draining lymphoid organ and to home to distal sites, thus disseminating the immune response. In the case of the memory cell it has usually been assumed that only the small mature cells are responsible for this phenomenon (69). However, recent evidence would suggest that a large memory cell may also be found in the TDL of immune animals (116). Strober found that when TDL from a recently immunized rat were fractionated by velocity sedimentation, the large-cell fraction (sedimentation velocity, 4.0 mm/hr) was enriched for memory cells when transferred to an adoptive recipient. Using essentially the same techniques, Hunt et al. (69) found only small memory cells. Strober (116) attempted to explain this apparent dichotomy on the basis that Hunt et al. (69) made no attempt to ensure adequate levels of T cells in each of their fractionated cell populations and thus may have failed to observe a large memory-cell population because of insufficient T cells. Alternatively, Strober and Gowans (personal communication) have

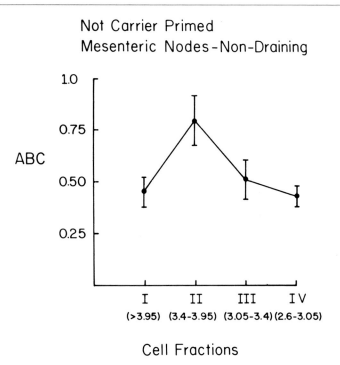

Fig. 3. *Adoptive secondary response of memory cells separated by velocity sedimentation.* The mesenteric lymph nodes were removed from an LBN rat immunized one month earlier by intraperitoneal injection of 1 mg DNP–BGG, alum precipitated, and 2 × 10⁹ killed *B. pertussis* organisms. The cells were separated by unit gravity velocity sedimentation and injected into syngeneic recipients which had been irradiated 24 hours earlier with 500 R whole-body X-irradiation. The recipients were challenged 24 hours later with 1 mg DNP-BGG given in saline and administered intravenously. Each recipient was given 6 × 10⁶ lymphocytes and three recipients were used for each cell population. The average antibody response (*ABC* = antigen binding capacity of 1 ml whole serum determined by the Farr technique), plus and minus one standard deviation is shown for each cell fraction. The brackets indicate the average sedimentation velocities for each cell fraction.

suggested that the difference may have been due to the circulating pattern of the large memory cell. Thus, using footpad immunization (116), lymphocytes leaving the draining popliteal nodes would be readily found in the thoracic duct when cannulation was performed in the abdomen (124). Using intraperitoneal injections (69), the draining lymph nodes should be the parathymics (124), and lymphocytes emigrating from these nodes do not appear in the thoracic duct unless they are truly recirculating cells.

Recent work in our own laboratory would seem to resolve these problems (Feldbush, unpublished observations). Rats were immunized with DNP-BGG either intraperitoneally or in the footpad, and different lymph nodes were removed one month later. Cell suspensions were made and fractionated into four groups based upon their sedimentation velocity at unit gravity in a 5–30% fetal calf serum gradient (69, 115). Group I cells show the fastest sedimentation velocity, Groups II and III are intermediate

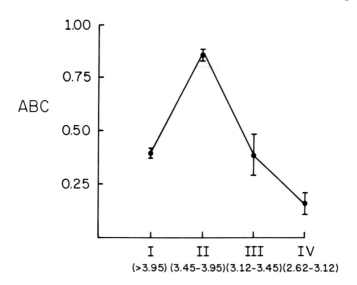

Cell Fractions

Fig. 4. *Adoptive secondary responses of memory cells separated by velocity sedimentation and transferred to carrier primed recipients. The methodology is the same as that described in Figure 3 except the recipients were primed with 1 mg alum-precipitated BGG two weeks before irradiation.*

and Group IV contains the smallest cells with the slowest sedimentation rates. Approximately 5–7% of the total cells are found in Group I, 40–50% in Groups II and III and 15–20% in Group IV. In our initial experiments (Figs. 3 and 4) donor rats were immunized intraperitoneally, mesenteric nodes were removed, fractionated, and transferred to both carrier-primed irradiated recipients (Fig. 4) and noncarrier-primed irradiated recipients (Fig. 3). If the first hypothesis were correct and T cells were limiting, a difference should be seen between the two groups, inasmuch as the carrier-primed irradiated recipients possess excess numbers of T cells. Furthermore, the use of mesenteric nodes, which do not drain the peritonium, should mimic the experiments of Hunt et al. (69) using TDL and intraperitoneal immunization. As can be seen in both Figures 3 and 4, only the smaller lymphocytes were capable of transferring memory, thus

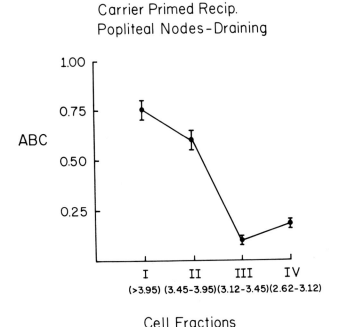

Cell Fractions

Fig. 5. *Adoptive secondary responses of memory cells collected from the drain-ing lymph nodes, separated by velocity sedimentation, and transferred to carrier-primed recipients. Memory cells were prepared from the popliteal lymph nodes one month after footpad immunization with 1 mg alum-precipitated DNP–BGG. The remainder of the methodology is the same as that described in Figures 3 and 4.*

confirming the results of Hunt *et al.* (69) and indicating that limiting numbers of T cells was not a problem.

In the next two experiments, rats were immunized in the footpad and the draining popliteal nodes removed (Fig. 5) or intraperitoneally with the parathymics removed (Fig. 6). Following fractionation and transfer to carrier-primed irradiated recipients, the large-cell fraction was found to be enriched for memory cells. Thus, the physical characteristics of the memory cell populations depend upon the area from which they have been isolated. From these data we would propose that following antigenic stimulation a large immature memory cell is formed in the draining lymphoid organs and that some of these cells may leave the stimulated nodes and enter the efferent lymphatics (116). These cells do not recirculate (69)

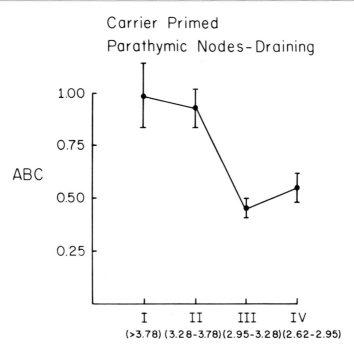

Fig. 6. *Adoptive secondary responses of memory cells collected from the draining lymph nodes, separated by velocity sedimentation, and transferred to carrier-primed recipients. The techniques used were the same as those described in Figure 5 except that the donors were immunized intraperitoneally and the parathymic lymph nodes were removed.*

but instead probably home into distal lymphoid organs and there presumably mature into small lymphocytes. We would further propose that the small cells are then capable of leaving the nodes and joining the recirculating pool. Thus, the large memory cell represents an intermediate step in the generation of the mature memory cells much as the basophilic cell of Hall et al. (59) represents an intermediate stage in the generation of plasma cells. It is even possible that these two cells are the same, but this conclusion must await further characterization of the cell population.

The above series of events may also have a parallel in the effector T cell system. Sprent and Miller (108, 109) have shown that alloantigen-activated T blast cells (T.TDL) can be found in the TDL of animals undergoing a GvH reaction. While some (0.4%) of these cells are capable of recirculation, others appear to home into lymph nodes, undergo division, and then rejoin the recirculating pool in expanded numbers.

VII. EFFECT OF TUMORS ON LYMPHOCYTE RECIRCULATION

In light of the previous discussion regarding the effect of antigens and adjuvants upon lymphocyte recirculation, it would seem worthwhile to consider the effects that tumors may have upon this process. A discussion of this nature is, however, complicated by the fact that an immune response can have a variety of effects upon tumor growth. On the one hand, it can effectively retard the tumor, while on the other it can in fact promote tumor growth by means of "blocking factors." In addition, tumors are known to possess varying degrees of antigenicity, conferred upon them by the neoantigens that appear upon the cell surfaces after malignant transformation; thus the response of hosts to different tumors may vary drastically.

With these observations in mind, one might consider the effect of tumors upon the homing patterns of lymphoid cells. Delorme et al. (14) showed that the appearance of lymphoblasts in the thoracic duct following antigenic challenge could be used as a measure of the immunologic reactivity of the host, and that a syngeneic tumor cell challenge could provoke the appearance of such cells in the lymph. However, in progressive subcutaneous implants of these tumors, the equivalent rise in immunoblasts was not seen (1) unless the tumors were excised. Histologically, the draining lymph node gave evidence of a vigorous immune response. The responses of these lymph nodes to other antigens were essentially normal, as were the responses of distal lymph nodes. These investigators theorized that the "trapping" phenomenon they observed was due to continual bombardment with antigen.

Such trapping has been investigated further using the ^{51}Cr-labeled lymphoid cell technique described earlier. Under normal circumstances, 24 hours after injection of labeled spleen cells, one finds 8–10% of the injected radioactivity localized in the lymph nodes, 20% in the spleen and 20–25% in the liver (136). As has been discussed previously, antigenic stimuli or the injection of adjuvants results in a temporary increase in the number of lymphoid cells localizing in the draining lymph nodes or spleen, depending upon the route of injection (17, 121, 137). Gershon and Fightlin (34) investigated the effect of two chemically induced transplantable tumors upon the phenomenon of lymphocyte recruitment. In mice differing from the tumor at the H-2 locus, a gradual rise in trapping in the draining lymph node was observed, peaking at day 4 and subsequently dropping off. In general, higher tumor cell doses maintained lymph node trapping for longer periods of time. Where histocompatibility differences did not exist, significant trapping occurred early in the response but was not maintained. The spleens exhibited modest amounts of trapping. The enhanced trapping observed with increasing antigenic disparity between host and tumor reinforced the contention that this was indeed a measure of an immune phenomenon. Zatz et al. (139) found, in addition, that the greater the antigenic disparity, the less the contribution of splenic trapping to the altered kinetics of lymphocyte recirculation. These results may reflect the efficacy of a localized immune response in situations where the antigenic stimulus is adequate to recruit and sensitize lymphocytes in the draining lymph node.

Gillette and Bellanti (39) studied the effect of a transplantable lymphosarcoma (6C3HED) upon lymphocyte trapping in C3H/J mice. They found up to a 20-fold increase in the number of cells present in the ipsilateral, draining lymph nodes as compared with the contralateral nodes in tumor-bearing animals. On the other hand, the migration of lymphoid cells obtained from tumor-bearing mice and transferred to normal mice decreased as a function of tumor progression. An enhanced migration of cells to the liver was noted, possibly due to an increased number of macrophages in the injected suspension (37, 123). The localization of normal lymphoid cells derived from either the spleen or lymph node in tumor-bearing mice was shown to occur predominantly in the ipsilateral draining lymph node. Secondary migration studies confirmed that cells localizing in the draining lymph node were indeed recirculating cells, identical to those localizing in normal lymph nodes.

The Moloney sarcoma, virus-induced rhabdosarcoma of mice, has the interesting feature of undergoing spontaneous regression in an immunologically intact host (83), so it formed a useful model in which to quantitate changes in lymphocyte traffic. Zatz et al. (139) found that maximal lymphocyte trapping by the draining lymph node occurred at a time corresponding to tumor regression, and that no equivalent trapping was observed in the other lymph nodes or the spleen. Interestingly, these workers found a biphasic response in the draining lymph node. The exact reason for this has not been established. However, it has been suggested that the initial response is due to the original antigenic stimulus introduced upon injection of tumor cells, while the latter is due to the response to growing tumors. An alternative possibility may be one based upon the observations of Romball and Weigle (93). These investigators observed a cycling effect in the plaque-forming cell responses of popliteal lymph nodes upon concomitant immunization in the footpad and intravenously. Footpad immunization alone did not produce such cycling. An explanation given for this phenomenon was the immunoregulatory role of the spleen, possibly mediated via suppressor cells. It may be that a similar cycling of the trapping phenomenon can occur when antigen escapes the regional lymph node and thus is able to stimulate the splenic immunoregulatory functions.

Gillette and Boone (36) studied the effect of a progressively growing fibrosarcoma upon lymphocyte homing. They consistently found a decreased homing of normal lymphoid cells to the bone-marrow compartment of tumor-bearing animals and an increase in migration to the spleen, with concomitant splenomegaly. Migration to and reactivity of peripheral lymphoid cell populations remained essentially normal. These workers champion the importance of the spleen in host responses to tumors and in this study did not look at the effect upon draining lymph nodes specifically.

The importance of splenic regulation of lymphocyte trapping has been further investigated by Fightlin et al. (21). In the presence of both H-2-compatible and H-2-incompatible tumor grafts an increased localization of ^{51}Cr-labeled lymphoid cells was seen in the regional lymph nodes and spleens. In allogeneic situations trapping in draining lymph nodes was shown to decline at the time of tumor rejection and concomitant trapping in the contralateral node was not seen. In syngeneic instances trapping was again seen, but to a lesser degree, and this persisted until animals succumbed to the tumor. The degree of trapping in the spleen was equivalent in each situation. Initially, splenectomy did not have a significant effect upon lymph node trapping—at best a marginal increase was observed. Later in the response, however, a significant decrease in lymph node trapping was seen in splenectomized animals. Tumor resection resulted in a decrease in trapping in the regional lymph nodes. A reduction in trapping in the spleen was only seen when resection was performed nine days after initiation of tumor growth, which was just prior to the time at which tumor rejection would occur. If splenectomy was performed in addition to tumor resection, a marked increase in lymphocyte trapping in the draining lymph node was observed, suggesting that the spleen has the capacity to modulate the response of the draining lymph node. The most likely explanation for such a phenomenon would be a specific regulatory effect of the spleen, perhaps via suppressor cells.

The above-mentioned results have all been obtained with solid tumors. Other work has shown that ascites tumors may in fact have a different effect upon lymphocyte trapping. Frost and Lance (32), for example, have observed defective trapping in animals bearing ascitic tumors, an effect which could be transferred to normal animals via injections of cell-free ascitic fluid. Upon intraperitoneal injection of S37 or Meth/A sarcoma cells into mice, a short-lived localization of labeled cells was observed in the spleen, but by the third day the levels were not significantly different from controls. Upon subcutaneous implantation of the tumor, however, there was augmented localization of the labelled cells in the draining lymph node, and this was continually present for the duration of the study, that is, while the tumor persisted. Interestingly, the presence of the ascitic tumors appeared to abrogate the trapping response to other unrelated antigens such as sheep erythrocytes, keyhole limpet haemocyanin and Salmonella H antigen, while solid tumors did not have this effect. This ruled out the possibility that minimal trapping was due to tolerance induction to the tumor antigen since tolerance has indeed been shown to abrogate trapping (138). In addition, treatment of normal animals with cell-free ascitic fluids prevented the trapping of lymphocytes normally observed upon subcutaneous challenge with antigen.

Mongini and Rosenberg (84) extended these studies, using a variety of cell-free ascitic fluids, namely, that from a spontaneous lymphatic leukemia, that from a Gross virus-induced lymphoma, and that from an ascites tumor with no known viral association. These workers also found that cell-free ascitic fluid ablated the trapping phenomenon in antigen-draining lymph nodes in most cases. Contrary to Frost and Lance (32), however, they demonstrated a failure of allogeneic cell-free ascitic fluids to diminish a trapping response elicited by antigen.

An immunosuppressive effect caused by cell-free ascitic fluids from Ehrlich ascites tumors has been investigated fairly extensively (75, 78, 85, 87, 132), as has that from TA3-Ha tumors (50). Although the immunosuppressive capacities have not been studied in terms of lymphocyte trapping, it has been shown that an important mechanism functional early in the immune response is the localization of lymphocytes in the draining lymph node and that an immunosuppressive action can be exerted by ablating the accumulation of lymphocytes in the vicinity of antigen. The mechanism for this is unknown. However, it may be that the cell-free ascitic fluids serve as a good source of soluble tumor antigen and that the widespread presence of antigen somehow exerts an immunosuppressive effect. Widespread circulating antigen would certainly diminish the efficacy of regional lymphocyte trapping. The observation of Frost and Lance (32) that the immunosuppression was not antigen-specific does present problems in interpretation, however. Several studies have shown that antigenic overload can have an immunosuppressive effect, for example, Paranjpe and Boone (89) caused specific depression of antitumor cellular immune responses with an intraperitoneal injection of tumor homogenate. Also, Jaroslow et al. (70) effected in vitro suppression of immunocompetent cells using lymphomas from spleens of aging mice. In the latter case they too were able to produce nonantigen-specific suppression.

In view of the possible immunosuppressive effects of agents capable of abrogating lymphocyte trapping it may be of interest to briefly consider the immunopotentiating effects of certain adjuvants such as BCG. Lieberman et al. (76) described the immunologic and histopathologic changes in patients with malignant melanomas upon treatment with BCG. Their results suggested that intralesional BCG administration stimulated both specific and nonspecific immune responses, thereby enhancing tumor regression. Similar results have been obtained by various other laboratories (3, 4, 95). Furthermore, certain retrospective studies have shown that "experiments of nature" have similar results. For example, Ruckdeschel et al. (97) found that patients who developed empyema, following surgical resection of carcinoma of the lung, had improved survival rates when compared with patients that did not develop the infection. The results were most marked in patients whose tumors had been limited to the lung and its draining regional lymph nodes.

Ogura et al. (88) investigated the kinetics of lymphoid cells in tumor-bearing animals as affected by BCG administration. Inoculation of BCG fractions together with tumor cells resulted in a suppression of tumor growth. This procedure also augmented lymphocyte trapping in the draining lymph node relative to animals not treated with BCG. Furthermore, in rats inoculated with oil-attached BCG cell wall, the phytohaemagglutinin (PHA) responses of lymphocytes derived from both draining and distal lymph nodes were elevated, indicative of enhanced T cell responses. This treatment also appeared to abrogate the formation of lymph node metastases as compared with control animals. The adjuvant therefore has an effect upon the recruitment of lymphocytes into draining lymph nodes in the presence of tumor—a phenomenon presumably important for the potentiation of an immune response directed against the tumor.

As discussed earlier, some controversy exists regarding the nature of the trapping phenomenon, and the cells involved. Clearly this is an important consideration since the efficacy of the phenomenon in the immunoregulation of tumor growth would depend upon the cells "recruited" and their capacity to deal with the tumor. The control of lymphocyte migration has been ascribed to at least three systems: T cells (134), macrophages (33), and a radiation-resistant mechanism (8). These factors may not, of course, be mutually exclusive since T cells are known to produce soluble factors which mediate their effects, and indeed some have been described which act directly upon macrophages (5, 13). In either event it would appear that tumor immunity could be effected by sensitization of cells upon entrapment in the draining lymph node. Cytotoxic T cells emanating from stimulated lymph nodes have been described by numerous workers (15, 30, 62) and these presumably would play a role in tumor immunity. On the other hand Hibbs (63, 64) has described a system in which macrophages act as cytotoxic effector cells. He demonstrated that antigen persistence in the locale of the macrophages was necessary for maintenance of resistance to tumor growth. In this system it should be noted that specificity of activation depends upon immune lymphocytes. One final mechanism depends upon antibody-dependent cytolytic effector lymphocytes or K cells (91). Such antibody production would clearly be dependent upon T and B cell interactions in the draining lymph nodes.

An important practical consideration in the clinical area relates to the role of the regional lymph node in the immune response to tumors and consequently the wisdom of lymph node removal during surgical resection of tumors. In this area too, somewhat conflicting evidence has accumulated. Guillou (51) devised a test to measure the immune reactivity (macrophage inhibition factor release) of lymphocytes in lymph nodes draining colorectal tumors. He did not show preferential sensitization of draining lymph nodes and saw no ground for abandoning lymph node resection in the management of colorectal cancer. Fisher and Fisher (22), on the other hand, found that spontaneous C3H mammary tumors grew better after removal of the draining lymph nodes (while methyl-cholanthrene-induced tumors did not). Their data indicated that, in the case of mammary tumors, the draining lymph nodes play a major role in resistance, especially to tumors with low antigenicity. In experimental cancer Goldfarb and Hardy (40) showed that the regional lymph nodes served as the initial recognition site of tumor antigen, and that it was a relay point for transfer of immunity to the central immunologic system by means of sensitized lymphocytes or soluble mediators. Ellis et al. (18), using the leukocyte migration assay to evaluate immune competence, demonstrated that cellular reactivity to tumor antigens was more marked in the lymph node lymphocytes than in peripheral blood lymphocytes. Similar results were obtained by Dheodhar et al. (16) except in instances of metastatic involvement when reactivity was minimized, and

Berlinger et al. (6) showed that patients with active immune responsive lymphocytes in regional lymph nodes in head and neck cancer had better prognosis than patients with unstimulated nodes.

In conclusion, these studies clearly indicate that an investigation into the immune capacities of draining lymph nodes is not purely an esoteric pursuit, but does indeed have direct implications in the human disease state. It appears that lymphocyte trapping in the draining lymph node occurs as a result of prolonged antigenic bombardment, and subsides upon spontaneous regression of the tumor or surgical resection thereof. The lymph node therefore forms an important primary filter responsible for tumor surveillance. If tumor cells manage to escape this mechanism, the spleen becomes sensitized and acts in a modulatory capacity. Once antigen has become disseminated, as in the development of metastatic lesions, the draining lymph node becomes less important since the immune mechanism has been essentially overwhelmed. Data concerning these phenomena—the mechanisms and importance of lymphocyte trapping—are rather sparse and, certainly in the field of tumor immunology, inconclusive. Perhaps we would be well advised to give these matters more attention.

VIII. CONCLUSIONS

From the preceding discussion it is apparent that an important aspect of the microenvironment of the immune system is the dynamic flux of lymphocytes through the lymph nodes and spleen. There is no question that the passage of specific lymphocytes through the antigen-stimulated lymphoid tissue is necessary for the development of an immune response. There is also no question that both antigen and adjuvant can alter this recirculation, resulting in the accumulation of both antigen-specific and -nonspecific lymphocytes in the stimulated lymph nodes or spleen. This localization appears to enhance the efficiency of antigen triggering and cellular cooperation, which apparently takes place in the outer zone of the PALS in the spleen and the paracortex of the lymph nodes. However, there is a significant number of questions regarding this microenvironment that is not yet resolved. For example, we do not yet fully understand the complex factors which control the selective migration of T and B cells through the PCV and the different areas of the lymph nodes and spleen. We also do not totally comprehend the differential homing of known lymphocyte subpopulations. Experiments utilizing agents which do not produce gross alterations of the cell surface and the evaluation of such agents on specific lymphocyte subpopulations should add greatly to our understanding of lymphocyte recirculation.

Since we know that antigen-specific lymphocytes recirculate and that this recirculation is necessary for the development of immune responses, it would seem logical that a large number of the antigen-triggered lymphocytes are recruited from the recirculating population. However, we have presented evidence which questions the ability of virgin T and B cells to recirculate. At present it is not possible to resolve this controversy, but several generalizations can be made. (1) The nonantigen-experienced T_1 cells do not recirculate. (2) Some virgin B cells, such as those specific for tetanus toxoid, diphtheria toxoid, and horse spleen ferritin, do not recirculate, while precursors for SRBC, flagellin, DNP, and BSA may indeed recirculate. (3) All of the antigen-experienced memory T and B cells have been shown to recirculate. (4) In at least one case in which virgin B cells are apparently found to be recirculating, there is evidence that these may be memory cells stimulated by environmental antigens. (5) Finally, in those circumstances in which antigen can drive the precursor cells to become recirculating memory cells, there appears to be an intermediate large cell stage which is capable of leaving the antigen stimulated node, circulating to other nodes, and there presumably converting into the small recirculating memory cell population. Because of these apparently divergent facts, it would seem to us that before it is possible to completely understand the contribution of recirculating and sessile lymphocytes to the microenvironment of the immune system, one must first know what role these cells play in both primary and secondary responses. For example, one could theorize that in some primary antibody responses, the B cell precursor is sessile while the antigen-experienced T_2 cell is recruited from the recirculating pool. In secondary responses, both cell populations are recruited from the recirculation.

Because of the relative paucity of information regarding the influence of tumors on draining lymph nodes and lymphocyte recirculation, it is difficult to arrive at any definitive conclusion. It would appear that the regional lymph nodes are affected differently, depending upon the nature of the tumor, its immunogenicity and its site and state of growth. Included in the latter would be the differential effects of ascites and solid tumors, the size of the tumor mass and its degree of metastasis. The most important aspect of draining lymph node involvement is its possible therapeutic value and its prognostic potential. A good deal of evidence supports the notion that T cell proliferation in the deep cortex of the draining node is of benefit to the host and indicative of a good prognosis. These observations may question the routine practice of removing regional lymph nodes upon tumor resection.

REFERENCES

1. Alexander, P., Bensted, J., Delorme, E. J., Hall, J. G., and Hodgett, J. 1969. The cellular immune response to primary sarcomata in rats. II. Abnormal responses of nodes draining the tumour. *Proc. Roy. Soc. B.* 174: 237.

2. Araneo, B. A., Marrack (Hunter), P. C., and Kappler, J. W. 1975. Functional heterogeneity among the T-derived lymphocytes of the mouse. II. Sensitivity of subpopulations to anti-thymocyte serum. *J. Immunol.* 114: 747.

3. Bast, R. C., Zbar, B., Borsos, T., and Rapp, H. J. 1974. BCG and Cancer. *N. Engl. J. Med.* 290: 1413.

4. Bast, R. C., Zbar, B., Borsos, T., and Rapp, H. J. 1974. BCG and Cancer. *N. Engl. J. Med.* 290: 1458.

5. Bennett, B., and Bloom, B. R. 1968. Reactions *in vivo* and *in vitro* produced by a soluble substance associated with delayed-type hypersensitivity. *Proc. Natl. Acad. Sci.* 58: 756.

6. Berlinger, N. T., Tsakrakides, V., Pollak, K., Adams, G. L., Yang, M., and Good, R. A. 1976. Immunologic assessment of regional lymph node histology in relation to survival in head and neck carcinoma. *Cancer* 37: 697.

7. Billingham, R. E. and Brent, L. 1959. Quantitative studies on tissue transplantation immunity. IV. Induction of tolerance in newborn mice and studies on the phenomenon of runt disease. *Philos. Trans. Roy. Soc., London* 242: 439.

8. Black, S. J. 1975. Antigen-induced changes in lymphocyte circulatory patterns. *Eur. J. Immunol.* 5: 170.

9. Cahill, R. N. P., Frost, H., and Trnka, Z. 1976. The effects of antigen on the migration of recirculating lymphocytes through single lymph nodes. *J. Exp. Med.* 143: 870.

10. Cantor, H., Simpson, E., Sato, V. L., Fathman, C. G., and Herzenberg, L. A. 1975. Characterization of subpopulations of T lymphocytes. I. Separation and functional studies of peripheral T-cells binding different amounts of fluorescent anti-thy 1.2 (Theta) antibody using a fluorescence-activated cell sorter (FACS). *Cell. Immunol.* 15: 180.

11. Crouse, D. A., Feldbush, T. L., and Evans, T. C. 1976. Radiation-induced alterations in murine lymphocyte homing patterns. I. Radiolabeling studies. *Cell. Immunol.* 27: 131.

12. Currie, G. A. and Basham, C. 1972. Serum mediated inhibition of the immunological reactions of the patient to his own cancer: A possible role for circulating antigen. *Brit. J. Cancer* 26: 427.

13. David, J. R. 1966. Delayed hypersensitivity *in vitro*: its mediation by cell-free substances formed by lymphoid cell-antigen interaction. *Proc. Natl. Acad. Sci.* 56: 72.

14. Delorme, E. J., Hodgett, J. G., and Alexander, P. 1969. The cellular immune response to primary sarcomata in rats. I. The significance of large basophilic cells in the thoracic duct lymph following antigenic challenge. *Proc. Roy. Soc. B.* 174: 229.

15. Denham, S., Wrathmell, A. B., and Alexander, P. 1975. Evidence of cytotoxic T and B immunoblasts in the thoracic ducts of rats bearing tumour grafts. *Transplantation* 19 (2): 102.

16. Dheodhar, S. D., Crile, G., and Esselstyn, C. B. 1972. Study of the tumor cell-lymphocyte interaction in patients with breast cancer. *Cancer* 29: 1321.

17. Dresser, D. W., Taub, R. N., and Krantz, A. R. 1970. The effect of localized injection of adjuvant material on the draining lymph node. II. Circulating lymphocytes. *Immunology* 18: 663.

18. Ellis, R. J., Wernick, G., Zabriskie, J. B., and Goldman, L. I. 1975. Immunologic competence of regional lymph nodes in patients with breast cancer. *Cancer* 35: 655.

19. Everett, N. B., and Tyler, R. W. 1967. Lymphopoiesis in the thymus and other tissues: functional implications. *Int. Rev. Cytol.* 22: 205.

20. Feldbush, T. L., and Gowans, J. L. 1971. Antigen modulation of the immune response. The effect of delayed challenge on the affinity of anti-dinitrophenylated bovine gamma globulin antibody produced in adoptive recipients. *J. Exp. Med.* 134: 1453.

21. Fightlin, R. S., Lytton, B., and Gershon, R. K. 1975. Splenic regulation of lymphocyte trapping in lymph nodes draining tumor grafts. *J. Immunol.* 115: 345.

22. Fisher, B., and Fisher, E. R. 1972. Studies concerning the regional lymph node in cancer. II. Maintenance of immunity. *Cancer* 29: 1496.

23. Ford, W. L. 1969. The kinetics of lymphocyte recirculation within the rat spleen. *Cell Tissue Kinet.* 2: 171.

24. Ford, W. L. 1969. The immunological and migratory properties of the lymphocytes recirculating through the rat spleen. *Brit. J. Exp. Path.* 50: 257.

25. Ford, W. L. 1972. The recruitment of recirculating lymphocytes in the antigenically stimulated spleen, specific and nonspecific consequences of initiating a secondary antibody response. *Clin. Exp. Immunol.* 12: 243.

26. Ford, W. L. 1975. Lymphocyte migration and immune responses. *Progress in Allergy*, Vol. 19, p. 1. Karger, Basel.

27. Ford, W. L., and Atkins, R. C. 1971. Specific unresponsiveness of recirculating lymphocytes after exposure to histocompatibility antigen in F_1 hybrid rats. *Nature New Biol.* 234: 178.

28. Ford, W. L., and Gowans, J. L. 1969. The traffic of lymphocytes. *Sem. Haemat.* 6: 67.

29. Ford, W. L., and Simmonds, S. J. 1972. The tempo of lymphocyte recirculation from blood to lymph in the rat. *Cell. Tissue Kinet.* 5: 175.

30. Fossati, G., Canevari, S., Della Porta, G., Balzarini, G. P., and Veronesi, U. 1972. Cellular immunity to human breast carcinoma. *Int. J. Cancer* 10: 391.

31. Freitas, A. A., and deSousa, M. 1976. Control mechanisms of lymphocyte traffic. Modification of the traffic of ^{51}Cr-labeled mouse lymph node cells by treatment with plant lectins in intact and splenectomized hosts. *Eur. J. Immunol.* 5: 831.

32. Frost, P., and Lance, E. M. 1973. Abrogation of lymphocyte trapping by ascitic tumors. *Nature* 240: 101.

33. Frost, P., and Lance, E. M. 1974. The cellular origin of the lymphocyte trap. *Immunology* 26: 175.

34. Gershon, R. K., and Fightlin, R. S. 1973. Recruitment of lymphocytes in response to tumor growth, *in* S. Garrottini and G. Franch (ed.), *Chemotherapy of Cancer Dissemination and Metastasis 1973*, p. 139–147. Raven Press, NY.

35. Gesner, B. M., and Ginsburg, V. 1964. Effect of glycosidases on the fate of transfused lymphocytes. *Proc. Natl. Acad. Sci.* 52: 750.

36. Gillette, R. W., and Boone, C. W. 1974. Changes in the homing properties of labeled lymphoid cells caused by solid tumor growth. *Cell. Immunol.* 12: 363.

37. Gillette, R. W., and Lance, E. M. 1971. Kinetic studies of macrophages. I. Distributional characteristics of radio-labeled peritoneal cells. *J. Reticuloendoth. Soc.* 10: 223.

38. Gillette, R. W., McKenzie, G. O., and Swanson, M. H. 1973. Effect of concanavalin A on the homing of labeled T lymphocytes. *J. Immunol.* 111: 1902.

39. Gillette, S., and Bellanti, J. A. 1973. Kinetics of lymphoid cells in tumor-bearing mice. *Cell. Immunol.* 8: 311.

40. Goldfarb, P. M., and Hardy, M. A. 1975. The immunologic responsiveness of regional lymphocytes in experimental cancer. *Cancer* 35: 778.

41. Goldschneider, I., and McGregor, D. O. 1968. Migration of lymphocytes and thymocytes in the rat. I. The route of migration from blood to spleen and lymph nodes. *J. Exp. Med.* 127: 155.

42. Gowans, J. L. 1957. The effect of the continuous reinfusion of lymph and lymphocytes on the output of lymphocytes from the thoracic duct of unanaesthetized rats. *Brit. J. Exp. Path.* 38: 67.

43. Gowans, J. L. 1959. The recirculation of lymphocytes from blood to lymph in the rat. *J. Physiol., Lond.* 146: 54.

44. Gowans, J. L. 1962. The fate of parental strain lymphocytes in F_1 hybrid rats. *Ann. N.Y. Acad. Sci.* 99: 335.

45. Gowans, J. L. 1966. Life-span, recirculation and transformation of lymphocytes. *Int. Rev. Exp. Path.* 5: 1.

46. Gowans, J. L. 1970. Lymphocytes. Harvey Lectures, Series 64: 87.

47. Gowans, J. L., and Knight, E. J. 1964. The route of recirculation of lymphocytes in the rat. *Proc. Roy. Soc. B.* 159: 257.

48. Gowans, J. L., and Uhr, J. W. 1966. The carriage of immunological memory by small lymphocytes in the rat. *J. Exp. Med.* 124: 1017.

49. Greaves, M. F., Owen, J. J. T., and Raff, M. C. 1974. T and B lymphocytes. Origins, properties and roles in immune responses. (Elsevier-Excerpta Medica-North Holland, Amsterdam 1974).

50. Grohsman, J., and Nowotny, J. 1972. The immune recognition of TA3 tumors, its facilitation by endotoxin and abrogation by ascites fluid. *J. Immunol.* 109: 1090.

51. Guillou, P. J. 1975. A study of lymph nodes draining colorectal cancer using a two-stage inhibition of leucocyte migration technique. *Gut* 16 (4): 290.

52. Gutman, G. A., and Weissman, I. L. 1973. Homing properties of thymus-independent follicular lymphocytes. *Transplantation* 16 (6): 621.

53. Gutman, G. A., and Weissman, I. L. 1975. Evidence that uridine incorporation is not a selective marker for mouse lymphocyte subclasses. *J. Immunol.* 115 (3): 739.

54. Hall, J. G., and Morris, B. 1962. The output of cells in lymph from the popliteal node of sheep. *Quart. J. Exp. Physiol.* 47: 360.

55. Hall, J. G., and Morris, B. 1963. The lymph-borne cells of the immune response. *Quart. J. Exp. Physiol.* 48: 235.

56. Hall, J. G., and Morris, B. 1964. Effect of X-irradiation of the popliteal lymph-node on its output of lymphocytes and immunological unresponsiveness. *Lancet* i: 1077.

57. Hall, J. G., and Morris, B. 1965. The immediate effect of antigens on the cell output of a node. *Brit. J. Exp. Path.* 46: 450.

58. Hall, J. G., and Morris, B. 1965. Origin of the cells in the efferent lymph from a single lymph node. *J. Exp. Med.* 121: 901.

59. Hall, J. G., Morris, B., Moreno, G. D., and Bessis, M. C. 1967. The ultrastructure and function of the cells in lymph following antigenic stimulation. *J. Exp. Med.* 125: 91.

60. Hall, J., Scollay, R., and Smith, M. 1976. Studies on the lymphocytes of sheep. I. Recirculation of lymphocytes through peripheral lymph nodes and tissues. *Eur. J. Immunol.* 6: 117.

61. Hay, J. B., Cahill, R. N. P., and Trnka, Z. 1974. The kinetics of antigen-reactive cells during lymphocyte recruitment. *Cell. Immunol.* 10: 145.

62. Henney, C. S. 1975. T cell mediated cytolysis: consideration of the role of a soluble mediator. *J. Reticuloend. Soc.* 17: 231.

63. Hibbs, J. B. 1975. Activated macrophages as cytotoxic effector cells. I. Inhibition of specific and non-specific tumor resistance by Trypan Blue. *Transplantation* 19: 77.

64. Hibbs, J. B. 1975. Activated macrophages as cytotoxic effector cells. II. Requirement for local persistance of inducing antigen. *Transplantation* 19: 81.

65. Hollingsworth, J. W., Carr, J., and Ford, W. L. 1972. Lymphopenia produced by polyethylene-^{32}P strip applied to the rabbit appendix. *Cell. Immunol.* 4: 407.

66. Howard, J. C. 1972. The life-span and recirculation of marrow-derived small lymphocytes from rat thoracic duct. *J. Exp. Med.* 135: 185.

67. Howard, J. C., Hunt, S. V., and Gowans, J. L. 1972. Identification of marrow-derived and thymus-derived small lymphocytes in the lymphoid tissue and thoracic duct lymph of normal rats. *J. Exp. Med.* 135: 200.

68. Howard, J. C., and Scott, D. W. 1972. The role or recirculating lymphocytes in the immunological competence of rat bone marrow cells. *Cell. Immunol.* 3: 421.

69. Hunt, S. V., Ellis, S. T., and Gowans, J. L. 1972. The role of lymphocytes in antibody formation. IV. Carriage of immunological memory by lymphocyte fractions separated by velocity sedimentation and on glass bead columns. *Proc. Roy. Soc. B.* 182: 211.

70. Jaroslow, B. N., Suhrbier, K. M., Fry, R. J. M., and Tyler, S. A. 1975. In vitro suppression of immunocompetent cells by lymphomas from aging mice. *J. Natl. Cancer Inst.* 54: 1427.

71. Klinman, N. R., and Press, J. L. 1975. The B cell specificity repertoire: its relationship to definable subpopulations. *Transplant. Rev.* 24: 41.

72. Koburg, E. 1967. Cell production and cell migration in the tonsil *in* H. Cottler, N. Odentchenko, R. Schindler, C. C. Congdon (eds.), *Germinal Centers in Immune Responses*, p. 176. Springer, Berlin.

73. Koster, F. T., McGregor, D. D., and Mackaness, G. B. 1971. The mediator of cellular immunity. II. Migration of immunologically committed lymphocytes

into inflammatory exudates. *J. Exp. Med.* 133: 400.

74. Koster, F. T., and McGregor, D. D. 1971. The mediator of cellular immunity. III. Lymphocyte traffic from the blood into the inflamed peritoneal cavity. *J. Exp. Med.* 133: 864.

75. Laurence, J. C., Hamaoki, T., and Kitagawa, M. 1976. Proliferative responses of T lymphocytes to allogeneic tumor without generation of killer T lymphocytes in the presence of Ehrlich ascites tumor fluid. *Gann* 67: 417.

76. Lieberman, R., Wybran, J., and Epstein, W. 1975. The immunologic and histopathologic changes of BCG-mediated tumor regression in patients with malignant melanoma. *Cancer* 35: 756.

77. Lubaroff, D. M. 1973. Cellular requirements for the rejection of skin allografts in rats. *J. Exp. Med.* 138: 331.

78. McCarthy, R. E., Coffin, J. M., and Gates, S. L. 1968. Selective inhibition of the secondary immune response to mouse skin allografts by cell-free Ehrlich ascites carcinoma fluid. *Transplantation* 6: 737.

79. McGregor, D. D., and Gowans, J. L. 1963. The antibody response of rats depleted of lymphocytes by chronic drainage from the thoracic duct. *J. Exp. Med.* 117: 303.

80. McGregor, D. D., Koster, F. T., and MacKaness, G. B. 1971. The mediator of cellular immunity. I. The life-span and circulation dynamics of the immunologically committed lymphocyte. *J. Exp. Med.* 133: 389.

81. Miller, J. F. A. P., and Mitchell, G. F. 1971. Antigen-induced selective recruitment of circulating lymphocytes. *Cell. Immunol.* 2: 171.

82. Mitchell, J. 1973. Lymphocyte circulation in the spleen. Marginal zone bridging channels and their possible role in cell traffic. *Immunol., Lond.* 24: 93.

83. Moloney, J. B. 1966. Virus-induced rhabdomyosarcoma of mice. *Natl. Cancer Inst. Monogr.* 22: 139.

84. Mongini, P. K. A., and Rosenberg, L. T. 1975. Inhibition of lymphocyte trapping by cell-free ascitic fluids cultivated in syngeneic mice. *J. Immunol.* 114: 650.

85. Motoki, H., Kamo, I., Kikuchi, M., Ono, V., and Ishida, N. 1974. Purification of an immunosuppressive principle derived from Ehrlich carcinoma cells. *Gann* 65: 269.

86. Nieuwenhuis, P., and Ford, W. L. 1976. Comparative migration of B- and T-lymphocytes in the rat spleen and lymph nodes. *Cell. Immunol.* 23: 254.

87. Nitta, K., and Umezawa, H. 1975. Presence of immunosuppressive agents with various activities in Ehrlich ascites fluid. *Gann* 66: 459.

88. Ogura, T., Azuma, I., Nishikawa, H., Namba, M., Hirao, F., and Yamamura, Y. 1975. Effect of oil-attached BCG cell wall on the kinetics of lymphocytes in the draining lymph node. *Gann* 66: 349.

89. Paranjpe, M. S., and Boone, C. W. 1975. Specific depression of the antitumor cellular immune response with autologous tumor homogenate. *Cancer Res.* 35: 1205.

90. Parish, C. R., and Hayward, J. A. 1974. The lymphocyte surface. II. Separation of Fc receptor, C3 receptor and surface Ig-bearing lymphocytes. *Proc. Roy. Soc. B.* 181: 65.

91. Perlmann, P., Perlmann, H., Larsson, A., and Wahlin, B. 1975. Antibody

dependent cytolytic effector lymphocytes (K cells) in human blood. *J. Reticuloendoth. Soc.* 17: 241.

92. Raff, M. C., and Cantor, H. 1971. Subpopulation of thymus cells and thymus derived lymphocytes, *in* B. Amos (ed.), *Progress in Immunology*, Vol. 1, p. 83. Academic Press, New York.

93. Romball, C. G., and Weigle, W. O. 1976. Modulation of regulatory mechanisms operative in the cyclical production of antibody. *J. Exp. Med.* 143: 497.

94. Ropke, C., Hougen, H. P., and Everett, N. B. 1975. Long-lived T and B lymphocytes in the bone marrow and thoracic duct lymph of the mouse. *Cell. Immunol.* 15: 82.

95. Roth, J. A., Golub, S. H., Holmes, E. C., and Morton, D. L. 1975. Effect of Bacillus Calmette-Guerin immunotherapy on tumor antigen-induced lymphocyte stimulated protein synthesis in melanoma patients. *Surgery* 78: 66.

96. Rowley, D. A., Gowans, J. L., Atkins, R. C., Ford, W. L., and Smith, M. E. 1972. The specific selection of recirculating lymphocytes by antigen in normal and pre-immunized rats. *J. Exp. Med.* 136: 499.

97. Ruckdeschel, J. C., Codish, S. D., Stranahan, A., and McKneally, M. F. 1972. Postoperative empyema improves survival in lung cancer. *N. Engl. J. Med.* 287: 1013.

98. Schrader, J. W., and Vadas, M. 1976. Differences between virgin and memory IgM-antibody-forming cell precursor B-cells, and correlations with the heterogeneity present in B-cell populations from un-immunized mice. *Cell. Immunol.* 21: 217.

99. Scott, D. W., and Howard, J. C. 1972. Collaboration between thymus-derived and marrow-derived thoracic duct lymphocytes in the hemolysin response of the rat. *Cell. Immunol.* 3: 430.

100. Severson, C. D., Blaschke, J. W., and Thompson, J. S. 1976. Isolation of human B cells utilizing dextran to enhance T cell rosette formation. *Transplantation* 21: 340.

101. Shellam, G. R. 1971. Mechanism of induction of immunological tolerance. VII. Studies of adoptive tolerance to flagellin. *Int. Arch. Allergy* 40: 507.

102. Simic, M. M., and Petrovic, M. Z. 1967. Effects of local irradiation of the spleen on the primary response in rats, *in* H. Cottier, N. Odentchenko, R. Schindler, C. C. Congdon (eds.), *Germinal Centers in the Immune Response*, p. 240, Springer-Verlag, New York.

103. Simpson, E., and Cantor, H. 1975. Regulation of the immune response by subclasses of T lymphocytes. II. The effect of adult thymectomy upon humoral and cellular responses in mice. *Eur. J. Immunol.* 5: 337.

104. Sprent, J. 1973. Migration of T and B lymphocytes in the mouse. I. Migratory properties. *Cell. Immunol.* 7: 10.

105. Sprent, J. 1976. Fate of H2-activated T lymphocytes in syngeneic hosts. I. Fate in lymphoid tissues and intestines traced with ³H-thymidine, ¹²⁵I-deoxyuridine and ⁵¹chromium. *Cell. Immunol.* 21: 278.

106. Sprent, J., and Lefkovits, I. 1976. Effect of recent antigen priming on adoptive immune responses. IV. Antigen-induced selective recruitment of recirculating lymphocytes to the spleen demonstrable with a microculture system. *J.*

Exp. Med. 143: 1289.

107. Sprent, J., and Miller, J. F. A. P. 1973. Effect of recent antigen priming on adoptive immune responses. I. Specific unresponsiveness of cells from lymphoid organs of mice primed with heterologous erythrocytes. *J. Exp. Med.* 138: 143.

108. Sprent, J., and Miller, J. F. A. P. 1976. Fate of H2-activated T lymphocytes in syngeneic hosts. II. Residence in recirculating lymphocyte pool and capacity to migrate to allografts. *Cell. Immunol.* 21: 303.

109. Sprent, J., and Miller, J. F. A. P. 1976. Fate of H2-activated T lymphocytes in syngeneic hosts. III. Differentiation into long-lived recirculating memory cells. *Cell. Immunol.* 21: 314.

110. Sprent, J., Miller, J. F. A. P., and Mitchell, G. F. 1971. Antigen induced selective recruitment of recirculating lymphocytes. *Cell. Immunol.* 2: 171.

111. Strober, S. 1969. Initiation of antibody responses by different classes of lymphocytes. I. Types of thoracic duct lymphocytes involved in primary antibody responses of rats. *J. Exp. Med.* 130 (4): 895.

112. Strober, S. 1970. Initiation of antibody responses by different classes of lymphocytes. III. Differences in the proliferative rates of TDL involved in primary and secondary responses. *J. Immunol.* 105: 734.

113. Strober, S. 1972. Initiation of antibody responses by different classes of lymphocytes. V. Fundamental changes in the physiological characteristics of virgin thymus-independent ("B") lymphocytes and "B" memory cells. *J. Exp. Med.* 136: 851.

114. Strober, S. 1975. Immune function, cell surface characteristics and maturation of B cell subpopulations. *Transplant. Rev.* 24: 84.

115. Strober, S. 1975. Maturation of B lymphocytes in the rat. II. Subpopulations of virgin B lymphocytes in the spleen and thoracic duct lymph. *J. Immunol.* 114: 877.

116. Strober, S. 1976. Maturation of B lymphocytes in rats. III. Two subpopulations of memory B cells in the thoracic duct lymph differ by size, turnover rate, and surface immunoglobulin. *J. Immunol.* 117: 1288.

117. Strober, S., and Dilley, J. 1973. Biological characteristics of T and B memory lymphocytes in the rat. *J. Exp. Med.* 137: 1275.

118. Strober, S., and Dilley, J. 1973. Maturation of B lymphocytes in the rat. I. Migration pattern, tissue distribution and turnover rate of unprimed and primed B lymphocytes involved in antidintrophenyl response. *J. Exp. Med.* 138: 1331.

119. Strober, S., and Law, L. W. 1971. Initiation of antibody responses by different classes of lymphocytes. IV. Lymphocytes involved in the primary antibody response to a Hapten-protein conjugate. *Immunol.* 20: 831.

120. Taliaferro, W. H., and Taliaferro, L. G. 1956. X-ray effects on hemolysin formation in rabbits with spleen shielded or irradiated. *J. Infect. Dis.* 99: 109.

121. Taub, R. N., and Gershon, R. K. 1972. The effect of localized injection of adjuvant material on the draining lymph node. III. Thymus dependence. *J. Immunol.* 108: 377.

122. Taub, R. N., Krantz, A. R., and Dresser, D. W. 1970. The effect of localized injection of adjuvant material on the draining lymph node. I. Histology. *Immunology* 18: 171.

123. Taub, R. N., and Lance, E. M. 1968. Effects of heterologous anti-lymphocyte serum on the distribution of ^{51}Cr-labeled lymph node cells in mice. *Immunology* 15: 633.

124. Tilney, N. L. 1971. Patterns of lymphatic drainage in the adult laboratory rat. *J. Anat.* 109: 369.

125. Waksman, B. H. 1973. The homing pattern of thymus-derived lymphocytes in calf and neonatal mouse Peyer's patches. *J. Immunol.* 111: 878.

126. Werdelin, O., Foley, P. S., Rose, N. R., and McCluskey, R. T. 1971. The growth of the cell population in the draining popliteal lymph node of rats injected with rat adrenal in Freund's adjuvant. *Immunol.* 21: 1054.

127. Woodruff, J. J. 1974. Role of lymphocyte surface determinants in lymph node homing. *Cell. Immunol.* 13: 378.

128. Woodruff, J., and Gesner, B. M. 1968. Lymphocytes: Circulation altered by trypsin. *Science* 161: 176.

129. Woodruff, J. J., and Gesner, B. M. 1969. The effect of neuraminidase on the fate of transfused lymphocytes. *J. Exp. Med.* 129: 551.

130. Woodruff, J. F., and Woodruff, J. J. 1972. Virus-induced alterations of lymphoid tissues. II. Lymphocyte receptors for Newcastle disease virus. *Cell. Immunol.* 5: 296.

131. Woodruff, J. J., and Woodruff, J. F. 1972. Virus-induced alterations of lymphoid tissues. III. Fate of radiolabelled thoracic duct lymphocytes in rats inoculated with Newcastle disease virus. *Cell. Immunol.* 5: 307.

132. Yamazaki, H., Nitta, K., and Umezawa, H. 1973. Immunosuppression induced with cell-free fluid of Ehrlich carcinoma ascites and its fractions. *Gann* 64: 83.

133. Zatz, M. M. 1976. Effects of BGG on lymphocyte trapping. *J. Immunol.* 116: 1587.

134. Zatz, M. M., and Gershon, R. K. 1974. Thymus dependence of lymphocyte trapping. *J. Immunol.* 112: 101.

135. Zatz, M. M., and Gershon, R. K. 1975. Regulation of lymphocyte trapping: the negative trap. *J. Immunol.* 115: 450.

136. Zatz, M. M., and Lance, E. M. 1970. The distribution of chromium ^{51}Cr-labelled lymphoid cells in the mouse: a survey of anatomical compartments. *Cell. Immunol.* 1: 3.

137. Zatz, M. M., and Lance, E. M. 1971. The distribution of ^{51}Cr-labelled lymphocytes into antigen-stimulated mice, lymphocyte trapping. *J. Exp. Med.* 134: 224.

138. Zatz, M. M., and Lance, E. M. 1971. Lymphocyte trapping in tolerant mice. *Nature New Biol.* 234: 253.

139. Zatz, M. M., White, A., and Goldstein, A. L. 1973. Alterations in lymphocyte populations during tumorigenesis. I. Lymphocyte trapping. *J. Immunol.* 111: 706.

CHAPTER 6

EVIDENCE FOR ORGAN SPECIFICITY OF DEFENSES AGAINST TUMORS

Arnold E. Reif

Mallory Institute of Pathology
Boston City Hospital
and the Department of Pathology
Boston University School of Medicine
Boston, Massachusetts 02118

An understanding of defenses against initiation of tumors is basic both for prevention and for therapy of cancer. Burnet and Good have maintained that immune surveillance eliminates most incipient cancer clones. Prehn believes that immune surveillance is ineffective in clinically relevant situations. This apparent contradiction can be resolved by the concept that immune defenses against tumors may be either systemic, or organ specific, or both. Systemic effects can be directed against viral or against tumor cell-associated antigens. Organ-specific immunity against tumors, possible since most organs possess private as well as systemic defenses, appears more important.

Then I beheld all the work of God:
... Though a wise man think to know it
Yet shall he not be able to find it.

—Ecclesiastes 8: 17

Historical

As recently as 1958, the leading theory of cancer causation was somatic mutation (266). Today, somatic mutation is still accepted as a possible mechanism for radiation carcinogenesis, but chemical carcinogenesis is thought to occur more usually by the direct interaction of the "ultimate" carcinogen with DNA, and possibly even with RNA (211, 281). Further, the role of DNA and RNA viruses in the causation of certain mammalian neoplasms in species other than man is almost universally accepted (53, 126, 189). In the future, contemporary hypotheses on immune surveillance against tumors seem likely to suffer the same fate as the theory of somatic mutation. No matter, as long as these hypotheses have elicited new experimental work or new ideas that will eventually prove useful for the prevention or therapy of cancer.

ORIGINS OF THE THEORY OF IMMUNE SURVEILLANCE.
Paul Ehrlich in 1909 first proposed the concept that the host possesses immune surveillance against cells or tissues which, arising newly in the body, are recognized as foreign and destroyed (77). Fifty years later, Lewis Thomas reintroduced this concept (316). Despite the paucity of hard experimental data available, few subjects have been reviewed as frequently in the modern medical literature. For it is virtually impossible to review tumor immunology without touching upon the central question of immune surveillance.

GREEN'S IMMUNOLOGICAL THEORY OF CANCER. I still
remember seeing Professor Green browsing through the bookstore at Moscow's Ukraine Hotel during the 8th International Cancer Congress in 1962. A studious, slight, and reticent man ahead of his time, his immunological theory of cancer largely failed to win the recognition it deserved, at least during his lifetime. First proposed by him in 1954 (122) and elaborated in his posthumous book of 1967, coauthored by Anthony,

Baldwin, and Westrop (123), his theory's central theme was that "malignant cells *are* malignant because they have lost tissue-specific antigens and are no longer subject to tissue-homeostatic control mechanisms" (123).

As it turned out, Green was partly right. Since then, few types of tumors have been studied antigenically without finding the diminution or lack of some of the antigens present in the normal tissue of origin (181, 230, 274, 300, 346). One reason for this loss of antigens could be dedifferentiation of cells, and this would have exactly the effect Green proposed. Another reason not mentioned by Green could be the development of neoplastic potential in a single cell type that differs both functionally and antigenically from cells that appear to be identical when examined under the microscope; this is certainly true for globulins produced by plasmacytomas. In fact, we have only become aware of the kaleidoscopic diversity of normal plasma cells through the study of plasma cell clones that have been vastly expanded because they have become malignant (23). Thirdly, antigenic loss in tumor cells could also occur because of tumor development in a stem cell, which may be a likely event (243): the stem cell may not yet have differentiated sufficiently to acquire an adult complement of tissue-specific antigens.

FURTH'S THEORY OF HORMONAL PROMOTION.   An early and influential view of neoplasia was suggested by Furth as early as 1953 (99). Furth, working with mice, found that destruction of the thyroid causes pituitary tumors. Such tumors resembled normal cells both histologically and functionally. After several passages, the tumor cells lost their responsiveness to growth inhibition by thyroid hormone and acquired the ability to grow continuously without it (autonomy). He believed hormones acted merely as powerful promoters (or, on occasion, as inhibitors) of neoplasia, which made possible the emergence of latent tumor cells that had already undergone the primary carcinogenic change in their DNA (100, 101).

THEORIES OF NORMAL GROWTH CONTROL AND TUMOR DEVELOPMENT.   By 1967, Green and his collaborators had incorporated into their thinking most of the intervening conceptual advances (137, 140, 145, 171, 229, 305, 346, 347). Perhaps the most interesting of these were theories that accounted for normal growth control, and included tumor development as a special case. These have recently been reviewed in detail by Burch (37). A brief description is necessary to gain a full understanding of contemporary thinking.

Tyler suggested in 1946 that growth was analogous to antibody formation as depicted by the instructive theory, which was in vogue at that time (324). According to Tyler, each cell contains both "antigens" and "antibodies." While all "antigens" are present in all cells, the quantities differ greatly, depending upon the location of the cell and the organ in which it is found. Differences in rate of production of "antigens" cause the differentiation of a given tissue. While these details may sound unconvincing today, his theory of cancer is still of great interest: he believed that aberrant (mutated) cells attack the host (324, 325). The same idea has been advanced recently to explain the development of neoplasia in *lymphoid* cells (112, 286). Also, the concept that nonlymphoid cells can mount an attack on other cells is again in fashion. Tumor cells have long been known to produce "toxohormone." In modern terms, this means that tumor cells shed antigens that block lymphoid responses to the tumor, plus proteolytic or fibrinolytic enzymes (and enzyme activators such as plasminogen activator) which can facilitate invasion by tumor cells. Also, we now know that certain nonlymphoid cells, such as fibroblasts, and kidney and lung cells, can secrete plasminogen activator.

In his later theory of cancer, Tyler supposed that tumor cells arise from a single cell that has lost a gene which specifies one or more cell surface antigens. Since in his theory *all* cells are immunocompetent, the mutated cell is continuously immunostimulated by the cell surface antigens it has lost (and now recognizes as "foreign" in its host). This immunostimulation causes continuous growth of the tumor cell (216, 326).

Weiss' template-antitemplate theory of growth of 1950 differed from Tyler's theory principally in assuming that cell "antigens" (now called "templates") are diffusible, a property that Tyler already assumed to hold for antibodies (now called "antitemplates"). In Weiss' theory, growth stops when intra- and extra-cellular concentrations of antitemplates are in equilibrium. The theory invoked the concept of negative feedback for control of normal growth (323).

Druckrey's theory of 1959 for the first time included the idea that "higher" regulating centers can produce *stimulators* of growth, in addition to assuming that the *deficiency* of an *inhibitor* alone can stimulate growth (75). Experimental evidence that mitotic inhibitors ("chalones") exist *in vivo* was later provided by Bullough *et al.* (34, 36).

Burwell in 1963 advanced a theory of growth (47) that was later developed with Burch into a unified theory of growth and disease (38, 47). The basic suggestion was that lymphoid cells are the "central" tissue that control the growth of all body cells. The complicated details of Burwell's early theory (47) have recently been simplified by Burch (37). Burch's theory (37) represents yet another step forward in our understanding of growth and cancer, yet it still falls short of explaining these mysteries satisfactorily.

KLEIN'S SURVEILLANCE SYSTEM. By 1965, Klein had used the term "surveillance system" for mechanisms involved with inhibition or elimination of aberrant cells (123). At that point, he was not convinced of their immunologic nature, although he thought that surface recognition factors were of fundamental importance. He did not think it was possible to draw a clear line of distinction between the types of recognition involved in mitotic control, in elimination of aberrant cells, in cellular reactivity and in antibody production (123, 170).

GREEN'S LATER IMMUNOLOGICAL THEORY OF CANCER.

By 1967, Green and collaborators had incorporated into their thinking (123) the ideas and new experimental findings of the intervening years (see above). Green believed that, under normal conditions, the presence of tumor-specific antigens on some types of tumor cells would inhibit the outgrowth of the tumor cells, which is a basic tenet of later theories of immune surveillance. He also foreshadowed Prehn's later point of view (13, 251, 258) with the remark that "under some conditions, an immune reaction (to an antigenic alteration of a cell component altered during the course of carcinogenesis) may *hasten* carcinogenesis by stimulating the adaptive loss of the component concerned, in much the same way as bacteria adapt to a hostile environment" (123). This latter idea was later expanded into the concept of antigenic modulation by Old and Boyse (231). The views of Green and his collaborators on autoimmunity and cancer (123) were, first, that autoimmune diseases are precancerous and predispose to malignancy; this concept has since been refined by Schwartz to apply only to lymphoid neoplasms (260, 284). Secondly, Green and his collaborators (123) maintained that tumors may be accompanied by lesions at distant sites unaffected by metastases, lesions that are allergic in nature and represent host response to the tumor—an idea that has since been confirmed, at least in one system (69).

BURNET'S THEORY OF IMMUNOLOGICAL SURVEILLANCE.

Following a number of outstanding reviews between 1964 and 1970 (69, 137, 140, 145, 171, 172, 174, 192, 209, 229, 299, 305, 306, 346, 347), interest in immune surveillance peaked in 1970 with the publication of Burnet's book (44), as well as the proceedings of a symposium on this topic (300). Burnet's theory explains surveillance as follows.

Tumors are initiated in hosts with inadequate immune status through one or more random genetic changes that take place in somatic cells. If viruses are the causative agent for the genetic change, virus-specific cell surface changes are induced. If the initiating agent is chemical or radiation, the presence of minor antigens restricted to individual or to a few cells of the host permits these antigens to be recognized as aberrant as soon as their concentration rises above a threshold necessary for their immunologic detection, as the tumor cells multiply. The normal course of events is the elimination of these aberrant cells by a mechanism essentially identical with delayed hypersensitivity. Thymus-dependent (T) lymphocytes control this mechanism. As the thymus atrophies with increasing age, or if the tumor cells have a low degree of antigenicity, immune surveillance may prove insufficient to prevent the escape of tumor cells and the development of overt malignancy.

Burnet's theory has been criticized strongly by a number of investigators including Prehn (13, 251, 252, 253, 254, 255, 256, 258) and Schwartz (286) for assuming that systemic immune surveillance is highly effective in prevention of tumors, which they believe is false. Burch feels that Burnet has failed to discuss how surveillance is possible in the numerous tissues that lie behind blood-tissue barriers (37). An extensive discussion of Burnet's theory is available (300).

BURWELL-BURCH THEORY OF NORMAL GROWTH, DISEASE, AND CANCER.

In its most recent form developed in Burch's book of 1976, the Burwell-Burch theory has grown into an ambitious attempt to arrive at a unified concept that will explain both normal growth and its abnormal manifestations, namely various diseases and cancer (37). As in previous theories, the principal assumption is that growth is regulated by feedback mechanisms that are comprised of antibodies and antigens (324, 343). It is assumed that antibodies (now called mitotic-control proteins, or MCPs) are elaborated only by the central control system (which is assumed to be the lymphoid cell system), rather than by all somatic cells as previously thought (75, 324). The antigens (now called tissue coding factors, or TCFs) are presumed to be present on the surface of all somatic cells (75, 324, 343). The same genes that code for a given antigen (TCF) also code for the corresponding specific antibody (MCP). Growth control is exercised by the same type of mechanism assumed to act in the previous theories: MCPs *inhibit* growth by binding to the target TCFs on somatic tissue cells; tissue cells secrete TCFs that bind to MCPs on the surface of the central control cells (lymphoid cells) and thereby *stimulate* the division of these cells, and thereby the output of MCPs. Homeostasis is maintained by such negative and positive feedback. The possibility that some TCFs can *stimulate* rather than inhibit the growth of target tissues is included in the theory, which therefore becomes sufficiently flexible that almost any biologic event can be accounted for. Autoimmune diseases are explained in current conventional terms (338, 339) as due to the reaction of immune competent lymphoid cells with normal body constituents that have undergone a slight antigenic change, but this explanation is couched in terms of TCFs and MCPs. Consideration of the age and sex distribution of various non-malignant diseases and of cancer cause Burch to conclude that they are identical processes that depend upon heritable genetic changes in stem cells or in other somatic cells for their initiation.

Burch's key concept is that nature generally chooses a single simple all-inclusive mechanism to accomplish her goals, rather than a multitude of different complicated ones. He has found that the age-related incidence of degenerative diseases is quite similar or identical with that of neoplastic diseases. Therefore, he thinks that the mechanism of the two types of diseases may be the same. Here he may have a brilliant point. The very latest data on the origin of atherosclerosis from the laboratory of E. P. Benditt indicates that atherosclerotic plaques from human arteries are composed of smooth muscle cells and often monoclonal in nature (16A). If such monoclonal growths are indeed benign tumors initiated by contact with carcinogens present in the circulation, as Benditt believes, then this degenerative disease is caused by a benign tumor and should indeed have the same age incidence as do other tumors. Burch, however, goes further. Based on a set of assumptions, he has evolved a mathematical model of the age incidence of tumors that will fit the human data. He tacitly assumes that such agreement proves his assumptions and his model are correct. This is false logic. In fact, a limitless number of mathematical models, each based on a different set of assumptions, can be invented to give equally good agreement with the data. All that we can be sure of is that no mechanism that *fails* to lead to the actual age-incidence relationship can be valid; but agreement validates neither the mechanism assumed nor the assumptions made (72). Further, Burch dismisses other theories because they will not fit the data; but it is Burch who makes the assumptions necessary to test these theories, and one wonders whether his assumptions are appropriate.

Finally, Burch assumes that the central lymphoid system controls the *growth* of *all* somatic cells, as well as *differentiation* and *surveillance* (37). We know too much regarding the complexities of hormonal growth control, and of hormonal interactions between different endocrine systems (198) to imagine that lymphoid cells could exercise dominant growth control, at least in endocrine organs. While lymphoid cells may have surveillance functions regarding the *extent* of differentiation in a given organ (see below), the actual *process* of differentiation seems to be concerned primarily with stem cells and hormonal control, not with lymphoid cells (58, 167). Few scientists remain who doubt that lymphoid cells are not concerned to some degree, at least, in surveillance. However, Burch dismisses other cancer theories because they will not fit his mathematical analysis. Here again, the additional assumptions he has made to construct a model that will test a given hypothesis may be wrong, and therefore his test would be invalid.

ATTACKS ON IMMUNE SURVEILLANCE. During the early 1970s, Klein (177, 178, 180, 181, 182) and Good (2, 105, 116, 117, 118) were the main proponents of the theory of immune surveillance against tumors, while Prehn began to play the role of the devil's advocate. His main thesis, which is discussed later, was that tumor-specific antigens may represent laboratory artifacts, and immunity to them may stimulate rather than retard tumors. Further, he believed that the antigenicity of most clinically relevant tumors was very low, and doubted that immune surveillance could play a major role in the destruction of incipient tumor clones (13, 251, 253, 254, 255, 256, 258). Many other reviewers have contributed much to a better understanding of host defenses against tumors (22, 29, 45, 46, 61, 132, 136, 165, 206, 213, 225, 227, 230, 301, 341). Still, the main disparities remain largely unresolved. A different hypothesis is here suggested to reconcile discordant views.

Organ-Specific Defenses Against Tumors

The suggestion that the main host defenses against the initiation of tumors might be organ-specific rather than systemic was presented as a lecture in 1973.[1] An outline of this concept was published in 1975 (268). A more thorough description is given here. It represents an attempt to provide a coherent explanation for the variety of evidence presently available that bears on host defenses against the initiation of tumors.

ORGAN SPECIFICITY OF LYMPHOID CELLS. Systemic immunity may be one of the main factors that determines whether a person develops cancer from opportunistic infections of certain oncogenic viruses, as suggested by the evidence accruing from cancer development in patients who have received long-term immunosuppressive therapy following a kidney allotransplant (see below). However, systemic immunity against many types of tumors that develop in man or are the subject of experimentation is surprisingly low (251, 252, 253, 254, 255, 256, 258). If it is agreed that the lymphoid system provides surveillance against living matter foreign to the genetic blueprint of the host (and there seems to be general agreement on this point), then we must take into account new evidence on the organ specificity of lymphocytes.

We now have firm evidence that both mouse and man possess many different types of lymphocytes (121, 183, 289). Studies of immunoglobulins secreted by plasma cells that have become neoplastic indicate that normal plasma cells secrete many distinct types of immunoglobulins (23) and it is only rarely, if ever, that a single plasma cell can be shown to secrete more than one type of immunoglobulin (296, 308). This indicates that many clones of plasma cells with distinct properties but apparently identical morphology exist in the body. More importantly, there is now incontrovertible evidence that different types of lymphocytes are present not only in lymphoid organs (115, 121, 318), but in many other organs (308, 318). Similarly, there is increasing evidence that there exists not one single type of macrophage, but several different types of macrophages or macrophage-like cells in lung, liver, peritoneal cavity, spleen, bone marrow and infiltrating tumors (321). Behind the blood-brain barrier, even brain has its own resident macrophages (28).

The evidence on heterogeneity in types of lymphocytes, plasma cells, and macrophages in the body points to the existence of organ-specific defense systems. The evidence that such organ-specific or "local" immunity really exists is now firmly established relative to organs where a specific immunoglobulin is locally synthesized, and local and peripheral levels of this immunoglobulin can be accurately measured. This is the case for IgA, which is secreted by local lymphoid cells in the salivary gland, lung, stomach, intestine, uterine tubes, endometrium, and cervix (319), and for IgE, which is secreted in the lymphoid tissues of tonsil, adenoid, bronchus and respiratory epithelium, gastrointestinal mucosa, spleen, and subcutaneous tissue (158). After infections of certain organs such as the respiratory tract, the local concentration of IgA far exceeds systemic concentrations (222, 318). IgE is the major, or perhaps only, human immunoglobulin capable of mediating reaginic hypersensitivity reactions, and is synthesized by lymphoid cells located in or adjacent to the body surfaces with which the sensitizing antigen makes first contact (158).

Perhaps more obviously, different organs possess quite different architecture. The spacial distribution of both the systemic lymphatic system and of the local lymphoid cells that may reside permanently in that organ also are characteristic for different organs. One possible interrelation between leukocytes in the *peripheral circulation,* in the *lymphatics,* and in *local* residence may be as follows. The prime function of the *circulation* is oxygen and metabolite transport; leukocytes are present in low proportion (approximately 1:1,000 erythrocytes) to maintain sterility. Because of the high rate of blood flow in some organs, and the low concentration of leukocytes, the *lymphatics* are necessary to permit inter-organ transport of leukocytes in sufficiently high concentration and at a sufficiently slow rate, to permit the proper "servicing" of the lymph nodes in the various organs. The *locally* resident leukocytes must fulfill the specialized functions that meet a particular organ's needs (as, for instance, IgA or IgE synthesis).

With regard to the surveillance function of locally resident lymphocytes (which may well include a portion of lymphocytes in the organ's lymph nodes), it seems to make good sense in terms of what we now know about tissue-specific antigens, that organ-adapted lymphoid cells would be required to detect aberrant cells in a given organ. A wide range of organ-specific antigens are now known to exist (161, 210). Further, histocompatibility antigens that play a major role in allograft rejection, H-2 in the mouse and HLA in man, have widely different organ distributions, as do the many other known alloantigens in mouse or man (161, 302, 303). Given a very slight antigenic alteration relative to surrounding cells, the probability that this would be detected by lymphoid surveillance cells already attuned to the local organ-specific antigenic environment seems far higher, than if circulating lymphoid cells were required to be effectors. Circulating lymphoid cells would be exposed to a multitude of different antigenicities in their passage through the body. Normally, they would not recognize any organ-specific antigens as "foreign," since they would be tolerant to them (338, 339). But the degree of antigenic aberration for this tolerance to be broken (17) would certainly be far smaller in locally acclimatized ("resident") lymphoid cells.

Evidence that delayed hypersensitivity and the arming of monocytes may take place within the tumor site comes from experimental studies (92, 93, 139). It is supported by increasing evidence that the lymph nodes that drain a tumor have a definite function with regard to limiting the metastasis of tumors (19, 92, 94, 103, 331). One of the responses of the host to malignant cells in the gastrointestinal tract is indeed an increase in the local secretion of IgA (195).

If lymphocytes are composed partly of resident and partly of systemic cells (and all gradations in between), then one would expect lymphocytes to home to non-lymphoid tissues. This has in fact been reported, giving further support to the concept of organ specific defenses (119).

ORGAN SPECIFICITY OF ONCOGENIC AGENTS. Much is known about the specificity of various oncogenic agents, and the reasons for such specificity is beginning to be understood. In the case of chemical carcinogens, the cause of the tissue specificity may be the preferential organ localization of the carcinogenic chemical or of the "ultimate carcinogen," or else the *presence* of carcinogen-activating enzymes, or the *absence* of carcinogen-inactivating enzymes in the susceptible organs (86, 211, 280, 281, 340). In the case of oncogenic viruses, organ specificity seems to be due to the preferential infection of certain cell types by certain oncogenic viruses (40, 126, 165). Once generated, metastases of chemically and virally induced leukemias tend to localize (or home) in the respective tissue of origin (155). This suggests that they are recognized as foreign and destroyed in other tissues by the resident lymphoid cells. The same inference comes from studies of tumor metastasis: far more tumor cells are shed into the circulation than establish "foreign colonies."

EFFECT OF DAMAGE TO INTEGRITY OF ORGAN ARCHITECTURE. If organ-specific immunity plays an important role in the initiation of many types of tumors, then disruption of the normal architecture of the organ, or the specific killing of "resident" lymphoid cells, should promote carcinogenesis. One type of disruption of normal architecture is implantation of a simple plastic film (foreign-body tumorigenesis). The process of tumorigenesis involves four distinct phases: (a) formation of a capsule around the foreign body, (b) fibrosis of the capsule, (c) dormancy of phagocytes attached to the foreign body, and (d) proliferation of preneoplastic cells on the surface of the foreign body (33, 96). The important point is that stage (c) involves inactivity of the macrophages. While the reasons for this inactivity are unknown, possible mechanisms might include constraint of movement through the fibrotic capsule, restriction to attack on a 2π- rather than 4π-front, or surface changes in preneoplastic cells following attachment to a flat surface.

In human beings, there is considerable evidence that bronchogenic carcinoma tends to develop at the site of repeated injury, for instance the bifurcation of bronchi or bronchioles against which inhaled aerosols impinge (32, 67). A combination of tissue damage and carcinogen has been shown to be optimal for experimental induction of bronchogenic carcinoma (190). Particularly effective for the induction of lung cancer in man is the combination of two types of carcinogens, each introducing its own characteristic tissue damage as well as its particular carcinogenic action. For instance, asbestos inhalation plus cigarette smoking (290), or uranium mining plus cigarette smoking (8, 9) are remarkably potent for carcinogenesis, and act synergistically.

Similar findings have been made for hepatoma. This cancer develops with relatively high frequency in persons with alcoholic cirrhosis, and generally begins within cirrhotic nodules (14). In experimental liver carcinogenesis with aflatoxin, damage to the liver architecture precedes the development even of preneoplastic foci and nodules (163).

In line with the above considerations, a typical sequence of events in chemical carcinogenesis consists of several stages, the first of which is degenerative (52). During this degenerative stage, relatively extensive necrosis proceeds in the area surrounding the implanted pellet. In this case, also, destruction of tissue architecture precedes the development of preneoplastic and eventually of neoplastic cells. A typical example of this is the implantation of a pellet of 9,10-dimethyl-1,2-benzanthracene (DMBA) in a rat salivary gland (51, 52).

Whether the target cells in *radiation carcinogenesis* are transformed by viruses or by radiation-induced mutation of DNA, at least at higher radiation doses the initial changes include disruption of normal tissue architecture. For instance, in dogs fed the bone-seeking radioisotopes radium (^{226}Ra) or else strontium-90 (^{90}Sr), the initial changes in bone are cortical sclerosis and thickening, fractures, osteolytic lesions and trabecular coarsening (214). These lesions parallel the changes seen following radium administration in man (84). Similar initial changes are observed in other types of radiation carcinogenesis (333). Because lymphoid cells are one of the most radiation-sensitive cells in the body, very significant eradication of "resident" lymphoid cells must take place at target organ doses above 1,000 rad (233, 327). This may explain why radiation, destructive both of organ architecture and of lymphoid cells, is an effective carcinogen in so many instances (56, 311, 328).

Do *oncogenic viruses* cause disruption of cell architecture or inactivation of "resident" lymphoid cells prior to oncogenesis? The thymic leukemia that is initiated by the Gross virus in AKR mice starts unilaterally in 95% of the mice that develop this neoplasm. First one lobe atrophies, while the other enlarges slightly. Most interesting for the present thesis, thymic leukemia *always* begins in the lobe that has atrophied (295). The same is true for thymic leukemias induced by the Friend and by the Rauscher virus (295). The closest candidate for a virally induced neoplasm in man is Burkitt's lymphoma (179). Damage to the reticuloendothelial system by an attack of malaria may be a necessary predisposition for the development of Bukitt's leukemia prior to infection with a nearly ubiquitous virus such as the herpes virus EBV, which may prove to be the etiologic agent (41, 179, 273). In this connection, it is relevant that *complete* herpes viruses have been claimed to be invariably lethal to the cells in which they multiply (273); this certainly suggests that such viruses possess the capability to damage the lymphoid system.

Causation of tumors as a result of *trauma* is a controversial subject (78, 104, 282). There can be no question, though, that "the potentiality of a burn scar to undergo malignant neoplastic degeneration, and the type of epithelioma resulting, are related to the extent of the surface involved and the depth of the burn" (104, 322). In terms of the present discussion, this fits well with the concept that the more severe the disruption of tissue architecture, the higher the possibility for tumor development. Based on a study of over 2,000 cases of skin cancer, 2% of all epidermoid carcinomas and 0.3% of all basal cell carcinomas originate on skin subjected to thermal injury (104, 322). The kangri burn cancer of the Indians and the kairo burn cancer of the Japanese are examples of chronic dermatitis due to contact with heated body-warmers that, in an appreciable number of persons, progress to frank neoplasm (104).

CELLS INVOLVED IN ORGAN-SPECIFIC DEFENSES. If the host defenses against many types of tumors are organ-specific rather than systemic, what are the mechanisms involved? Which are the effector cells or soluble factors? Is immunity involved or not? At present, it is not possible to give conclusive answers to these questions. However, simply the presence of many types of lymphoid cells in most tumors (21) strongly suggests that the effector cells are lymphoid cells.

A tumor is a complex structure consisting of malignant cells supported by stroma and by a vascular system, both made up of normal cells; in addition, normal inflammatory cells such as lymphocytes, polymorphonuclear leucocytes and macrophages are present (3). Also, a variety of other cells involved with inflammation or the repair of tissue injury may be present within or surrounding the tumor (21). Because of the tremendous complexity and diversity of different body tissues, it seems unlikely that precisely the same mechanism is active in all tissues. But various lines of evidence suggest that the macrophage (histiocyte), or rather the organ-specific resident macrophage (321), is an important effector cell for defense against initiation of tumors (21, 60, 71, 114, 139, 149, 245, 248).

ARE ORGAN-SPECIFIC DEFENSES IMMUNE OR NONIMMUNE? Experimental work suggests that even when macrophages have been activated *nonspecifically*, they kill neoplastic cells but not normal cells. This finding was made after *in vitro* stimulation of macrophages (83, 245), as well as after *in vivo* activation with a tumor plus BCG. In the latter situation, the macrophages were then nonspecifically cytotoxic against tumor other than that used for stimulation (83, 149). In contrast, recognition factors seem to be essential for macrophage surveillance (71, 83). In some instances, at least, such factors may be antibodies capable of "arming" macrophages or monocytes for specific reactivity against the tumor (3, 114, 139). In other systems, the recognition factors are heat-labile α_2-globulins (71). There is extensive evidence that such globulins can serve as immunoregulatory agents (60, 110).

In support of the above thesis, adjuvants such as BCG have been found to eradicate tumors as "innocent bystanders" (63). The opposite may also be true: immune destruction of tumor cells (mediated specifically) can leave unrelated "bystander" tumor cells intact (344). It therefore seems likely that specific antitumor attack is a more effective mechanism (if it can be invoked) than nonspecific attack, even for surveillance against incipient tumor cells.

NATURAL ANTIBODIES. We have seen that normal adult sera contain antibodies to Burkitt's lymphoma cells. These are presumably the result of specific immunization. Further, American blacks possess strong serum cytotoxicity against melanoma cells (143, 144); it seems possible that this antibody serves for prevention of melanoma, and is actively acquired. Any antibody that seems to appear fortuitously, in the sense that we are not sure how it was derived, is classified as a natural antibody. Such antibodies could perform surveillance functions by "arming" macrophages or other lymphoid cells.

Terasaki et al. have described natural antibodies in heterologous mammalian sera that react against the lymphocytes of other mammalian species (314). Such antibodies might result from stimulation by microbial antigens, which crossreact with the histocompatibility antigens of other species (314). Of even greater interest are natural antibodies that are present in inbred mouse strains and react against isologous tumor cells (16, 194, 244, 313).

Also of great interest are natural antibodies in human sera that bind to human tumor cells (25, 26, 157, 275). However, human sera may contain anti-HLA reactive antibodies which could produce the reactivity that is seen. Since such normal sera cannot be tested against isologous tumor, the precise meaning of such natural antibodies remains in doubt.

Thus, the results on the presence of natural antibodies to tumors in mice have not yet been duplicated in man. The tumors involved in the mouse work are leukemias (16, 244) or else RNA-virus-induced (194). before natural antibodies can be recognized as present. Thus, neuraminidase treatment of the target tumor cells, to increase their antigenicity, may be necessary to reveal the presence of natural antibodies (120, 147, 276, 292).

NATURAL CYTOTOXICITY OF LYMPHOCYTES. Several reports have claimed that lymphocytes show natural cytotoxicity against isologous tumors (124, 226, 291, 352). As in the case of natural antibodies, most of the reports involve leukemias as target cells (226, 291, 352). In some instances, this cytotoxicity may be due to lymphotoxin-like mediators that are not immunoglobulins (241).

EFFECT OF LOCAL IMMUNOSUPPRESSION OR IMMUNO-STIMULATION. If organ-specific immune defenses play a large role in the genesis of tumors, then organ-specific immune suppression should be effective in inducing tumors, and organ-specific immune stimulation should be effective protection against initiation of tumors or (possibly) against outgrowth of tumors. In this connection, the appearance of reticulum cell sarcoma at the site of injection of antilymphocyte globulin has been reported (62). Further, BCG, DNCB, and many other adjuvants presently used for immunotherapy of tumors are relatively ineffective unless applied at or close to the site of the tumor (31, 63, 169).

OTHER DEFENSE MECHANISMS.   Beyond cellular defenses against initiation of tumors—and these include not only lymphoid but fibroblastic cells responsible for walling off nests of certain tumors—a variety of noncellular defense mechanisms are relevant (7). These include tissue-specific chalones capable of inhibiting the mitotic activity of a given cell type, oncolytic α_1-lipoprotein with some specificity against transformed cells, as well as a number of nonspecific chemicals that promote the metabolism of the ultimate carcinogen or inhibit the action of carcinogens by capturing free radicals (7). Hormones, most of which show a high degree of tissue specificity, can be very effective in modifying the growth rate of sensitive tumors that have not yet progressed beyond response to the particular hormone (54, 208).

Systemic Defenses Against Tumors

The evidence for immune defenses against tumors can be broadly divided into the effects of immune deprivation, the effects of immune (or nonspecific) stimulation, and relevant information obtained from studies of the immunobiology of tumors. Perhaps the most definitive evidence concerns the effects of immune deprivation. The multifaceted data on immune deprivation in experimental animals and in man include the following subjects, which are taken up in order below: immune suppression of transplant recipients, immune suppression for other medical reasons, immune deficiency diseases, experimental immune deficiency, effects of young or old age, and systemic aspects of chemical and physical carcinogenesis. A summary of this data for man has been made previously (20, 48, 238, 240, 268, 271, 309, 334).

IMMUNE-SUPPRESSED PATIENTS.   Recipients of kidney allografts (homotransplants) receive immunosuppression to prevent rejection of the graft. Four to six percent of these patients develop lymphoid or epithelial tumors within 3 years (20, 48, 238, 240, 268, 271, 309, 334).

There is a 30-fold higher incidence of lymphomas and leukemias in transplant recipients compared to age-matched normal control subjects.

This incidence has been explained to be the result of chronic stimulation of the host's immune system by the foreign tissue introduced as the transplant (113, 254, 255, 284, 326). This seems to be a reasonable explanation; in fact, one of the reasons for the natural incidence of lymphoreticular neoplasms in the general population may be chronic immune stimulation, perhaps caused by long-standing infections (268). Both in the general population and in transplant recipients, infection by a virus with oncogenic potential and genetic predisposition seem to be additional requirements for tumor development (284, 113). Immune stimulation may serve to provide an adequate supply of target cells appropriate for oncogenic conversion by a latent virus, as well as a growth stimulus that will ensure the outgrowth of incipient neoplastic cells (111, 112, 113, 286).

Epithelial tumors and sarcomas are found about 50 times more frequently in transplant patients than in matched controls. This includes tumors of the skin, lip, cervix and abdominal organs. With chronic exposure to sun, a 14% incidence of skin cancers develops in transplant recipients (187, 334). This is over 100-fold higher than normal. The high incidence of epithelial tumors has been explained as an artifact due to incomplete reporting of incipient neoplasms in the general population, coupled with intense observation of transplant recipients (254, 255, 286). Such reasoning seems hardly sufficient to explain a 50-fold increase. Another attempt to explain this increase as unrelated to immune surveillance consists of maintaining that even untreated patients with kidney disease have a higher incidence of neoplasms: This argument founders on the probability that chronic kidney disease is of itself associated with reduced immune function. Another line of argument is to question why the incidence of sarcomas is so very high in renal transplant patients, yet the incidence of the commonest neoplasm of women, breast cancer, is not increased (286).

The present view that immune surveillance against tumors is primarily organ specific provides satisfactory answers to a surprising number of these questions. The increased incidence of leukemias and lymphomas has already been reasonably well explained by current theories (see above).

A novel explanation provided by the present view is that *the tissue in which immune suppression is taking place is the lymphoid tissue, and therefore primarily tumors of the lymphoid tissue would be expected to arise.* This is in fact what occurs (20, 48, 79, 113, 148, 238, 240, 254, 255, 271, 284, 310, 326, 334). With regard to the high incidence of sarcomas, reticulum cell sarcomas are really a form of malignant lymphoma, and therefore fall under the heading of lymphoid tumors (270). That only leaves the increased incidence of epithelial tumors for which to account. The current concept is that these tumors may be caused by "opportunistic" viruses, such as those of the Herpes family, which are very common in transplant recipients (240). Surveillance against opportunistic infection by such viruses would certainly be systemic in nature, and would be expected to be reduced by systemic immunosuppression. This explains the higher incidence of epithelial neoplasms. There would be little or no effect on immunity already established against viruses present before immunosuppression began; in mice, at least, breast tumor viruses are generally transmitted vertically.

An additional possibility is that systemic immunosuppression also causes organ-specific immune depletion in a manner dependent upon the particular agent used. However, there is currently no evidence that the type of epithelial tumor that develops in transplant patients depends upon the mode of immunosuppression used (240). Hence, it is doubtful that this possibility plays an appreciable role. Finally, it should be mentioned that misdiagnosis of certain undifferentiated tumors as of epithelial origin, whereas in fact they are reticulum cell sarcomas or fibrosarcomas, is not uncommon (50).

Other facets of immunosuppression require explanation (112, 113, 193, 239, 267, 285, 286, 294). First of all, are not all immunosuppressive agents carcinogenic? If so, is not the increased incidence of tumors in immunosuppressed patients explained by it? In the case of anti-lymphocyte serum (ALS) which has been used in many of the patients who developed tumors (148, 240), there is agreement that it is only immunosuppressive, not carcinogenic. Yet present evidence suggests that there is no difference in the type and number of tumors that develop in transplant patients who have received ALS (240). Thus, the undoubted carcinogenic properties of many immunosuppressive agents are not alone responsible for the increased tumor incidence (267, 285, 287, 294). Nor has methotrexate therapy for patients with psoriasis been remarkably oncogenic (11); however, the *pattern* of malignancies that develop is essentially the same as in immunosuppressed transplant recipients (20, 48, 238, 240, 268, 271, 309, 334); this suggests a common etiology.

The above discussion leaves in doubt whether the 4–6% incidence of tumors in transplant recipients is not due in part to the carcinogenic effects of the immunosuppressive drugs rather than systemic immunosuppression. What is the situation in cancer patients treated by chemotherapy with the same type of drugs? Here again, the situation is not clear-cut. Patients cured of squamous carcinomas possess a persisting high incidence of impaired cellular immunity (323). Further, the risk of second tumors in survivors of childhood cancer can be 20 times higher than normal (196); most of these survivors had had radiation, or treatment with a radiomimetic drug for therapy of their first cancer. Subsequent neoplasia developing in patients with chronic lymphocytic leukemia who had been treated with standard chemotherapeutic agents was approximately threefold that for age- and sex-matched controls (202).

Patients with leprosy have depressed immune reactivity. This is indicated by a decrease in circulating T lymphocytes, depressed lymphocyte transformation by phytohemagglutinin and depletion of lymphocytes in their lymph nodes. If systemic surveillance were a significant factor in tumor development, one might expect a higher tumor incidence in such patients (111, 112, 113, 261, 268). In a series of leprosy patients, most of whom were United States citizens, a precisely normal incidence of 16.9% tumors was claimed (261). In another series that (in contrast to the above study) included approximately 50% of patients with tuberculoid rather than just lepromatous leprosy, a questionably elevated 30% incidence of tumors was found (102). The present interpretation of these data is that leprosy patients do show an increased tumor incidence. The authors of the United States study (261) failed to correct for the fact that their subjects dying from diseases other than cancer averaged 60 years at death, compared to 72 years for the American population (329). The percentage of the United States population who dies of neoplasms (including lymphoid and hematopoietic tumors) before the age of 60 is 5.3% and before the age of 65 is 7.4%, compared to an overall incidence of 16.5% for all deaths in 1968 (329). Thus, the incidence of tumors in the U.S. study of leprosy patients (261) was at least twice that expected when a rough correction for the earlier age of deaths in leprosy patients is made. The much higher incidence of cancer deaths in the Japanese study (30%) also becomes more significant, since also in that study a comparison with age-matched controls was omitted (102). Finally, it should not be forgotten that the leprosy bacillus is closely related to the tubercle bacillus and BCG, which are immunostimulants.

The conclusion from the above data is that systemic immunosuppression has an appreciable (though by no means dramatic) effect on the incidence of tumors. Tumors develop at 20 to 50 or more times the normal rate in the tissue that is immunosuppressed, namely the lymphoid tissue. The cause may well be the derangement of normal feedback inhibition of cell proliferation. In addition, epithelial tumors are more frequent. The cause for this increase may be decreased systemic surveillance against infection by opportunistic oncogenic viruses.

TUMOR INCIDENCE IN ATHYMIC (NUDE) MICE. Those who argue against the reality of immune surveillance against tumors use data on athymic (nude) mice as a cornerstone of their position (31, 199, 204, 312). Their major errors seem to be: failure to take into account the short lifespan of athymic (nu/nu) mice, the question of whether athymic mice born to heterozygous (nu/+) mothers have not been exposed to thymic hormone during fetal life and, as a consequence, possess rudimentary thymus tissue, and the question of whether systemic T cell deficiency is of necessity relevant for organ-specific defenses against the initiation of tumors.

Regarding tumor development in nude mice, in a study "*equivalent* to lifetime observation in 1,700 mice," it was reported that no malignant neoplasms developed (279). The authors actually observed 2900 mice over the whole of their life span (approximately 7 months), and 7900 mice from birth to 3 months of age! Nevertheless, they concluded that their observations invalidated the theory of immune surveillance against tumors, since nude mice accept skin grafts from other mice, indicating a severe deficiency in delayed hypersensitivity reactions (279). Since the mean lifespan of bred females for 7 inbred mouse strains for which data are available for the latest period recorded, 1960–62 (278) was 582 days, the lifespan observed for the 2,900 mice that lived 7 months was equivalent to under 37% of the lifespan for normal mice. Since the number of people who develop tumors during the first 40% of their lifespan (by age 29) is under 0.5%, the authors' conclusion does not seem to be justified. In fact, a rudimentary T cell lymphocyte has been described in athymic mice, even in those born to nu/nu mothers. This suggests that the crucial step of differentiation by which multipotential stem cells become committed to the T pathway takes place outside the thymus and does not require its presence (272, 283). Further, athymic mice possess activated macrophages that are surprisingly effective for resistance to facultative intracellular bacteria such as *Brucella abortus* and *Listeria monocytogenes* (55). Thus, a variety of experimental findings regarding nude mice can be explained by the hypothesis that anti-tumor defenses against many types of tumors are mediated by null cells (147) or macrophages (150). Such findings include tumor induction with 3-methyl-cholanthrene, which proceeds at the same rate in athymic as in intact mice (312); low circulating antibody production to sheep erythrocytes in athymic mice (205); and nongenetic variability in susceptibility to oncogenesis (257). The last finding might be due to the presence of variable numbers of "activated" macrophages, depending upon individual exposure to bacteria and viruses endemic in the animal colony. As expertise in prolonging the life of athymic mice is obtained, the expected findings of greatly increased lymphoid neoplasms together with an only slightly increased epithelial tumor incidence may well be realized; such findings would then correspond to those in immunosuppressed transplant patients (see above), or to people with immune deficiency diseases (see below). The data obtained in athymic mice are valuable in ruling out conventional delayed hypersensitivity as a major mechanism by which mice reject incipient nonlymphoid neoplasia (30), and with it the likelihood that Burnet's theory of T cell dependent systemic surveillance has extensive relevance for defenses against tumors.

IMMUNE-DEFICIENCY DISEASES. Immune deficiency diseases include Bruton-type agammaglobulinemia, Hodgkin's disease, ataxia-telangiectasia, Wiskott-Aldrich syndrome, common variable immunodeficiency, Chediak-Higashi anomaly, DiGeorge syndrome, and others (2, 105, 116, 118). The incidence of leukemias and lymphomas is about 10%, and of epithelial tumors and sarcomas approximately 1% overall in these diseases (73, 106). Because this subject has been reviewed with exceptional depth and clarity (loc. cit.), the data will be examined here mainly for fit or misfit to the general hypothesis, that the risk of malignancy increases primarily in the tissue in which immune defenses have been disrupted.

As in the discussion of tumors in nude mice, the incidence of neoplasms in immune deficiency diseases is meaningless unless it is compared with incidence in age- and sex-matched controls. Because many of the patients live for less than twenty years, Gatti and Good have estimated that the incidence of malignancy in patients with primary immunodeficiencies is roughly 10,000 times that of the general population (106). In view of these statistics, a closer look at two of the above deficiency diseases seems in order.

Patients with infantile X-linked (Bruton-type) agammaglobulinemia lack humoral immunity (106). They do not make circulating antibodies in response to immunization with diphtheria, tetanus or typhoid antigens, and their immunoglobulin levels are extremely low. On the other hand, cell-mediated immunity and delayed hypersensitivity reactions are essentially normal (106, 116). Up to 1972, only some 50 patients with this type of disease had been discovered, and five of these (about 10%) had developed leukemia (116). Perhaps remarkable is the variability in cell type of these five leukemias: acute lymphocytic, lymphatic, chronic monomyelogenous, malignant lymphoma, and thymoma (106). Such different leukemias might result from chronic infection with viruses with oncogenic potential, against which antibodies constitute the usual host defense. If a particular type of differentiated lymphocyte responded to a particular infectious agent without being able to limit the agent's multiplication, the stage would be set for the continuous growth of that type of lymphocyte. This would constitute lymphoid neoplasia, and could occur in young patients—and most of these patients do die young. In contrast, an increase in epithelial tumors would be expected only if antibodies played the major role in protection against epithelial tumors, which is apparently not the case.

In contrast, ataxia-telangiectasia is a neurologic disease of childhood, which often begins with loss of muscular coordination as early as 6 months of age. The children with this disease usually have low IgA levels and varying inadequacies of their cell-mediated immunity (106). At least 10% of such children die with malignancies, of which epithelial tumors associated with organs that have resident IgA-producing lymphocytes constitute approximately half; the other half die with lymphomas (106, 131). In terms of the discussion of tumors in immunosuppressed patients, this is exactly what would be expected if this genetically mediated immune deficiency disease was functionally identical to medication-mediated immune deficiency.

TUMOR DEVELOPMENT IN THE YOUNG. Seven types of tumors have peak incidences between 2 and 5 years in early childhood: an epithelial tumor (Wilm's tumor), 3 types of sarcoma (embryonal rhabdomyosarcoma, neuroblastoma and osteogenic sarcoma), and 3 types of lymphoid tumors (acute lymphocytic leukemia, malignant lymphoma, and Burkitt's lymphoma). What is responsible for these age-related incidences?

First, animal experiments (201, 345) indicate that the very young have a strongly repressed primary and secondary antibody response (Fig. 1). Thus, infants are susceptible to infection by those bacteria or viruses, against which antibody response is a major defense (153, 249). This increased susceptibility relative to adults holds true for first contact with any antigen that has not previously been encountered.

Secondly, infants pass through a phase during the first few months or even years of life, during which they are particularly vulnerable to opportunistic infections. Protective antibodies pass from the circulation of the mother into the fetus, and protect the newborn. As such antibodies decline in the months after birth, they aid the infant to become actively immunized on contact with agents against which they react or cross-react. Until such active immunity against a variety of infectious agents has been produced, the infant is more susceptible to infection than at any other time in life. An illustration of acquisition of active immunity to an endemic virus is provided by the data on yellow fever (Table 1). Similarly, the data on serum antibody to Burkitt's lymphoma in the United States (Table 2) illustrate the fact that immunity (or cross-reacting immunity) to virally induced cell surface antigens is reduced in children. Interesting data on antibody to neuroblastoma cells are also available (144, 152, 234).

Thirdly, infants and adolescents are still growing and their tissues are still under the influence of hormones mediating development. Bone growth is particularly active during adolescence. It therefore seems more than coincidental that the early peak in osteogenic sarcoma incidence falls during this period of active bone growth (Fig. 2).

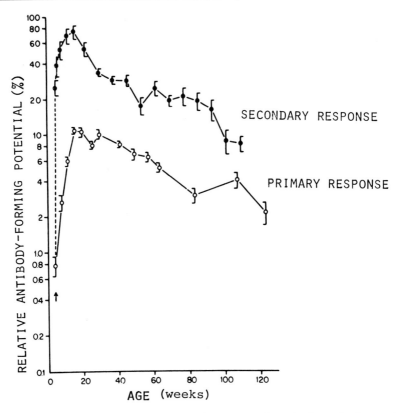

Fig. 1.   Change in the relative potential for formation of antibody with change in age of an inbred mouse strain (201). Reprinted by permission of Academic Press from Developmental Biology, Vol. 14: pgs. 96–111, Makinodan, T. and Peterson, W. J., © 1966, "Secondary anti-body forming potential."

Table 1.   Immunity to yellow fever in African lowlands[a]

Age, years	0–1	1–2	2–3	3–4	4–5
Per cent immune	0	2	20	45	70

a. Data of G. W. A. Dick, quoted by Haddow (130). From Burkitt, D. P. and Wright, D. H., 19–0 Burkitt Lymphoma, 1st Edition, Edinburgh, Churchill Livingstone.

Table 2.   Serum antibody to Burkitt's lymphoma cells in U.S.[a]

	Normal Children	Normal Adults	Burkitt's Lymphoma Patients
Fluorescent antibody, % positive	30–35	85–90	100
Complement fixation, % positive	15–20	60	92

a. Data of G. W. A. Dick, quoted by Haddow (130). From Burkitt, D. P., and Wright, D. H., 19–0 Burkitt Lymphoma, 1st Edition, Edinburgh, Churchill Livingstone.

The seven neoplasms mentioned above all have an early childhood peak and then increase again late in life, as do most neoplastic diseases (72). The biphasic age distribution of these tumors is a mirror image of the data on age distribution of antibody response (Fig. 1). Therefore, affected children may well possess a crucial immune defect or damage (41). Other lines of evidence support this possibility. Circumstantial evidence based on humoral and cellular immunity suggests that all the above "childhood tumors" may be of viral etiology (4, 5, 80, 81, 127, 128, 130, 162, 175, 176, 262, 263, 265). There is a large body of experimental evidence reviewed in the above references that indicates that immunosuppression greatly increases the likelihood of tumor development caused by infection with an oncogenic virus (for instance, 265). Further, oncogenic viruses per se may be immunodepressive (70).

Other lines of evidence that support the above view include evidence that many more infants develop incipient neoplasms of certain of the above tumors than eventually show clinical symptoms of disease. This would suggest that such tumors are relatively strong in antigenicity, and can therefore be rejected as a rule, acceptance being the exception. This explanation is supported by evidence on spontaneous remissions and regressions, and by the relative effectiveness of chemotherapy and immunotherapy (see below).

Autopsy studies done on infants who died for any reason between birth and 3 months of age show that incipient neuroblastomas occur 40 times more frequently than expected from clinical appearance of the disease (15). Thus, for every tumor that becomes clinically evident, there are 39 that disappear spontaneously or develop into a benign tumor (27).

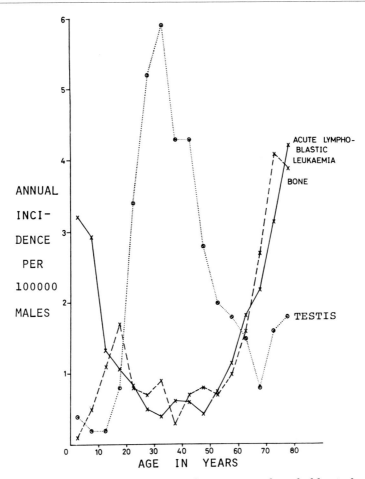

Fig. 2. Changes in cancer incidence with age: acute lymphoblastic leukemia, cancer of bone and testis. Data from England and Wales, 1960–62 (72). From *Cancer and Aging*, Skandia International Symposia (Almqvist & Wiksell International), Stockholm, 1968.

Thus, spontaneous regression of incipient neuroblastoma is frequent. As far as the spontaneous regression of *established* tumors is concerned, there have been 29 substantiated cases for Wilms tumor and 19 cases for various types of sarcomas, of which 8 were osteogenic sarcomas (85). The mean age of the 7 patients whose age was known was 19 years.

During the last five to ten years, dramatic improvements in survival of children and adolescents afflicted with each of the tumors mentioned

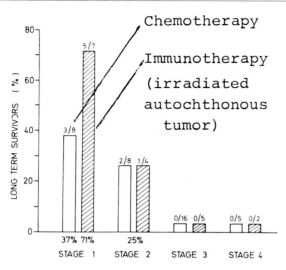

Fig. 3. Effect of chemotherapy alone, or chemotherapy plus immunotherapy, for treatment of Burkitt's lymphoma (57). From Burkitt, D. P. and Wright, D. H. *Burkitt Lymphoma,* First Edition, Edinburgh, Churchill Livingstone, Scotland.

above have been made (39, 57, 82, 146, 247, 320). Successful therapy has followed the general principle of reduction of tumor mass to the minimum possible (by use of surgery, or irradiation, or chemotherapy, as appropriate), followed at this point by intensive, aggressive courses of treatment with chemotherapy (sometimes intermittently with immunotherapy, as in Fig. 3), in an attempt to eradicate any remaining viable tumor cells (*loc. cit.*). A more likely mechanism for these successful cures is that the number of tumor cells that can be rejected successfully by the body (the "tumor rejection potential" [162]) is higher than for most types of *adult* malignancies. This would explain why very long-term remissions or outright cures in these childhood malignancies, when treated according to the above rationale, approximate 50%, while similarly aggressive treatment of adult malignancies is considerably less effective (*loc. cit.*). Nevertheless, there are several types of childhood tumors (myelocytic and monocytic leukemia, histiocytic lymphoma, malignant teratoma, and malignant brain tumors) that are still lethal in most children (247), possibly because they do not represent the relatively antigenic types that respond to aggressive therapy.

TUMOR DEVELOPMENT IN OLD AGE. In experimental animals, serum antibody production to a novel antigen is reduced in old age (see Fig. 1). The immunological defect responsible for this decreased humoral immunity in aged mice may be due to increased suppressor T cell activity (288). This may accord with an increase in thymus-derived cell frequency in senescent mice (259). The deficit in humoral immunity is apparently not due to B cell dysfunction (138). Old people possess increased levels of lymphocytotoxins (232).

With regard to cell-mediated immunity, lymphoid cells from aged mice give reduced graft-versus-host reactions (108, 168, 186, 336). Further, contact sensitivity to DNFB (2,4-dinitro-1-fluorobenzene) is not appreciably reduced in old BALB/c mice while it is impaired in old NZB/W mice (336). In line with these data, Gross has reported (125) a somewhat reduced response to skin sensitization with DNCB (2,4-dinitro-1-chlorobenzene) in old people (62% responders), compared to a control group 13 to 17 years old (97% responders).

Old age is accompanied by increase in certain immune phenomena such as autoantibody and immune complex disease (37, 200, 223). Hayflick has found that cultured embryonic tissue from mammalian species have a finite growth capacity that correlates well with mean maximum lifespan (141, 142). For human cells, this corresponds to about 50 population doublings. He believes that the ultimate death of a cell, or the loss or misdirection of its functional capacity, is a programmed event having a mean time of failure. Genetic instability as a cause of such age changes might include the progressive accumulation of faulty copying in dividing cells, or the accumulation of errors in information-containing molecules (141, 142).

In line with the above data and concepts, the incidence of tumors in old age can be explained by a combination of factors, including changes in tissue-specific defenses.

Carcinogens may well have a cumulative action (242) in the sense that stem cells (which may eventually become the progenitors of tumor cells [243]) may be caused to undergo heritable preneoplastic changes, producing cells more sensitive to later carcinogenic stimuli. Such changes may necessitate increased surveillance activity by resident lymphoid cells, which could be one reason for the finding of increased autoimmune reactions in aged animals and people. However, such surveillance would be less effective in aged tissues, because of (a) functional impairment of lymphoid cells by the type of cellular aging described by Hayflick, (b) physical impediment of macrophage movement by clogging of blood vessels, tissue scarring and cell depletion often associated with aging, and (c) formation of scar tissue somewhat analogous to the scar tissue that promotes foreign body carcinogesis, with the same end result. In addition, old age is associated with changes in hormone levels; recent work indicates that such changes serve to elicit outgrowth of hormone-unresponsive tumor cell clones (224).

If carcinogenesis is related to aging as described above, one would expect the application of a rapidly acting carinogen, such as DMBA (dimethylbenz-α-anthracene) to be more effective when painted on skin of old rather than of young mice. When DMBA was painted on skin grafted (either from old or from young mice) to young recipients, carcinomas developed on 39% of grafts from old donors and on 12% of grafts from young donors; also, the incidence of nonskin lymphoid tumors was highest in recipients bearing grafts from old donors (76). Similar results were obtained when a single dose of 3-methylcholanthrene was injected subcutaneously into C57BL mice of different ages: 100% of old mice, 96% of adult mice, but only 75% of weanling mice developed tumors at the site of injection (97). With regard to hormonal promotion of carcinogenesis by stimulating cell division, thereby facilitating the outgrowth of incipient neoplastic clones of cells, considerable evidence both in mouse and man supports this concept. For instance, mammary tumor induction by polycyclic aromatic hydrocarbons depends greatly on the frequency of mammary cell division at the time the carcinogen is applied (220).

Unhappily, such straightforward results (see above) are only obtained if relatively simple experimental systems are used. As soon as a carcinogen capable of tumorigenesis in a variety of tissues is chosen, and its action determined in mice of both sexes, various ages and several strains, complexities due to the interplay of many factors emerge. This is the case for ethylnitrosourea action, which generates a broad spectrum of tumors in mice (332). With this agent, newborn and infant mice responded more readily with liver, kidney and ovarian tumors than did young adults. Infants and young adults were more prone to stomach and lymphoreticular tumors than were newborns. Neurogenic tumors were observed most frequently in mice treated with carcinogen at birth. Mammary tumors developed most frequently in young adults, as did multiple lung tumors. Males developed liver tumors and females developed malignant lymphomas more frequently. The proportion of tumors that arose in different organs varied with the strain of mouse. The authors interpreted these results in terms entirely consistent with this review: that carcinogenesis is a multifaceted process, the outcome of which depends upon the interplay of a variety of modulating factors at the inception and/or during development of tumors. These factors included cell immaturity and replicating state, enzymatic competence if necessary for activation of the agent, hormonal environment, and finally the status of functional activity, genetic background, and immunological capability of the host (332).

The same type of complexities might well be expected to occur when the age at exposure to a carcinogen is varied in human beings. Most of the data available do show an increased risk with increase in age. Thus, the incidence of leukemia attributed to X-irradiation for treatment of ankylosing spondylitis rose from approximately 3 to 11 per 1000 patients, as the mean age at irradiation increased from 20 to 65 years (73). The incidence of cancer of the nasal sinuses from exposure at a nickel refinery rose fourfold between men whose age at first employment was 20 and those who were 35 or older. Similarly, increases in tumor incidence with age at first exposure have been noted for wart incidence from exposure to coal tar, lung cancer incidence in asbestos workers, and bladder cancer incidence from exposure to α- or β-naphthylamine or benzidine (73). On the other hand, leukemia incidence in the Japanese who survived the atomic bomb explosions at Hiroshima and Nagasaki was unrelated to age (73). Also, the risk of lung cancer development from cigarette smoking increases, the earlier smoking is started (134). However, the latter result is related to increased total carcinogen exposure, while the Japanese data suffer from uncertainties of dose estimation.

When the age incidence of various types of human tumors is examined, it is seen that cancer is generally a disease of old age. For tumors of the prostate, stomach, skin, rectum, pancreas, and esophagus, which are almost exclusively epithelial tumors or (in the real sense of the word) cancers, there is a dramatic increase of incidence with age (Fig. 4). This incidence can be represented by the equation

$$\text{incidence} = \text{const.} \times \text{age}^k$$

where the incidence is that which occurs at the stated age, and where k varies from 4.1 to 12.3 for these tumors (Fig. 5). The value of k is determined as the slope of log-log plots of incidence versus age (see Fig. 5). The above equation gives a more precisely linear relationship if "age" is corrected to "age at inception of tumor" by subtraction of the latent period, if this is known (72).

What is the reason for the steep increase in the incidence of epithelial tumors with age? The present answer (see above) is synergism between age-dependent processes and the accumulation of heritable changes induced by carcinogenic agents. Why, then, is the age-dependent rate of incidence, which is quantified by the factor k, so widely different in different organs? Three factors that may be of especial importance are the quantity of environmental carcinogen to which the population is exposed, the degree of recovery and repair of the target organ following delivery of the carcinogenic insult, and the hormonal factors operating (and their change with age) in the organ.

The low value of k for skin (4.1) may be due to a combination of relatively constant exposure to the main carcinogen (sunlight) throughout

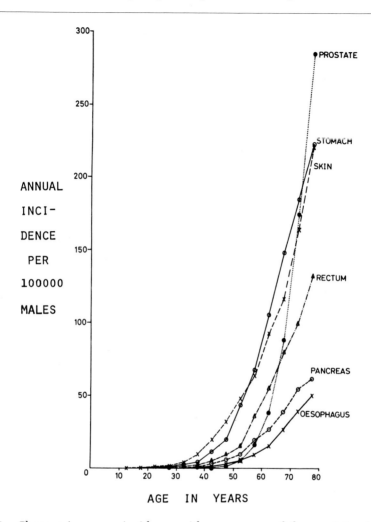

Fig. 4. Changes in cancer incidence with age: cancer of the prostate, stomach, skin, colon and rectum, pancreas, esophagus. Data from England and Wales, 1960–62 (72). From *Cancer and Aging*, Skandia International Symposia (Almqvist & Wiksell International), Stockholm, 1968.

life, relatively rapid repair of affected skin (as suggested by the rapid fading of sun tans) and a relatively low and constant hormonal milieu throughout life (129, 132, 159, 203, 277).

Cancer of the *colon* or *rectum* represents a more typical case as regards the increase of cancer incidence with age ($k = 6.3$). The precursor cells for colon or rectal cancer are adenomas, not hyperplastic nodules

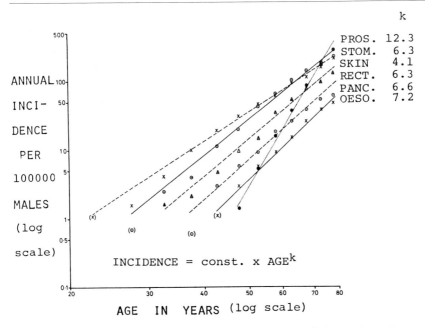

Fig. 5. Changes in logarithm of cancer incidence with logarithm of age. Data taken from Fig. 4 (72). From *Cancer and Aging*, Skandia International Symposia (Almqvist & Wiksell International), Stockholm, 1968.

(88, 216, 351). The normal colonic epithelium contains rapidly dividing cells, and is second only to lymphocytes in its sensitivity to the action of radiation (197). Therefore, cell repair probably also proceeds at a rapid rate. The normal colon has a bacterial flora that changes with diet. It seems probable that the bacterial flora can produce carcinogens from the diet, or from intestinal secretions such as bile acids (151). The composition of the diet may well determine both the quantities of carcinogen precursors and the composition of the bacterial flora which determines whether the precursors are converted into carcinogens (18, 42, 43, 151, 317, 348, 350). In addition, food additives such as sodium nitrite may be converted to carcinogens (in this case, nitrosamines) within the intestinal tract. A high-bulk diet may aid to guard against carcinogenesis by allowing less time for carcinogens to be produced within the colon, and less time for carcinogens that are produced to remain in contact with the colonic and rectal epithelium (42, 43, 298). Thus, low-fat (and possibly high-bulk) diets tend to reduce the incidence of colon and rectal cancer. The hormonal control of the colon and rectum do not seem to vary greatly throughout life, except in participating in the general gradual decrease in hormonal levels associated with aging (141, 142). Perhaps, then, the increased value of k for rectal cancer is due to an increased level of carcinogenic stimuli and increased turnover of cells relative to skin.

The exceptionally high value of k for *prostatic carcinoma*, namely 12.3 (72), indicates an extreme degree of dependence of the incidence rate on age. What is this due to? The United States population has a relatively very high incidence of this type of cancer. Japanese have about one-eighth the United States rate, and in general Orientals, rural workers, and unmarried men have lower rates than the general population (68, 219). Japanese in Hawaii have mortality rates from this disease that are more similar to the high rates of United States whites than to the low rates of Japanese natives (1). One explanation for these results is the relative level of testosterone (154) and other male androgens that may regulate cell division in the prostate. Traditionally, Japanese husbands mate with their wives rarely if at all after middle age. Compared to American males, Japanese males probably experience a greatly reduced androgenic stimulation of their prostate glands in old age, when prostatic cancer is such a threat in America. The possibility that androgenic stimulation plays an important role in the etiology of carcinoma of the prostate is strengthened by the biological evolution of prostatic carcinoma. The prostate gland in most American males continues to enlarge with age, so that relatively few males over the age of 60 do not have benign prostatic hypertrophy (335). Prostatic adenocarcinomas often develop as a nodule or as a diffuse mass in the posterior lobe of the gland (68). Microcarcinomas of the prostate were present in 26% of males aged 80 years and over, who died of unrelated causes (133). Given such a high frequency of nests of incipient carcinoma, it can be understood why growth stimulation of the gland with androgenic hormones might have a drastic effect on the outgrowth of these foci into clinical cancer (154, 191). While androgenic hormones may be the vital etiological factor, they might not be the primary cause. This may perhaps be an endemic oncogenic virus that may infect the prostate gland, much as bacteria cause chronic prostatitis.

In contrast to the age-incidence data for the above tumors (Figs. 4 and 5), carcinomas of the testis (Fig. 3), cervix, breast, and lung (Fig. 6) present a very different picture. The sharp peak in incidence of *testicular cancer* at 30 to 40 years of age may be due to the cumulative action of androgenic stimulation (possibly plus exposure to putative oncogenic viruses through coitus), with a rapidly declining incidence in middle age, as interest in sex declines. The reduction in the slope of the incidence rates for *carcinoma of the cervix and breast* (Fig. 6) occurs at or around the age of menopause. This strongly suggests that the change in estrogen hor-

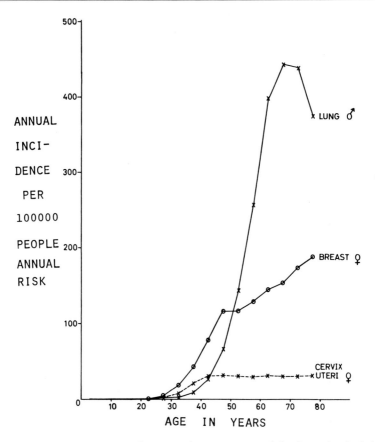

Fig. 6.   Changes in cancer incidence with age: cancer of the lung (males), breast, and cervix uteri (both females). Data from England and Wales, 1960–62 (72). From *Cancer and Aging*, Skandia International Symposia (Almqvist & Wiksell International), Stockholm, 1968.

mone balance that occurs at that time is responsible for the change. The "rounding off" of the *lung cancer* curve in old age (Fig. 6) is due to a far lower cumulative exposure to cigarette smoke in the age groups above 65 years old. Cigarette smoking was not yet a widely accepted practice in 1921, when the 65-year-old people in Doll's study were approximately 25 years old. If smoking had been a common habit in 1921, the data for lung cancer would probably conform to the more usual configuration (as in Figs. 4 and 5).

Cancer Biology

The current cancer research literature in the area of cancer biology is vast, and much of it has meaning when it is studied for clues to the defenses against the initiation of tumors. Paradoxically, most of the work deals with *systemic* immunity, and very little has relevance with regard to *organ* specific immunity. Since the (systemic) antigenicity of a tumor depends on the etiologic agent as well as on cell type, etiology is an important consideration, as is the process by which oncogenic agents act.

NECESSARY CONDITIONS FOR DEVELOPMENT OF TUMORS. Since cancer, both in man and in experimental animals, is comprised of a whole set of related diseases, any generalization is difficult. However, current concepts are that tumors cannot develop unless a combination of circumstances favorable for their emergence exists (22, 29, 45, 46, 61, 132, 136, 165, 206, 207, 213, 225, 227, 230, 268, 301, 341). Such necessary circumstances generally include some or all of the following conditions:

a. Presence of the carcinogenic agent in biologically active form.
b. Ability of the agent to gain access to a target cell sensitive to its oncogenic action.
c. Genetic susceptibility of the host.
d. Presence (then or later) of a mitotic or repair stimulus involving the cell or cells that have undergone oncogenic conversion.
e. Impairment of the normal defense systems of the target organ.

The target for carcinogenesis most likely to permit outgrowth into a frank tumor would seem to be those cells within a given organ that possess the highest growth potential; these are the "stem cells" responsible for normal cell replacement (243). For instance, there seems to be a strong consensus that the cells in which bronchogenic carcinoma develops most frequently are the cells at the base of the bronchial epithelium, which are most active in the normal regeneration of epithelial cells (10, 337).

ETIOLOGY AND ANTIGENIC STRENGTH OF TUMORS. The classical view used to be that many *physical agents* that cause tumors are mutagens and act as primary carcinogens (266). This may well be true under certain circumstances, since heritable changes in DNA are undoubtedly caused by many different types of radiation. In addition, some tumors induced by X-rays or bone-seeking radioisotopes can be transmitted by cell-free filtrates; this suggests that the true etiologic agent can be a virus (4, 5, 91, 165). Both types of mechanisms (primary carcinogenic action of radiation as compared to radiation damage permitting the expression of the oncogenic potential of a passenger virus) could well be active under different circumstances. For instance, given the presence of a highly active passenger virus in the vicinity of growing bone, it is easy to see how a bone-seeking radioisotope would produce the organ damage necessary for virally converted cells to survive and multiply. In contrast, the radiation–induced mutation of a somatic cell to a tumor cell may well represent a far more random event than specific viral oncogenesis, and be correspondingly more rare. Further, as Temin and Baltimore have shown, changes in RNA can induce heritable changes in cell DNA through mediation of the reverse (RNA–DNA) transcriptase.

A number of *DNA and RNA viruses* produce tumors in animals (4, 5, 53, 126, 189). Virtual proof of the viral etiology of such tumors has been obtained by injection of cell-free extracts of the tumor cells into newborn animals; when the same histological type of tumor develops rapidly in the injected animals, other explanations seem to be untenable. Work on the viral etiology of certain human tumors is of course hampered by an inability to perform this type of experiment.

Chemical carcinogens differ from viral agents in at least one important respect: individual tumors possess "private" antigens (268). These show antigenicity, as evidenced by the rejection (usually of a small number) of viable tumor cells by hosts previously immunized with sterilized tumor cells. Chemically induced tumors possess only very slight crossreactivity with other tumors induced by the same substance; even tumors induced in the same animal differ in this manner (173). This suggests that chemicals can act as true primary carcinogens, since all virally induced tumors crossreact with tumors induced by the same agent in different hosts of the same species (268).

The vital point with regard to the relative antigenic strengths of animal tumors (Table 3) is that these antigenic strengths are measured *systemically* in the conventional manner. Antigenic strength when measured in this way certainly has meaning when a particular tumor begins to grow in a particular organ, even though organ specific and not systemic immunity is then relevant. However, at this point we know very little about the relationship between local and systemic immunity, or their relative importance.

Experimental work on the antigenicity of tumors transplanted in isogenic hosts can be remarkably effective in cooling unwarranted enthusiasm regarding the antigenic strength of tumors. We recently completed experiments in which we attempted to induce *systemic* immunity to the DBA/2 leukemia L1210 and to the AKR leukemia BW-A in isogenic hosts by multiple preinjections with X-ray sterilized or iodoacetamide

Table 3. Relative antigenic strengths[a] of certain animal tumors[b]

Etiological Agent	Relative Antigenic Strength[a]	Cross-Reactivity of Tumors Induced:		
		As Other Primaries in the Same Individual	By the Same Agent in Other Individuals	By Other Agents in Other Individuals
DNA viruses	+ +	+ +	+ +	−
RNA viruses	+	+	+	−[c]
Chemical carcinogens	+ +	− (±)	− (±)	−
Radiation	−, ±	−, ±	−, ±	
"Spontaneous"	− (±)			

a. Even when the *relative* antigenic strength is high (+ +), the *absolute* antigenic strength compared to tissue alloantigens may be very low.

b. From Refs. 4, 5, 91, 126, 165, 268.

c. Cross-reactivity may be present within tumors induced by closely related viruses.

treated cells. Our results were consistently negative (Reif, Li, and Robinson, unpublished work). These results underline the fact that many tumor-associated antigens are remarkably weak compared to normal histocompatibility antigens (see footnote, Table 3).

ARE DEFENSES AGAINST ANTIGENIC TUMORS MORE EFFECTIVE? The question whether the antigenic strength of tumors plays a decisive role in acceptance or rejection of tumors was first addressed by Old et al. (228) and Johnson (160) using MCA (3-methylcholanthrene) as the carcinogen; then by Prehn (250) for tumors induced by subcutaneous (s.c.) implants of plastic film; and finally more definitively by Bartlett (12). Bartlett induced tumors in mice by s.c. implantation of 4-μg MCA in a paraffin disc. The antigenic strength of each tumor was determined by excising the tumor transplants from an experimental group of mice when the tumors had grown to 8–15 mm in diameter; at that point, fresh tumor tissue was injected by trocar into the experimental mice, as well as into a control group. Antigenic strength was measured by the ratio of mean diameter of tumors in control mice relative to experimental mice at a convenient endpoint (when two-thirds of the control mice had tumors 5 mm or greater in diameter). The latent period for each tumor was the time between administration of MCA and development of a progressively growing tumor at least 7 mm in diameter, which was then transplanted for determination of antigenic strength.

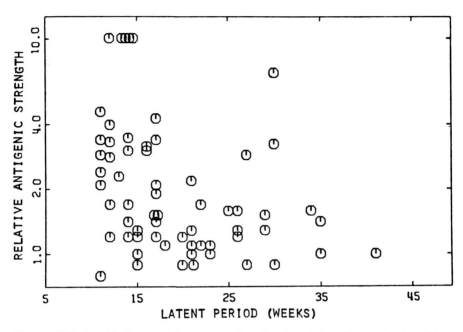

Fig. 7. Relationship between latent period and antigenicity of tumors induced by MCA in subcutaneous tissues of mice (12).

The relationship between antigenic strength and latent period obtained for 64 individual tumors in this way was found to be asymmetrical, due to a relative lack of tumors in the right top portion of the plot (Fig. 7). This deficiency corresponds to tumors with relatively high antigenicity that possess long latent periods. When Bartlett induced tumors with MCA in tissue placed in diffusion chambers (and therefore out of contact with the host's cellular defenses), the plot of antigenic strength against latent period became symmetrical (Fig. 8). This indicates that in the absence of host surveillance pressure, slowly growing tumors with relatively high antigenicity can survive. In contrast, such tumors must be presumed to have been rejected by the host (Fig. 7). Since Bartlett eliminated the possibility that there was a correlation between antigenicity and growth rate in a separate experiment, the data suggest that relatively highly antigenic tumors can only escape host defenses if they grow fast. Thus, the data indicate that immune defenses exist against tumors induced by MCA (12). It should be stressed that these immune defenses against tumors induced at relatively high local doses of MCA are not very effective: a comparison

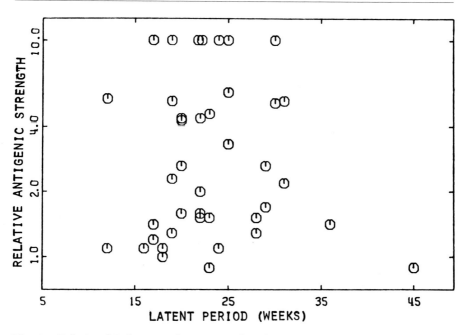

Fig. 8.   Relationship between latent period and antigenicity of tumors induced by MCA in mouse tissues in diffusion chambers (12).

of Figs. 7 and 8 suggests that at least half the tumors that began to grow *in vivo* managed to progress to frank tumors.

DEFENSES AGAINST VIRALLY INDUCED TUMORS.   Two types of immunity, often related, are involved with virally induced tumors: immunity against the virus, and immunity against the tumor cell induced by the virus. A brief account of the natural history of a relatively strongly antigenic DNA virus, such as the polyoma virus, leaves the impression that systemic immunity is of overriding importance for the determination of whether or not viral infection results in tumors.

In nature, polyoma virus abundantly infects wild mice. In a city such as New York, most mice carry both the virus and specific antibody to it. However, maternal antibody protects both the fetus and newborn mice, so that wild mice do not develop polyoma tumors as far as we are aware. Nevertheless, polyoma is highly effective for tumor production in the laboratory. However, in contrast to its presentation to mice in nature, a relatively *massive* dose of virus must be injected into *newborn* mice for tumors to result. In nature, the virus seems able to multiply in mouse tissues without producing tumors. Thus, it is possible to view tumor incidence from injection of polyoma virus as a laboratory tool, or even as a laboratory artifact (4, 5, 40, 126, 264, 315). However, it seems possible to draw a parallel between its natural and experimental history, and that of Burkitt's lymphoma.

In the United States, the bulk of the adult population possesses antibody to Burkitt lymphoma cells (Table 2), and the incidence of the tumor is rare. In contrast, in low-lying hot and wet portions of Africa, a lower percentage of the adult population possesses antibody to Burkitt lymphoma cells than in the United States and the incidence of the tumor is less rare (175). The additional etiologic factor in Africa seems to be a functional immunodeficiency caused by malaria. Perhaps, if we screened the wild mice in New York City with as much care as we devote to sick human beings, we would also find an occasional wild mouse in New York City that developed a polyoma tumor. If we knew for certain that such mice really do not exist in nature, then we would also feel assured that tumors induced by polyoma are more antigenic than those induced by the etiological agent responsible for Burkitt's lymphoma.

DEFENSES AGAINST RADIATION-INDUCED TUMORS. Moore and Williams have recently investigated the antigenicity of osteosarcomas induced in CBA mice with strontium-90 (215). Antigenicity could only be detected in less than half of the osteosarcomas that arose. Even this antigenicity was very weak. For its demonstration, a sensitive test system was required, in which small numbers of tumor cells were inoculated into hosts preirradiated with 400 rad of total-body X-irradiation. The authors suggested that immunoselection during the long latent period might be responsible for the low antigenicity of such tumors (215). These results are typical for work on the antigenicity of radiation-induced tumors (Table 3).

EFFECT OF SYSTEMIC IMMUNOSUPPRESSION ON EX-PERIMENTAL CARCINOGENESIS. Carcinogenic agents by themselves are often systemic immunosuppressants. The evidence for immunosuppression by oncogenic viruses has been reviewed by Dent (70). Immunosuppression seems limited to RNA leukemogenic viruses; with few exceptions, DNA viruses and RNA sarcoma viruses have not been found to be systemically immunodepressive (70). With regard to chemical carcinogens, both urethane and N-nitrosomethylurea greatly reduce the primary immune response against sheep red blood cells in mice (236), while 7,12-dimethylbenz(α)anthracene exposure depresses both the homograft rejection and the graft-versus-host reactivity in the rat (136).

Radiation is immunosuppressive if it permeats all body organs in suffi-cient dose, as in total body radiation. Even partial-body X-irradiation, as given during radiation therapy of tumors, frequently causes a drop in the white cell count of blood (233).

Viral oncogenesis is generally greatly facilitated by immunosuppres-sion or by physiological immaturity of the lymphoid system. Thus, thymectomy, antilymphocyte serum, chemical immunosuppressants and use of newborn as recipients for virus injections can be highly effective for viral induction of tumors (135, 136, 174, 181, 192, 193). Indeed, in most experimental situations, the systemic immunity of normal hosts must be depressed or compromised to permit the oncogenic expression of the virus.

Chemical carcinogenesis is significantly (though not extensively) en-hanced by powerful systemic immunosuppression. Review of the litera-ture in a recent study of this question revealed nine other studies in which significant enhancement had been found, and two papers in which no effect was reported (109). The two latter studies were both criticized for one or more serious deficiencies.

Radiation carcinogenesis has apparently not been studied in conjunc-tion with chemical immunosuppression or ALS (antilymphocyte serum) administration. In the mouse, the usual target tissue for leukemogenic virus is the thymus, and removal of the thymus will therefore inhibit leukemogenesis (164). Since radiation can greatly enhance other modes of carcinogenesis (see above), systemic immunosuppression is probably also synergistic with radiation carcinogenesis.

TISSUE-SPECIFIC EFFECTS OF EXPERIMENTAL CARCINO-GENS.

The main thrust of the present report is that *the effects of the carcinogen on the target organ outweigh systemic effects for many types of oncogenesis.* In general, viral, chemical, and physical carcinogens cause at least the last of the necessary conditions for development of tumors (see above), namely, impairment of the normal defense systems of the target organ. This can be done by inactivation of "resident" lymphoid cells, or by disrupture of the normal architecture that makes surveillance possible. The potent enhancement of viral oncogenesis by irradiation of the target organ is one illustration of this effect (135). In addition, all rapidly acting carcinogens have the ability to induce mitosis of the target cells, whether by direct or indirect action, one the target cells have undergone oncogenic conversion.

BIOLOGICAL PROPERTIES OF TUMORS.

Perhaps the most obvious (yet least studied) property of tumors is their hardness. A tumor can be felt as a hard lump. To negate the attack of host surveillance cells, clones of tumor cells would benefit from being "tough and impenetrable." Judging from the hardness of tumor nodules, most types of tumors must be capable of laying down a tough ground substance that resists lysis by lymphoid surveillance cells. One of the principal components of this ground substance seems to be collagen (personal communication from J. A. Hayes). However, another possibility is that this ground substance is secreted by host fibrous tissue and represents an unsuccessful attempt to wall off the tumor tissue.

From in vitro attempts to dissociate clumps of tumor cells, we know that proteolytic enzymes such as trypsin and collagenase are partly effective for this purpose. Such enzymes are present on the surface of phagocytes, yet do not harm the phagocyte itself, perhaps because of inhibitors of proteolytic enzymes that are present within the cell. From the work of Reich, and of Christman and others, we know that such proteolytic enzymes are also copiously produced by tumor cells (264a). Further, both tumor cells and some normal cells (macrophages, fibroblasts, kidney and lung cells) can activate serum plasminogen to the proteolytic enzyme plasmin. This mobilization of proteolytic activity may help both circulating lymphocytes and also tumor cells to penetrate body organs. For normal lymphocytes, such penetration would aid phatocytosis and response to messages sent by chemotactic factors, while for tumor cells it would facilitate metastasis.

Certain types of tumor cells must meet minimal resistance from host lymphoid cells, or they would be unable to spread via the lymphatic channels. To survive the "extreme cheek" of passage right through the ranks of their heriditary foes, tumor cells must either have eliminated or hidden the recognition factors (antigens) present on their surface, or else must be able to inactivate any lymphoid cell that attempts to attack them. One way such inactivation can be effected is through the copious shedding of tumor cell antigen. This antigen would bind to the lymphoid cell surface and saturate sites with anti-tumor reactivity that, in the absence of shed tumor antigen, could be free for specific attachment to tumor cells (162).

From immunotherapy experiments in man, we know that immunotherapy is almost never effective when the amount of residual tumor tissue exceeds roughly 10^9 tumor cells, or 1 ml of tissue. From Folkman's work on tumor angiogenesis, we know that oxygen can diffuse only about 0.015 cm (150 microns) into tumor tissue (95a). Thus, it follows that tumor cells at the center of a spherical piece of tumor 0.015 cm in radius will begin to become necrotic, while tumor growth can still continue in a layer 0.915 cm thick around the periphery, even if the tumor is not vascularized. Experimental work has shown that, in the absnece of vascularization, tumor growth stops for most carcinomas when a diameter of between 0.1 and 0.3 cm has been reached (J. Folkman, private communication). The point we wish to make here is that the quantity of tumor tissue required for tumor vascularization to begin is roughly in accord with the amount of tumor tissue present at the point when immunotherapy is no longer effective. It is certainly true that the effectiveness of host destruction of tumor cells is greatly reduced when the tumor becomes vascularized. One reason, and this may be the deciding one, is that the supply of oxygen and nutrients to individual tumor cells is greatly increased, facilitating rapid growth (95a). But in addition, access of surveillance cells to the tumor becomes limited to systemic rather than organ-specific cells; this may well greatly reduce the possibility for a specific cell-mediated reaction against the tumor.

Contradicting Evidence on Immune Surveillance

In the past, there have been heated discussions between the proponents and opponents of the theory of immune surveillance (64, 65, 188, 193, 251, 252, 253, 254, 255, 256, 258). Can some of these be resolved by utilizing the concept that immune defenses are often tissue-specific rather than systemic?

EFFECT OF IMMUNE STIMULATION ON CARCINOGENESIS.
One of the main arguments used against the concept of immune surveillance against tumors is that immune stimulation can enhance carcinogenesis (loc. cit.). Of course it can. There is incontrovertible evidence that, under special conditions, immune stimulation can enhance rather than retard tumor growth (89, 90, 221, 235, 258, 297). At least three explanations are possible.

First, immune stimulation is not a simple phenomenon in which a single population of host cells responds to a given immunostimulator: in contrast, it is a highly complex inflammation reaction involving a multitude of cell types and lymphokinins that appear in a staged progression (59, 66, 237). Further, the inflammatory response is closely allied to tissue repair and hence contains mitotic stimulators (59, 237). This by itself would explain why immunostimulation could be enhancing under certain situations.

Secondly, there are few processes in biology that will not reverse their effect when the conditions of action are suitably changed. One illustration of this is active immunity as contrasted to immune tolerance (Fig. 9). The response to injection of increasing doses of certain antigens in many species can be triphasic: at very low doses, there is a partial suppression of an effective immune response ("low dose tolerance"); over what is usu-

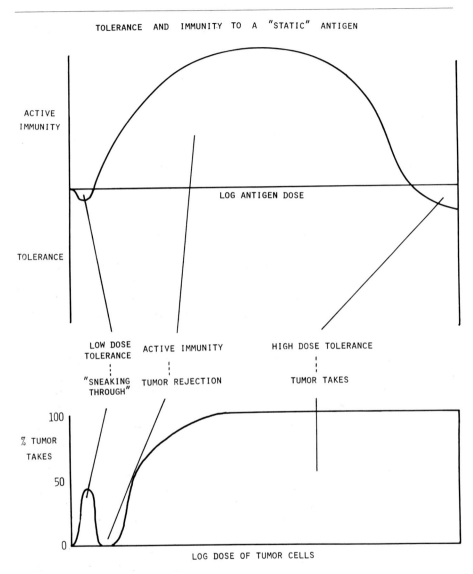

TOLERANCE AND IMMUNITY TO A "STATIC" ANTIGEN

ACTIVE IMMUNITY

LOG ANTIGEN DOSE

TOLERANCE

LOW DOSE TOLERANCE

ACTIVE IMMUNITY

HIGH DOSE TOLERANCE

"SNEAKING THROUGH"

TUMOR REJECTION

TUMOR TAKES

% TUMOR TAKES

LOG DOSE OF TUMOR CELLS

ESCAPE AND REJECTION OF TUMOR, A "DYNAMIC" COMPLEX ANTIGEN

Fig. 9. *Top:* Hypothetical relationship between immune response (active immunity or tolerance) and the logarithm of antigen dose for a conventional (static) antigen. *Bottom:* Hypothetical relationship between tumor take (% animals dying) and the logarithm of cells injected for a dynamic (growing) antigen complex (tumor cells).

ally a broad range of *intermediate concentrations* of antigen, injection of the antigen is followed by an effective immune response ("zone of active immunity"); at *high doses* of antigen, there can be a lack of immune response ("high dose tolerance") because of absorption of antibody by excess antigen still present in the body (74, 87, 166, 237, 268).

The same type of triphasic response (top portion, Fig. 9) to injection of various doses of antigens must equally apply to host reaction to a developing tumor (lower portion, Fig. 9). At *very low doses*, the tumor may escape effective immune elimination (the "sneaking through" phenomenon of Old and Boyse [227, 230]) by the cellular equivalent of low dose tolerance (227, 230); at *intermediate doses*, one would expect to find a zone of active immunity in which the tumor load is sufficiently small to permit an effective rejection response—except that the tumor differs from conventional antigens in being a "dynamic antigen complex": it is growing. It is this difference that presents the major problem of tumor control by the immune system. Very simply, only when the total host response (of resident lymphoid cells plus systemic cells marshalled to the site by an inflammation reaction or by other distress signals) is at a sufficient rate to overwhelm the mass of tumor cells at the rate they are multiplying, will the lymphoid defense response be effective for elimination of the tumor. Beyond this point, the tumor will outgrow any effective host response cells and overwhelm host defenses (high dose tolerance), which are then reduced to fighting a rear-guard action (bottom portion, Fig. 9).

However, it might be countered that the above considerations of active immunity and tolerance deal with antibodies rather than cells, and it is cellular reactivity that is of prime importance for defense against most types of tumors. Since antibodies are produced by lymphoid cells, at low levels of immunity, sensitization demonstrable *in vitro* is limited to cellular reactivity, probably mediated by cell-bound or cytophilic antibody (66, 87). Hence, essentially the same sequence of cell-mediated reactivity against tumor cells as depicted for antibodies (bottom portion, Fig. 9) would be expected to occur.

Thirdly, under most laboratory conditions, immune stimulation inhibits rather than enhances carcinogenesis. This holds true for chemical carcinogenesis (109). As for viral carcinogenesis, immune stimulation can strongly reduce or delay this process (192, 193).

EFFECT OF IMMUNE STIMULATION ON TUMOR GROWTH.

For the same reasons as set out above, immune stimulation can enhance tumor growth (98, 188). However, far more usually, immune stimulation is therapeutic. There is now a large and growing literature that suggests a mild efficacy for immunotherapy both in experimental animals and in man; this is reviewed elsewhere in this book. Many of the therapeutic procedures used to date are immunostimulatory (24, 136, 162, 307).

ARE DEFENSES AGAINST INITIATION OF TUMORS IMMUNE IN NATURE?

Prehn has argued vigorously that defenses against tumors are nonimmune and that immunity stimulates rather than inhibits tumor development (64, 65, 188, 251, 252, 253, 254, 255, 256, 258). Others have supported his thesis (64, 65, 188). How are these views reconciled with those which state that surveillance is both effective and immune in nature (45, 46, 193, 206, 207, 225, 227, 230, 305, 334)?

Let us begin by making exceptions of the childhood tumors that respond well to chemotherapy and of the more responsive adult neoplasms (antigenic group A discussed under "applications to man"). If, for other types of tumors, defenses against their initiation are largely *organ* specific, then we would not expect to see the development of systemic immunity to them until an extension into regional lymph nodes or beyond had occurred. Therefore, the absence of systemic immunity to initiation of such tumors says little or nothing about organ-specific mechanisms. The present viewpoint is therefore in agreement with the facts but not with the explanations given by the opponents of surveillance.

What sort of immunity would be expected from the "resident" lymphoid cells of an organ, that would be effective for immune defense against initiation of tumors? It would be immunity against any cell bearing antigens inappropriate to that organ. Such "inappropriate" cells would include the following: (a) cells from other organs, except those circulating cells (such as lymphoid cells or inflammatory cells or erythrocytes) which are recognized as normal or permitted, depending upon the physiological state of the organ; (b) cells more primitive than the stem cells necessary for normal cell replacement within the organ; and (c) cells bearing recognizably changed antigens. In support of the concept that organs can eliminate cells recognized as coming from other organs, one can cite the remarkable organ specificity of metastases (135, 342), which suggests that some organs possess defenses that prevent the invasion by cells from other organs. In line with this concept, we would expect organ-specific damage to aid metastasis formation in that organ, and systemic immunity to have relatively little effect on metastasis; both positive (49, 184, 185) and negative (156) reports have appeared on the latter subject. With regard to item (c), recognition of cells bearing changed antigens, the whole subject of autoimmune diseases bears witness to the fact that sensitization against changed cell surface antigens can occur (107, 338). Such sensitization, though always systemic when detected, must begin in the organ in which the cells with changed antigens reside. In the case of oncogenesis, this is the organ in which oncogenesis begins.

Past investigations have demonstrated that the cells involved in immune defenses against many experimental tumors are stimulated or antibody-armed macrophages and "null" cells, cells that do not have either T or B surface antigens (3, 64, 65, 71, 83, 114, 139). It is usually assumed that such "killer" cells function nonspecifically. However, such cells do show a particular type of specificity, since they attack neoplastic but not normal cells (245). If organ-specific defense is a reality, then such "nonspecific" killing represents immune killing. But the type of immunity is not what current assays are set up to measure. Whether or not they represent an immune event depends upon one's definition of what comprises "immunity" as contrasted with "recognition." If immunity is defined narrowly, in terms of conventional systemic immunity, then organ-specific immunity is largely nonimmune in nature. If immunity is defined to include the responses of lymphoid cells that follow recognition of a determinant, then organ-specific defenses are immune in nature. Thus, arguments remaining between proponents and opponents of immune surveillance on this particular point merely reduce to a matter of definition or of semantics.

OTHER MATTERS OF CONTENTION. As soon as it is acknowledged that immune defenses to many types of tumors are not sytemic in nature but organ specific, the main argument against acceptance of immune surveillance, the absence of an effective systemic immunity, is eliminated. Thus, the apparently conflicting evidence on tumor development in thymectomized, immunosuppressed or athymic animals is explained (see above). In addition, the questions regarding the specificity or nonspecificity of killer cell reactivity reduce to semantics (see above).

One final vital matter concerns Prehn's contention that immunity of any sort is irrelevant in tumor development (252, 253, 254, 255, 256, 258). A way of restating his hypothesis is that for most clinically evident tumors, immunity has little or nothing to do with tumor development, and may in fact be harmful; the most extreme form of this line of argument is "no immunity, no tumors" (personal communication). One justification for such points of view, even in terms of the evidence presented in this chapter, is that the degree of host control for most of the tumors discussed is relatively slim. Further, tumors that appear to be "more antigenic," such as the childhood tumors (see below), are relatively rare. The fact that any tumor becomes a clinical problem proves that it has escaped host control, and that this control has been ineffective. In rebuttal, Prehn's line of reasoning seems akin to "throwing out the baby with the bathwater." Indeed, host control over the most common tumors is slim; but this weak control is all we have to work with.

It behooves us to value what little control there is, and strive to understand, nourish, and strengthen it with all the ingenuity we can bring to bear. This may well represent the most meaningful objective in cancer research, and one of its greatest challenges.

Applications to Man

ANTIGENIC GROUPINGS. The data reviewed above suggest that systemic immunity may be very important in most of the childhood cancers. As with animal tumors (Table 3), human tumors can be ranked (in a very preliminary and approximate manner) by such criteria as (a) the number of substantiated cases of spontaneous regression, (b) the effectiveness of systemic chemotherapy or immunotherapy, and (c) evidence for antigenic crossreactivity for tumors of the same histologic type (268).

The above classification might well be modified here to include groups of tumors which, by the same criteria, seem to vary in antigenicity. Such variation in antigenicity may be due to the presence of subgroups of tumors, each with a characteristically different degree of antigenicity. The more antigenic tumors represent the most likely targets for successful therapy or even of prevention. Beginning with the relatively "more antigenic" group and ending with the least antigenic group, these groups tentatively comprise the following tumors:

a. Hypernephroma, choriocarcinoma, and the following tumors when they occur in childhood or adolescence: Wilms tumor, embryonal rhabdomyosarcoma, neuroblastoma, osteogenic sarcoma, acute lymphocytic leukemia, Hodgkin's disease and Burkitt's lymphoma.
b. Malignant melanoma, bladder cancer, sarcomas and certain types of leukemia when these occur in adult life, colon and rectal cancer, ovarian cancer, testicular cancer, breast cancer.
c. All other malignancies.

At this stage of our knowledge, which must be judged rudimentary, such a list still has some merit in directing attention to the likelihood of a parallel between experimental tumors (Table 3) and human tumors. As indicated (discussion of Table 3), such parallels can have important etiological and therapeutic connotations.

GENETIC AND ENVIRONMENTAL EFFECTS ON TUMOR DEVELOPMENT. There is presently a reasonably good consensus that tumors cannot develop unless a combination of circumstances favorable for their emergence exists (4, 5, 44, 123, 126, 162, 268, 300, 304). A list of these circumstances is set out above (see above, under Cancer Biology: Necessary Conditions for Development of Tumors). What meaning do these considerations have with regard to the development of tumors in people?

Obviously, any long-continued regimen of immunosuppression must be evaluated to decide whether a 4–6% risk of tumor development is justified. With regard to exposure to or immunization against oncogenic viruses, little can be done in that area at least until such viruses have been identified with reasonable certainty and isolated. With regard to genetics, this is something we cannot change. However, the identification of persons at high risk for cancer coupled with the protection of such people from carcinogenic stimuli to which they are particularly sensitive is a profitable area for future exploitation (6, 217, 246). Still, for the bulk of the population, the greatest benefit in terms of reduced cancer incidence will result from removal of environmental carcinogens or cocarcinogens.

An illustration of the above suggestion is given by the incidence of lung, laryngeal, oral, esophageal, bladder, pancreatic and renal cancer in cigarette smokers (268, 269, 330, 349). Mortality ratios for these cancers vary from over 11:1 to 2:1 for cigarette smokers relative to smokers. Because approximately 43% of the United States adult population smoke cigarettes, and have done so over many years, at least one quarter of the deaths from cancer during 1975 were "preventable" deaths caused by cigarette smoking; these figures are corrected for deaths from cancer that would have occurred even in the absence of cigarette smoking (269).

The scientific validity of the causation of lung cancer from smoking (which makes up two-thirds of the excess cancer deaths) is now as firmly established as any link between cause and effect involving human beings can ever be (268, 269, 330, 349). Nevertheless, Burch (a radiation physicist) has recently exhumed (37) the theory of Fisher (a brilliant statistician) that genetic background is more important than smoking history for development of lung cancer (95). Remarkably, both Fisher and Burk were perhaps more right than wrong in their scientific evaluation. In contrast, the conclusion that one might draw from it, namely that therefore one can smoke, is disastrously wrong. An explanation seems in order.

A definite genetic predisposition is necessary for the development of most types of tumors in animals as in man (6, 217, 218, 310). In experimental animals, different inbred strains have been developed within a single species (such as the mouse), each strain with widely different tumor incidences. This represents a compelling argument for the reality of genetic predisposition (303). In a highly heterogeneous population, as exists in most countries of the world, people with a whole spectrum of genetic predispositions to any particular type of tumor must exist. Even *without* exposure, some of the *most* susceptible individuals will escape competing causes of death and die from that particular tumor. Let us take lung cancer as an illustration. Looked at retrospectively, knowing that they developed lung cancer, we can be sure that nonsmokers who developed this disease (without vocational exposure) were highly susceptible. That means they would fall into the extreme right hand end of the distribution curve for human susceptibility to lung cancer (which might well be a "normal" or "Gaussian" distribution). Individuals whose susceptibility to lung cancer was still high, and who would find themselves plotted just short of the right hand end of this hypothetical distribution curve, would not develop lung cancer usually, but die from competing causes of death. Given, however, the additional stimulus of cigarette smoking, their high innate susceptibility would advance the time of development of lung cancer, and it would become overt before competing causes of death could take their toll.

To revert to Fisher and Burch's thesis: for any individual, the degree of genetic susceptibility to lung cancer may be the vital factor in whether or not lung cancer developed, quite independent of smoking. However, at present we are unable to evaluate susceptibility to lung cancer. If we could do this, those with low susceptibility could smoke like chimneys—unless, of course, they were susceptible to atherosclerosis, or emphysema, or chronic bronchitis. What we do know is that cigarette smoking increases one's chance of lung cancer by at least elevenfold.

ORGAN-SPECIFIC IMMUNITY AND CANCER PREVENTION. It has been known for a considerable time that two different carcinogens acting on the same organ are particularly vicious in their effectiveness. Such synergism has been described for uranium miners, who run the risk of lung cancer from inhalation of radioactive radon gas, a risk that is dramatically increased if they smoke in addition (290, 330). Precisely similar data hold for asbestos workers who inhale asbestos fibers and who also smoke (290, 330).

If organ-specific defenses are most important for development of many types of tumors, then any substance that damages an organ already the target of other carcinogens should be a most effective cocarcinogen. In line with this concept, it has long been known that alcoholic cirrhosis of the liver strongly predisposes to liver tumor. In fact, the asbestos fiber may be nothing more than a very effective cocarcinogen, that acts synergistically with environmental carcinogens whose target is the bronchial epithelium.

For purposes of prevention, then, it would seem particularly important that any person exposed to known industrial or environmental carcinogens be shielded from exposure to noncarcinogenic substances that are known to injure the target organ of the carcinogen.

ORGAN-SPECIFIC IMMUNITY AND IMMUNOTHERAPY. If organ-specific immunity is more important than systemic immunity for a given type of tumor, then organ-specific immunotherapy would be expected to be more effective for that tumor, at least while it remains localized in the tissue of origin. This is indeed what has been found to be true both experimentally and in the clinic. BCG is far more effective when given admixed with a tumor vaccine than if given systemically, and DNCB must be painted above or close to tumor nodules in the skin (24, 307).

How can the concept of organ specific immunity be used further for prevention and therapy? Once we have identified individuals susceptible to a particular organ-specific tumor, prevention by use of anticarcinogenic agents (7), especially when these have preferential localization in the target organ, will be possible. We already use some chemotherapeutic agents and immunotherapeutic agents that have specificity for the tissue of origin of the tumor. More purposeful design of such agents along these lines may offer hope for more rational and successful therapy in the future. Still prevention will always be more effective than cure.

ACKNOWLEDGMENTS

Best thanks are due to Miss Anne T. Fidler for help with the references. Overall support by contract EY-76-S-02-2539, from the United States Energy Research and Development Administration is gratefully acknowledged.

NOTE

1. Arnold E. Reif, *Evidence for Tissue Specificity of Immune Surveillance against Cancer*. Presented at the New York Academy of Sciences on October 17, 1973, under the aegis of the section of Microbiology.

REFERENCES

1. Akazaki, K., and Stemmermann, G. N. 1973. Comparative study of latent carcinoma of the prostate among Japanese in Japan and Hawaii. *J. Natl. Cancer Inst.* 50: 1137–1144.

2. Alexander, J. W., and Good, R. A. 1970. Cancer, *Immunobiology for Surgeons*, pp. 132–144. W. B. Saunders Co., Philadelphia.

3. Alexander, P., Eccles, S. A., and Gauci, C. L. L. 1976. The significance of macrophages in human and experimental tumors. *Ann. N.Y. Acad. Sci.* 276: 124–133.

4. Allen, D. W., and Cole, P. 1972. Viruses and human cancer. I. DNA viruses. *N. Engl. J. Med.* 286: 70–82.

5. Allen, D. W., and Cole, P. 1972. Viruses and human cancer. II. RNA viruses. *N. Engl. J. Med.* 286: 70–82.

6. Anderson, D. E. 1975. Familial susceptibility, in J. F. Fraumeni, Jr. (ed.), *Persons at High Risk of Cancer. An Approach to Cancer Etiology and Control*, pp. 39–54. Academic Press, New York.

7. Apffel, C. A. 1976. Nonimmunological host defenses: a review. *Cancer Res.* 36: 1527–1537.

8. Archer, V. E., Wagoner, J. K., and Lundin, F. E. 1973a. Lung cancer among uranium miners in the United States. *Health Phys.* 25: 351–371.

9. Archer, V. E., Wagoner, J. K., and Lundin, F. E. 1973b. Uranium mining and cigarette smoking effects on man. *J. Occup. Med.* 15: 204–211.

10. Auerbach, O., Hammond, E. C., and Garfinkel, L. 1971. Epithelial changes in ex-cigarette smokers. *Cancer Cytol.* 11: 5–12.

11. Bailin, P. L., Tindall, J. P., Roenigk, Jr., H. H., and Hogan, M. D. 1975. Is methotrexate therapy for psoriasis carcinogenic? A modified retrospective-prospective analysis. *JAMA* 232: 359–362.

12. Bartlett, G. L. 1972. Effect of host immunity on the antigenic strength of primary tumors. *J. Natl. Cancer Inst.* 49: 493–504.

13. Basombrío, M. A., and Prehn, R. T. 1972. Studies on the basis for diversity and time of appearance of antigens in chemically induced tumors. *Natl. Cancer Inst. Monogr.* 35: 117–124.

14. Becker, F. F. 1974. Hepatoma: nature's model tumor. A review. *Amer. J. Path.* 74: 179–210.

15. Beckwith, J. B., and Perrin, E. V. 1963. In situ neuroblastoma: a contribution to the natural history of neural crest tumors. *Amer. J. Pathol.* 43: 1089–1104.

16. Bencinelli, M., Nardini, L., and Campa, M. 1974. Neutralization of Friend leukemia virus by sera of unimmunized animals. *J. Gen. Virol.* 22: 207–214.

16a. Benditt, E. P. 1977. The origin of atherosclerosis. *Sci. Amer.* 236: no. 2, 74–85.

17. Benjamin, D. C., and Weigle, W. O. 1970. The termination of immunological unresponsiveness to bovine serum albumin in rabbits. I. Quantitative and qualitative response to cross-reacting albumins. *J. Exp. Med.* 132: 66–76.

18. Berg, J. W., and Howell, M. A. 1974. The geographic pathology of bowel cancer. *Cancer* 34: 807–814.

19. Berg, J. W., Huvos, A. G., Axtell, L. M., and Robbins, G. F. 1973. A new sign of favorable prognosis in mammary cancer: hyperplastic reactive lymph nodes in the apex of the axilla. *Ann. Surg.* 117: 8–12.

20. Bergan, J. J. 1976. Quotation on kidney transplantation and cancer. *JAMA* 235: 1195–1199.

21. Berman, L. B. 1975. Immune parameters in the host response to neoplasia: morphological considerations, in A. E. Reif (ed.), *Immunity and Cancer in Man: An Introduction*, pp. 103–117. Marcel Dekker, New York.

22. Bernstein, I. D. 1973. Immunologic defenses against cancer. *J. Pediat.* 83: 906–918.

23. Bersagel, D. E. 1973. Plasma cell neoplasms, in J. F. Holland and E. Frei (eds.), *Cancer Medicine*, p. 1330–1358. Lea and Febiger, Philadelphia.

24. Biano, G. 1975. Clinical aspects of cancer immunotherapy, in A. E. Reif (ed.), *Immunity and Cancer in Man: An Introduction*, pp. 47–79. Marcel Dekker, Inc., New York.

25. Bias, W. B., Santos, G. W., Burke, P. J., Mullins, G. M., and Hymphrey, R. L. 1972. Cytotoxic antibody in normal human serums reactive with tumor cells from acute lymphocytic leukemia. *Science* 178: 304–306.

26. Bias, W. B., Santos, G. W., Burke, P. J., Mullins, G. M., and Hymphrey, R. L. 1973. Normal human sera with cytotoxic reactivity to acute lymphocytic leukemia cells. *Transplant. Proc.* 5: 949 952.

27. Bill, Jr., A. J. 1968. The regression of neuroblastoma. *J. Pediat. Surg.* 3: 103–106.

28. Bleier, R., Albrecht, R., and Cruce, J. A. 1975. Supraependymal cells of hypothalamic third ventricle: identification as resident phagocytes of the brain. *Science* 189: 299–301.

29. Bloom, B. R. 1972. Introductory remarks on immunology and oncology. *Front. Rad. Ther. Onc.* 7: 1–2.

30. Bonmassar, E., Campanile, F., Houchens, D., Crino, L., and Goldin, A. 1975. Impaired growth of a radiation-induced lymphoma in intact or lethally irradiated allogeneic athymic (nude) mice. *Transplantation* 20: 343–346.

31. Boros, T., and Rapp, H. J. (eds.). 1972. Conference on the use of BCG in therapy of cancer. *Natl. Cancer Inst. Monogr.* 39.

32. Boucot, K. R., Cooper, D. A., Weiss, W., et al. 1964. The natural history of lung cancer. *Amer. Rev. Resp. Dis.* 89: 519–527.

33. Brand, K. G., Buoen, L. C., Johnson, K. H., and Brand, I. 1975. Etiological factors, stages, and the role of the foreign body in foreign body tumorigenesis: a review. *Cancer Res.* 35: 279–286.

34. Bullough, W. S. 1965. Mitotic and functional homeostasis: a speculative review. *Cancer Res.* 25: 1683–1727.

35. Bullough, W. S., Lawrence, E. B., Iverson, O. H., and Elgjo, K. 1967. The vertabrate epidermal chalone. *Nature (London)* 214: 578–580.

36. Bullough, W. S., and Rytomaa, T. 1965. Mitotic homeostasis. *Nature (London)* 205: 573–578.

37. Burch, P. R. J. 1976. *The Biology of Cancer: A New Approach*. MTP Press Ltd., Lancaster, England.

38. Burch, P. R. J., and Burwell, R. G. 1965. Self and not-self: a clonal induction approach to immunology. *Quart. Rev. Biol.* 40: 252–279.

39. Burchenal, J. H. 1973. Hematologic neoplasms. Introduction, in J. F. Holland and E. Frei (eds.), *Cancer Medicine*, pp. 1167–1173. Lea and Febiger, Philadelphia.

40. Burdette, W. J. (ed.). 1966. *Viruses Inducing Cancer. Implications for Therapy*. University of Utah Press, Salt Lake City, Utah.

41. Burkitt, D. P. 1970. An alternative hypothesis to a vectored virus, in D. P. Burkitt and D. H. Wright (eds.), *Burkitt's Lymphoma*, p. 210–214. E and S Livingstone, Edinburgh and London.

42. Burkitt, D. P. 1975. Epidemiology and etiology. *JAMA* 231: 517–518.

43. Burkitt, D. P. 1975. Large-bowel cancer: an epidemiologic jigsaw puzzle.

J. Natl. Cancer Inst. 54: 3–6.

44. Burnet, F. M. 1970. *Immunological Surveillance*. Pergamon Press, New York.

45. Burnet, F. M. 1971. Immunological surveillance in neoplasia. *Transplant. Rev.* 7: 3–25.

46. Burnet, F. M. 1971. Implications of immunological surveillance for cancer therapy. *Israel J. Med. Sci.* 7: 9–16.

47. Burwell, R. G. 1963. The role of lymphoid tissue in morphostasis. *Lancet* 2: 69–74.

48. Caprini, J. A. 1974. Risk of cancer in renal-transplant recipients. *Surg. Gynec. Obstet.* 138: 516.

49. Carnaud, C., Hoch, B., and Trainin, N. 1974. Influence of immunologic competence of the host on metastases induced by the 3LL Lewis tumor in mice. *J. Natl. Cancer Inst.* 52: 395–399.

50. Castleman, B., Scully, R. E., and McNeely, B. U. (eds.). 1972. Case records of the Massachusetts General Hospital. Case 52-1972. *N. Engl. J. Med.* 287: 1343–1350.

51. Cataldo, E., and Shklar, G. 1964. Chemical carcinogenesis in the hamster submaxillary gland. *J. Dent. Res.* 43: 568–579.

52. Cataldo, E., Shklar, G., and Chauncey, H. H. 1964. Experimental submaxillary gland tumors in rats. *Arch. Path.* 77: 305–316.

53. Ceglowski, W. S., and Friedman, H. (eds.). 1973. *Virus Tumorigenesis and Immunogenesis*. Academic Press, New York.

54. Chan, L., and O'Malley, B. W. 1976. Mechanism of action of the sex steroid hormones. *N. Engl. J. Med.* 294: 1430–1437.

55. Cheers, C., and Waller, R. 1975. Activated macrophages in congenitally athymic "nude" mice and in lethally irradiated mice. *J. Immunol.* 115: 844–847.

56. Clapp, N. K., and Yuhas, J. M. 1973. Suggested correlation between radiation-induced immunosuppression and radiogenic leukemia in mice. *J. Natl. Cancer Inst.* 51: 1211–1215.

57. Clifford, P. 1970. Treatment-response to particular chemotherapeutic and other agents and treatment of CNS involvement, *in* D. P. Burkitt and D. H. Wright (eds.), *Burkitt's Lymphoma*, pp. 52–63. E and S Livingstone. Edinburgh and London.

58. Coggin, Jr., J. H., and Anderson, N. G. 1974. Cancer, differentiation and embryonic antigens: some central problems, *in* G. Klein and S. Weinhouse (eds.), *Advances in Cancer Research*, Volume 19, pp. 105–165. Academic Press, New York.

59. Cooperband, S. R. 1972. Humoral factors in the stimulation and inhibition of lymphopoiesis, *in* R. L. Goss (ed.), *Regulation of Organ and Tissue Growth*, pp. 159–186. Academic Press, New York.

60. Cooperband, S. R., Badger, A. N., Davis, R. C., Schmid, K., and Mannick, J. A. 1972. The effect of immunoregulatory α-globulin (IRA) on lymphocyte stimulation *in vitro. J. Immunol.* 109: 153–163.

61. Cottier, H., Hess, M. W., Keller, H. U., Luscieti, P., and Sordat, B. 1974. Immunological deficiency states and malignancy, *in* V. P. Bond, S. Hellman, S. E. Order, H. D. Suit and H. R. Withers (eds.), *Interaction of Radiation and Host*

Immune Defense Mechanisms in Malignancy, pp. 30–51. National Technical Information Service, U.S. Dept. of Commerce. Springfield, Virginia.

62. Cotton, J. R., Sarles, H. E., Remmers, Jr., A. R., Lindley, J. D., Beathard, G. A., Cottom, D. L., Fish, J. C., Townsend, Jr., C. M., and Ritzmann, S. E. 1972. The appearance of reticulum cell sarcoma at the site of antilymphocyte globulin injection. *Transplantation* 16: 154–157.

63. Crispen, R. G. (ed.). 1975. *Neoplasm Immunity: Theory and Application.* I T R, Chicago.

64. Currie, G. A. 1974. *Cancer and the Immune Response.* The Williams and Wilkins Company, Baltimore.

65. Currie, G. 1976. Immunological aspects of host resistance to the development and growth of cancer. *Biochem. Biophys. Acta* 458: 135–165.

66. David, J. R. 1971. Lymphocyte factors in cellular hypersensitivity, in R. A. Good and D. W. Fisher (eds.), *Immunobiology*, pp. 146–156. Sinauer Associates, Inc., Stamford, Conn.

67. Davis, A. M. 1976. Bronchogenic carcinoma in chronic obstructive pulmonary disease. *JAMA* 235: 621–622.

68. del Regato, J. A. 1976. Cancer of the prostate. *JAMA* 235: 1727–1730.

69. Del Villano, B. C., Croker, B. P., McConahey, P. J., and Dixon, F. J. 1976. Immunopathogenicity and oncogenicity of murine leukemia viruses. *Amer. J. Pathol.* 82: 299–314.

70. Dent, P. B. 1972. Immunodepression by oncogenic viruses. *Progr. Med. Virol.* 14: 1–35.

71. DiLuzio, N. R., McNamee, R., Olcay, I., Kitahama, A., and Miller, R. H. 1974. Inhibition of tumor growth by recognition factors (37800). *Proc. Soc. Exp. Biol. Med.* 145: 311–315.

72. Doll, R. 1968. The age distribution of cancer in man, in A. Engel and T. Larsson (eds.), *Cancer and Aging*, pp. 15–40. Nordiska Bokhandelns Förlag, Stockholm.

73. Doll, R., and Kinlen, L. 1970. Immunosurveillance and cancer: epidemiological evidence. *Brit. Med. J.* 4: 420–422.

74. Dresser, D. W., and Mitchison, N. A. 1968. The mechanism of immunological paralysis, in F. J. Dixon, Jr., and H. G. Kunkel (eds.), *Advances in Immunology*, Vol. 8, pp. 129–181. Academic Press, New York.

75. Druckery, H. 1959. Pharmacological approach to carcinogenesis, in G. E. W. Wolstenhome and M. O'Connor (eds.), *Ciba Foundation Symposium on Carcinogenesis. Mechanisms of Action*, pp. 110–127. J. and A. Churchill Ltd., London.

76. Ebbeson, P. 1974. Aging increases susceptibility of mouse skin to DMBA carcinogenesis independent of general immune status. *Science* 183: 217–218.

77. Ehrlich, P. 1909. Ueber den jetzigen stand der Karzinomferschung. Nederlandsch Tijdschrift voor Geneeskunde, Earste Helft No. 5.

78. Eisenbud, E., and Walter, R. M. 1975. Cancer at insulin injection site. *JAMA* 233: 985.

79. Enderlin, F., and Guisan, Y. 1973. Malignant tumors developing during immunosuppressive therapy: a new problem in the recipients of transplants. *Helv. Chir. Acta* 40: 773–776.

80. Essex, M. 1976. Immunity to leukemia, lymphoma, and fibrosarcoma in cats: a case for immunosurveillance, in M. G. Hanna and F. Rapp (eds.), Contemporary Topics in Immunobiology, pp. 71–106. Plenum Press, New York.

81. Essex, M., Sliski, A., Cotter, S. M., Jakowski, R. M., and Hardy, Jr., W. D. 1975. Immunosurveillance of naturally occurring feline leukemia. Science 190: 790–792.

82. Evans, A. E. 1975. The success and failure of multimodal therapy for cancer in children. Cancer 35: 48–54.

83. Evans, R., and Alexander, P. 1976. Mechanisms of extracellular killing of nucleated mammalian cells by macrophages, in D. S. Nelson (ed.), Immunobiology of the Macrophage, pp. 535–576. Academic Press, New York.

84. Evans, R. D., Keane, A. T., Kolenkow, R. J., Neal, W. R., and Shanahan, M. M. 1969. Radiogenic tumors in the radium and mesothorium cases studied at M. I. T., in C. W. Mays, W. S. S. Jee, R. D. Lloyd, B. J. Stover, J. H. Dougherty and G. H. Taylor (eds.), Delayed Effects of Bone-Seeking Radionuclides, pp. 157–194. University of Utah Press, Salt Lake City, Utah.

85. Everson, T. C., and Cole, W. H. 1966. Spontaneous Regression of Cancer. W. B. Saunders Company, Philadelphia.

86. Farber, E. 1973. Carcinogenesis-cellular evolution as a unifying thread: presidential address. Cancer Res. 33: 2537–2550.

87. Feldman, J. D. 1972. Immunological enhancement: a study of blocking antibodies, in F. J. Dixon and H. G. Kunkel (eds.), Advances in Immunology, Volume 15, p. 167–214.

88. Fenoglio, C. M., and Lane, N. 1974. The anatomical precursor of colorectal carcinoma. Cancer 34: 819–823.

89. Fidler, I. J. 1973. In vitro studies of cellular-mediated immunostimulation of tumor growth. J. Natl. Cancer Inst. 50: 1307–1312.

90. Fidler, I. J. 1974. Immune stimulation-inhibition of experimental cancer metastasis. Cancer Res. 34: 491–498.

91. Finkel, M. P., Biskis, B. O., and Jenkins, P. B. 1966. Virus induction of osteosarcomas in mice. Science 151: 698–701.

92. Fisher, B. 1975. Immune parameters in the surgery of cancer, in A. E. Reif (ed.), Immunity and Cancer in Man: An Introduction, pp. 81–90. Marcel Dekker, New York.

93. Fisher, B., and Fisher, E. R. 1972. Studies concerning the regional lymph node in cancer. II. Maintenance of immunity. Cancer 29: 1496–1501.

94. Fisher, B., Saffer, E. A., and Fisher, E. R. 1972. Studies concerning the regional lymph node in cancer. III. Response of regional lymph node cells from breast and colon cancer patients to PHA stimulation. Cancer 30: 1202–1215.

95. Fisher, R. A. 1959. Smoking. The Cancer Controversy. Some Attempts to Assess the Evidence. Oliver and Boyd, Edinburgh.

95a. Folkman, J. 1976. The vascularization of tumors. Sci. Amer. 243:58–73.

96. Folkman, J., and Greenspan, H. P. 1975. Influence of geometry on control of cell growth. Biochem. Biophys. Acta 417: 211–236.

97. Franks, L. M., and Carbonell, A. W. 1974. Effect of age on tumor induction in C57BL mice. J. Natl. Cancer Inst. 52: 565–566.

98. Froese, G., Berczi, I., and Sehon, A. H. 1974. Brief communication:

Neuraminidase-induced enhancement of tumor growth in mice. *J. Natl. Cancer Inst.* 52: 1905–1908.

99. Furth, J. 1953. Condition and autonomous neoplasms: a review. *Cancer Res.* 13: 477–492.

100. Furth, J. 1963. Influence of host factors on the growth of neoplastic cells. *Cancer Res.* 23: 21–34.

101. Furth, J. 1969. Pituitary cybernetics and neoplasia, *in The Harvey Lectures, Series 63,* pp. 47–71. Academic Press, New York.

102. Furuta, M., Ozaki, M., Harada, N., Takahashi, S., Matsumoto, S., and Murakami, M. 1972. Malignant tumors in leprosy patients-autopsy report from OKU-KOMYO-EN. *Lepro (Tokyo)* 41: 76–77.

103. Futrell, J. W., and Myers, Jr., G. H. 1973. Regional Lymphatics and cancer immunity. *Ann. Surg.* 117: 1–7.

104. Gaeta, J. F. 1973. Trauma and inflammation, *in* J. F. Holland and E. Frei (eds.), *Cancer Medicine,* pp. 102–106. Lea and Febiger, Philadelphia.

105. Gatti, R. A., and Good, R. A. 1970. The immunological deficiency diseases. *Med. Clin. N. Amer.* 54: 281–307.

106. Gatti, R. A., and Good, R. A. 1971. Occurence of malignancy in immunodeficiency diseases. *Cancer* 28: 89–98.

107. Gell, P. G. H., and Coombs, R. R. A. (eds.). 1962. *Clinical Aspects of Immunology.* Blackwell Scientific Publications, Oxford.

108. Gerbase-DeLima, M., Meredith, P., and Walford, R. L. 1975. Age-related changes, including synergy and suppression, in the mixed lymphocyte reaction in long-lived mice. *Fed. Proc.* 34: 159–161.

109. Giunta, J. L., Reif, A. E., and Shklar, G. 1974. Bacillus Calmette-Guérin and antilymphocyte serum in carcinogenesis. Effects on the hamster pouch. *Arch. Pathol.* 98: 237–240.

110. Glasgow, A. H., Cooperband, S. R., Occhino, J. A., Schmid, K., and Mannick, J. A. 1971. Inhibition of secondary immune responses *in vivo* by immunoregulatory α-globulin (IRA). *Proc. Soc. Exp. Biol. Med.* 138: 753–757.

111. Gleichmann, E., Gleichmann, H., and Schwartz, R. S. 1972. Immunologic induction of malignant lymphoma: genetic factors in the graft-versus-host model. *J. Natl. Cancer Inst.* 49: 793–804.

112. Gleichmann, E., and Gleichmann, H. 1973. Immunosuppression and neoplasia II. Is deficient immunosurveillance the only mechanism by which immunosuppression promotes neoplasia? A speculative review. *Klin. Wochschr.* 51: 260–265.

113. Gleichmann, H., and Gleichmann, E. 1973. Übersichten. Immunosuppression and neoplasia. *Klin. Wochschr.* 51: 255–265.

114. Goldrosen, M. H., and Dent, P. B. 1975. Significance of arming, potentiating and blocking factors as correlates of tumour-host interaction in the hamster SV40 system. *Brit. J. Cancer* 32: 667–677.

115. Good, R. A. (ed.). 1971. *Immunobiology.* Sinauer Associates, Stamford, Conn.

116. Good, R. A. 1972. Relations between immunity and malignancy. *Proc. Natl. Acad. Sci.* 69: 1026–1032.

117. Good, R. A. 1975. Clinical implications of the data base concerning the

tumor-host relationship, in R. T. Smith and M. Landy (eds.), Immunobiology of the Tumor-Host Relationship, pp. 277–301. Academic Press, New York.

118. Good, R. A., and Finstad, J. 1969. Essential relationship between the lymphoid system, immunity, and malignancy. Natl. Cancer Inst. Monogr. 31: 41–58.

119. Goudie, R. B., and MacFarlane, M. K. 1974. Homing of lymphocytes to non-lymphoid tissues. Lancet I: 292–293.

120. Gray, B. N. 1976. Naturally occurring human antibody to neuraminidase-treated human lymphocytes. J. Natl. Cancer Inst. 56: 211.

121. Greaves, M. F., Owen, J. J. T., and Raff, M. C. 1974. T and B Lymphocytes: Origins, Properties and Roles in Immune Responses. American Elsevier Publishing Co., Inc., New York.

122. Green, H. N. 1954. An immunological concept of cancer: a preliminary report. Brit. Med. J. 2: 1374–1380.

123. Green, H. N., Anthony, H. M., Baldwin, R. W., and Westrop, R. W. 1967. An Immunological Approach to Cancer. Appleton-Century-Crofts, New York.

124. Greenberg, A. H., and Playfair, J. H. L. 1974. Spontaneously arising cytotoxicity to the P-815-Y mastocytoma in NZB mice. Clin. Exp. Immunol. 16: 99–110.

125. Gross, L. 1965. Immunological defect in aged population and its relationship to cancer. Cancer 18: 201–204.

126. Gross, L. 1970. Oncogenic Viruses, 2nd ed. Pergamon Press, New York.

127. Gross, L. 1974. The role of viruses in the etiology of cancer and leukemia. JAMA 230: 1029–1032.

128. Gross, L. 1976. The role of C-type and other oncogenic virus particles in cancer and leukemia. N. Engl. J. Med. 294: 724–725.

129. Gumport, S. L., Harris, M. N., and Kopf, A. W. 1974. Diagnosis and management of common skin cancers. Ca. - A Cancer Journal for Clinicians 24: 218–228.

130. Haddow, A. J. 1970. Epidemiological evidence suggesting an infective element in the aetiology, in D. P. Burkitt and D. H. Wright (eds.), Burkitt's Lymphoma, pp. 198–209. E and S Livingstone, Edinburgh and London.

131. Haerer, A. F., Jackson, J. F., and Evers, C. G. 1969. Ataxia-telangiectasia with gastric adenocarcinoma. JAMA 210: 1884–1887.

132. Hall, T. C. 1974. Oncocognitive autoimmunity. Cancer Chemother. Rep., Part 1 58: 441–449.

133. Halpert, B., Sheehan, E. E., Schmalhorst, W. R., and Scott, Jr., R. 1963. Carcinoma of the prostate. A survey of 5,000 autopsies. Cancer 16: 737–742.

134. Hammond, E. C. 1966. Smoking in relation to the death rates of 1 million men and women. Natl. Cancer Inst. Monogr. 19: 127–204.

135. Haran-Ghera, N. 1971. Influence of host factors on leukemogenesis by the radiation leukemia virus. Israel J. Med. Sci. 7: 17–25.

136. Harris, J. E., and Sincovics, J. G. 1976. The Immunology of Malignant Disease, 2nd ed. C. V. Mosby Co., St. Louis.

137. Harris, R. J. C. (ed.). 1967. Specific Tumor Antigens. Medical Examination Publishing Co., Inc., Flushing, New York.

138. Harrison, D. E., and Doubleday, J. W. 1975. Normal function of im-

munologic stem cells from aged mice. *J. Immunol.* 114: 1314–1317.

139. Haskill, J. S., Yamamura, Y., Radov, L., and Parthenais, E. 1976. Discussion paper: Are peripheral and *in situ* tumor immunity related? *Ann. N.Y. Acad. Sci.* 276: 373–380.

140. Hattler, Jr., B., and Amos, B. 1966. The immunobiology of cancer: tumor antigens and the responsiveness of the host. *Monogr. Surg. Sci.* 3: 1–34.

141. Hayflick, L. 1975. Current theories of biological aging. *Fed. Proc.* 34: 9–13.

142. Hayflick, L. 1976. The cell biology of human aging. *N Engl J Med.* 295: 1302–1308.

143. Hellström, I., and Hellström, K. E. 1972. Some aspects of human tumor immunity and their possible implications for tumor prevention and therapy. *Front. Rad. Ther. Onc.* 7: 3–15.

144. Hellström, K. E., and Hellström, I. 1972. Immunity to neuroblastomas and melanomas. *Ann. Rev. Med.* 23: 19–37.

145. Hellström, K. E., and Möller, G. 1965. Immunological and immunogenetic aspects of tumor transplantation, *in* P. Kallós and B. H. Waksman (eds.), *Progress in Allergy*, Volume 9, pp. 158–245. S. Karger, Basel, New York.

146. Helson, L. 1975. Management of disseminated neuroblastoma. *Ca.-A Cancer Journal for Clinicians* 25: 264–277.

147. Herberman, R. B., Nunn, M. E., Holden, H. T., and Lavrin, D. H. 1975. Natural cytotoxic reactivity of mouse lymphoid cells against syngeneic and allogeneic tumors. II. Characterization of effector cells. *Internation. J. Cancer* 16: 230–239.

148. Hersh, E. M., Gutterman, J. U., Mavligit, G., McCredie, K. B., Bodey, G. P., Freireich, E. J., Rossen, R. D., and Butler, W. T. 1973. Host defense, chemical immunosuppression and the transplant recipient. Relative effects of intermittent versus continuous immunosuppressive therapy with reference to the objectives of treatment. *Transplant. Proc.* 5: 1191–1195.

149. Hibbs, Jr., J. B. 1975. Activated macrophages as cytotoxic effector cells. II. Requirement for local persistence of inducing antigen. *Transplantation* 19: 81–87.

150. Hibbs, Jr., J. B., Lambert, Jr., L. H., and Remington, J. S. 1972. Possible role of macrophage mediated nonspecific cytotoxicity in tumour resistance. *Nature New Biol.* 235: 48–50.

151. Hill, M. J. 1974. Bacteria and the etiology of colonic cancer. *Cancer* 34: 815–818.

152. Horn, L., and Horn, H. L. 1971. An immunological approach to the therapy of cancer? *Lancet* 2: 466–469.

153. Horsfall, Jr., F. L., and Tamm, I. (eds.). 1965. *Viral and Rickettsial Infections of Man.* J. B. Lippincott Company, Philadelphia.

154. Huggins, C., Stevens, R. E., and Hodges, C. N. 1941. Studies on prostatic cancer. II. The effect of castration on clinical patients with carcinoma of the prostate. *Arch. Surg.* 43: 209–223.

155. Ioachim, H. L., Pearse, A., and Keller, S. 1975. Patterns of metastases in viral and chemical leukemias: immunological correlations. *Proc. Amer. Assoc. Cancer Res.* 16: 106.

156. Ioachim, H. L., Pearse, A., and Keller, S. E. 1976. Role of immune mechanisms in metastatic patterns of hemopoietic tumors in rats. *Cancer Res.* 36: 2854–2862.

157. Irie, R. F., Irie, K., and Morton, D. L. 1974. Natural antibody in human serum to a neoantigen in human cultured cells grown in fetal bovine serum. *J. Natl. Cancer Inst.* 52: 1051–1058.

158. Ishizaka, K., Ishizaka, T., Tada, T., and Newcomb, R. W. 1970. Site of synthesis and function of gamma-E, in D. H. Dayton, P. A. Small, R. A. Chanock, H. E. Kaufman and T. B. Tomasi (eds.), *The Secretory Immunologic System*, pp. 71–80. U.S. Govt. Printing Office, Washington, D.C.

159. Jarrett, A. (ed.). 1973. *The Physiology and Pathophysiology of the skin*, Vol. 2: *The Nerves and Blood Vessels.* Academic Press, New York.

160. Johnson, S. 1968. The effect of thymectomy and of the dose of 3-methylcholanthrene on the induction and antigenic properties of sarcomas in C57Bl mice. *Brit. J. Cancer* 22: 93–104.

161. Kahan, B. D., and Reisfield, R. A. (eds.). 1972. *Transplantation Antigens. Markers of Biological Individuality.* Academic Press, New York.

162. Kaiser, C. W., and Reif, A. E. 1975. Immunological monitoring and adjuvant immunotherapy of selected cancer patients, in A. E. Reif (ed.), *Immunity and Cancer in Man: An Introduction*, pp. 19–46. Marcel Dekker, New York.

163. Kalengayi, M. M. R., and Desmet, V. J. 1975. Sequential histological and histochemical study of the rat liver during aflatoxin B_1-induced carcinogenesis. *Cancer Res.* 35: 2845–2852.

164. Kaplan, H. S. 1967. On the natural history of the murine leukemias: presidential address. *Cancer Res.* 27: 1325–1340.

165. Kaplan, H. S. 1971. Role of immunologic disturbance in human oncogenesis: some facts and fancies. *Brit. J. Cancer* 25: 620–627.

166. Katz, D. H., and Benacerraf, B. (eds.). 1974. *Immunological Tolerance. Mechanisms and Potential Therepeutic Applications.* Academic Press, New York.

167. King, T. J. (ed.). 1974. *Developmental Aspects of Carcinogenesis and Immunity.* Academic Press, New York.

168. Kishimoto, S., Shigemoto, S., and Yamamura, Y. 1973. Immune response in aged mice. Change of cell-mediated immunity with aging. *Transplantation* 15: 455–459.

169. Klein, E., and Holterman, O. A. 1972. Immunotherapeutic approaches to the management of neoplasms. *Natl. Cancer Inst. Monogr.* 35: 379–402.

170. Klein, G. 1965. Symposium summary, in J. Palm (ed.), *Isoantigens and Cell Interactions.* Wistar Inst. Press, Philadelphia.

171. Klein, G. 1966. Humoral and cell-mediated mechanisms for host defense in tumor immunity, in W. J. Burdette (ed.), *Viruses Inducing Cancer, Implications for Therapy*, pp. 323–349. University of Utah Press, Salt Lake City.

172. Klein, G. 1966. Recent trends in tumor immunology. *Israel J. Med. Sci.* 2: 135–142.

173. Klein, G. 1968. Tumor-specific transplantation antigens. *Cancer Res.* 28: 625–634.

174. Klein, G. 1969. Experimental studies in tumor immunology. *Fed. Proc.* 28: 1739–1753.

175. Klein, G. 1971. Immunological aspects of Burkitt's lymphoma, in F. J. Dixon and H. G. Kunkel (eds.), *Advances in Immunology*, Volume 14, pp. 187–250. Academic Press, New York.

176. Klein, G. 1972. Herpesviruses and oncogenesis. *Proc. Natl. Acad. Sci. USA* 69: 1056–1064.

177. Klein, G. 1972. Tumor immunology, in F. H. Bach and R. A. Good (eds.), *Clinical Immunobiology*, Vol. 1, pp. 219–241. Academic Press, New York.

178. Klein, G. 1973. Tumor immunology. *Transplant. Proc.* 5: 31–41.

179. Klein, G. 1975. The Epstein-Barr virus and neoplasia. *N. Engl. J. Med.* 293: 1353–1357.

180. Klein, G. 1975. Factors that interfere with or prevent effective destruction of tumors via immune mechanisms, in R. T. Smith and M. Landy (eds.), *Immunobiology of the Tumor-Host Relationship*, pp. 201–215. Academic Press, New York.

181. Klein, G. 1975. Immunological surveillance against neoplasia, in *The Harvey Lectures*, Series 69, pp. 71–102. Academic Press, New York.

182. Klein, G. 1976. Tumour immunology: a general appraisal, in T. Symington and R. L. Carter (eds.), *Scientific Foundations of Oncology*, pp. 497–504. William Heinemann Medical Books, London.

183. Kochwa, S., Terry, W. D., Capra, J. D., and Yang, N. L. 1971. Structural studies of immunoglobulin E. I. Physicochemical studies of the IgE molecule. *Ann. N.Y. Acad. Sci.* 190: 49–70.

184. Kodama, M., and Kodama, T. 1975. Enhancing effect of hydrocortisone on hematogenous metastasis of Ehrlich ascites tumor in mice. *Cancer Res.* 35: 1015–1021.

185. Kodama, T., Gotohda, E., Takeichi, N., Kuzumaki, N., and Kobayashi, H. 1975. Histopathology of regression of tumor metastasis in the lymph nodes. *Cancer Res.* 35: 1628–1636.

186. Konen, T. G., Smith, G. S., and Walford, R. L. 1973. Decline in mixed lymphocyte reactivity of spleen cells from aged mice of a long-lived strain. *J. Immunol.* 110: 216–1221.

187. Koranda, F. C., Dehmel, E. M., Kahn, G., and Penn, I. 1974. Cutaneous complications in immunosuppressed renal homograft recipients. *JAMA* 229: 419–424.

188. Kripke, M. L., and Borsos, T. 1974. Immune surveillance revisited. *J. Natl. Cancer Inst.* 52: 1393–1395.

189. Kurstak, E., and Maramorosch, K. (eds.). 1974. *Viruses, Evolution and Cancer*. Academic Press, New York.

190. Kuschner, M. 1968. The J. Burns Amberson lecture: The causes of lung cancer. *Amer. Rev. Resp. Dis.* 98: 573–590.

191. Landau, R. L. 1974. Does testosterone therapy for impotence increase risk of prostatic carcinoma? *JAMA* 229: 1357.

192. Law, L. W. 1969. Studies of the significance of tumor antigens in induction and repression of neoplastic diseases: presidential address. *Cancer Res.* 29: 1–21.

193. Law, L. W. 1975. Immune surveillance revisited. *J. Natl. Cancer Inst.* 54: 280–282.

194. Lee, J. C., and Ihle, J. N. 1975. Autogenous immunity to endogenous RNA tumor virus: reactivity of natural immune sera to antigenic determinants of several biologically distinct murine leukemia viruses. *J. Natl. Cancer Inst.* 55: 831–838.

195. Levy, M., Petreshock, E. P., Mandell, C., Deysine, M., Katzka, I., and Aufses, A. H. 1975. The response of the local immunoglobulin system to malignant lesions of the stomach: a new diagnostic test. *Cancer* 36: 1991–1995.

196. Li, F. P., Cassady, J. R., and Jaffe, N. 1975. Risk of second tumors in survivors of childhood cancer. *Cancer* 35: 1230–1235.

197. Lipkin, M. 1976. Biology of large bowel cancer. Present status and research frontiers. *Cancer* 36: 2319–2324.

198. Loeb, J. N. 1976. Corticosteroids and growth. *N. Engl. J. Med.* 295: 547–552.

199. Maguire, Jr., H., Outzen, H. C., Custer, R. P., and Prehn, R. T. 1976. Brief communication: invasion and metastasis of a xenogeneic tumor in nude mice. *J. Natl. Cancer Inst.* 57: 439–442.

200. Makinodan, T., and Adler, W. H. 1975. Effects of aging on the differentiation and proliferation potentials of cells of the immune system. *Fed. Proc.* 34: 153–158.

201. Makinodan, T., and Peterson, W. J. 1966. Secondary antibody-forming potential of mice in relation to age—its significance in senescence. *Devel. Biol.* 14: 96–111.

202. Manusow, D., and Weinerman, B. H. 1975. Subsequent neoplasia in chronic lymphocytic leukemia. *JAMA* 232: 267–269.

203. Marks, F. 1976. Epidermal growth control mechanisms, hyperplasia, and tumor promotion in the skin. *Cancer Res.* 36: 2636–2643.

204. Marx, J. L. 1974. Tumor immunology (I): the host's response to cancer. *Science* 184: 552–556.

205. McCann, R. L., and Sussdorf, D. H. 1974. Antibody responses in athymic ('nude') mice implanted with neonatal or adult allogeneic thymus (37808). *Proc. Soc. Exp. Biol. Med.* 145: 351–353.

206. McKhann, C. F. 1972. Immune surveillance and malignancy. *Front. Rad. Ther. Onc.* 7: 16–22.

207. McKhann, C. F., and Jagarlamoody, S. M. 1971. Evidence for immune reactivity against neoplasms. *Transplant. Rev.* 7: 55–77.

208. Milder, J. W. 1965. Conference on hormone-related tumors: introduction. *Cancer Res.* 25: 1056.

209. Milder, J. W. 1968. Introductory remarks: symposium on tumor antigens. *Cancer Res.* 28: 1279.

210. Milgrom, F. 1968. Autoimmunity in relation to transplantation, in F. T. Rapaport, F. T. and Dausset, J. (eds.), *Human Transplantation*, pp. 587–600. Grune and Stratton, New York.

211. Miller, J. A. 1970. Carcinogenesis by chemicals: an overview-G. H. A. Clowes memorial lecture. *Cancer Res.* 30: 559–576.

212. Mittal, K. K., Ferrone, S., Mickey, M. R., Pellegrino, M. A., Reisfeld, R. A., and Terasaki, P. I. 1973. Serological characterization of natural antihuman lymphocytotoxic antibodies in mammalian sera. *Transplantation* 16: 287–294.

213. Möller, G., and Möller, E. 1975. Considerations of some current concepts in cancer research. *J. Natl. Cancer Inst.* 55: 755–759.

214. Momeni, M. H., Williams, J. R., Jow, N., and Rosenblatt, L. S. 1976. Dose rates, dose, and time effects of ^{90}Sr + ^{90}Y and ^{226}Ra on beagle skeleton. *Health Phys.* 30: 381–390.

215. Moore, M., and Williams, D. E. 1973. Tumor-specific antigenicity of osteosarcomas induced in rodents by bone-seeking radionuclides, in C. L. Sanders, R. H. Busch, J. E. Ballou and D. D. Mahlum, *Radionuclide Carcinogenesis.* U.S. Atomic Energy Commission Symposium, Series 29, pp. 289–306. Tech. Inf. Center, Oak Ridge, Tenn.

216. Morson, B. C. 1974. Evolution of cancer of the colon and rectum. *Cancer* 34: 845–849.

217. Mulvihill, J. J. 1975. Congenital and genetic diseases, in J. F. Fraumeni, Jr. (ed.), *Persons at High Risk of Cancer. An Approach to Cancer Etiology and Control,* pp. 3–37. Academic Press, New York.

218. Murphy, D. P., and Abbey, H. 1959. *Cancer in Families.* Harvard University Press, Cambridge, Mass.

219. Murphy, G. P. 1974. Prostate cancer. *Ca.-A Cancer Journal for Clinicians* 24: 282–288.

220. Nagasawa, H., and Yanai, R. 1974. Brief communication: Frequency of mammary cell division in relation to age: its significance in the induction of mammary tumors by carcinogen in rats. *J. Natl. Cancer Inst.* 52: 609–610.

221. Nathan, C. F., and Terry, W. D. 1975. Differential stimulation of murine lymphoma growth in vitro by normal and BCG-activated macrophages. *J. Exp. Med.* 142: 887–902.

222. Newhouse, M., Sanchis, J., and Bienenstock, J. 1976. Lung Defense Mechanisms. *N. Engl. J. Med.* 295: 1045–1052.

223. Noar, D., Bonavida, B., and Walford, R. L. 1976. Autoimmunity and aging: the age-related response of mice of a long-lived strain to trinitrophenylated syngeneic mouse red blood cells. *J. Immunol.* 117: 2204–2208.

224. Noble, R. L. 1977. Hormonal control of growth and progression in tumors of Nb rats and a theory of action. *Cancer Res.* 37: 82–94.

225. Nossal, G. J. V. 1974. Lymphocyte differentiation and immune surveillance against cancer, in T. J. King (ed.), *Developmental Aspects of Carcinogenesis and Immunity,* pp. 205–213. Academic Press, New York.

226. Nunn, M. E., Djeu, J. Y., Glaser, M., Lavrin, D. H., and Herberman, R. B. 1976. Natural cytotoxic reactivity of rat lymphocytes against syngeneic Gross virus-induced lymphoma. *J. Natl. Cancer Inst.* 56: 393–399.

227. Oettgen, H. F., Old, L. J., and Boyse, E. A. 1971. Human tumor immunology. Symposium on medical aspects of cancer. *Med. Cl. N. Amer.* 55: 761–785.

228. Old, L. J., Boyse, E. J., Clarke, D. A., et al. 1962. Antigenic properties of chemically induced tumors. *Ann. N.Y. Acad. Sci.* 101: 80–106.

229. Old, L. J., and Boyse, E. A. 1964. Immunology of experimental tumors. *Ann. Rev. Med.* 15: 167–186.

230. Old, L. J., and Boyse, E. A. 1973. Current enigmas in cancer research, in *The Harvey Lectures, Series 67,* pp. 273–315. Academic Press, New York.

231. Old, L. J., Stockert, E., Boyse, E. A., and Kim, J. H. 1968. Antigenic

modulation: loss of T L antigen from cells exposed to T L antibody, study of the phenomenon in vitro. J. Exp. Med. 127: 523–539.

232. Ooi, B. S., Orlina, A. R., Masaitis, L., First, M. R., Pollack, V. E., and Ooi, Y. M. 1974. Lymphocytoxins in aging. Transplantation 18: 190–192.

233. Order, S. E. 1975. Immune parameters in the radiation therapy of cancer, in A. E. Reif (ed.), Immunity and Cancer in Man: An Introduction, pp. 91–102. Marcel Dekker, New York.

234. O'Toole, C., Perlmann, P., Unsgaard, B., Moberger, G., and Edsmyr, F. 1972. Cellular immunity to human urinary bladder carcinoma. I. Correlation to clinical stage and radiotherapy. Int. J. Cancer 10: 77–91.

235. Paranjpe, M. S., and Boone, C. W. 1974. Stimulated growth of syngeneic tumors at the site of an ongoing delayed-hypersensitivity reaction to tuberculin in BALB/c mice. J. Natl. Cancer Inst. 52: 1297–1299.

236. Parmiani, G., Colnaghi, M. I., and Della Porta, G. 1971. Immunodepression during urethane and N-nitrosomethylurea leukaemogenesis in mice. Brit. J. Cancer 25: 354–364.

237. Peacock, Jr., E. E., and Van Winkle, Jr., W. 1970. Surgery and Biology of Wound Repair. W.B. Saunders Company, Philadelphia.

238. Penn, I. 1974. Chemical immunosuppression and human cancer. Cancer 34: 1474–1480.

239. Penn, I. 1976. Second malignant neoplasms associated with immunosuppressive medications. Cancer 37: 1024–1032.

240. Penn, I., and Starzl, T. E. 1972. Malignant tumors arising de novo in immunosuppressed organ transplant recipients. Transplantation 14: 407–417.

241. Peter, H. H., Eife, R. F., and Kalden, J. R. 1976. Spontaneous cytotoxicity (SCMC) of normal human lymphocytes against a human melanoma cell line: a phenomenon due to a lymphotoxin-like mediator. J. Immunol. 116: 342–348.

242. Peto, R., Roe, F. J. C., Lee, P. N., Levy, L., and Clack, J. 1975. Cancer and aging in mice and men. Brit. J. Cancer 32: 411–426.

243. Pierce, G. B., and Johnson, L. D. 1971. Differentiation and cancer. In Vitro 7: 140–145.

244. Pierotti, M. A., and Colnaghi, M. I. 1975. Natural antibodies directed against murine lymphosarcoma cells. J. Natl. Cancer Inst. 55: 945–949.

245. Piessens, W. F., Churchill, Jr., W. H., and David, J. R. 1975. Macrophages activated in vitro with lymphocyte mediators kill neoplastic but not normal cells. J. Immunol. 114: 293–299.

246. Pike, M. C., Gordon, R. J., Henderson, B. E., Menck, H. R., and SooHoo, J. 1975. Air pollution, in J. F. Fraumeni (ed.), Persons at High Risk of Cancer. An Approach to Cancer Etiology and Control, pp. 225–239. Academic Press, New York.

247. Pinkel, D. 1976. Curability of childhood cancer. JAMA 235: 1049–1050.

248. Pisano, J. C., Jackson, J. P., DiLuzio, N. R., and Ichinose, H. 1972. Dimensions of humoral recognition factor depletion in carcinomatous patients. Cancer Res. 32: 11–15.

249. Plotkin, S. A. 1975. Immunoprophylaxis and immunotherapy of virus infections, in C. Koprowski and H. Koprowski (eds.), Viruses and Immunity, pp. 117–127. Academic Press, New York.

250. Prehn, R. T. 1963. The role of immune mechanisms in the biology of chemically and physically induced tumors, in Conceptual Advances in Immunology and Oncology, pp. 475–485. Harper and Row, New York.

251. Prehn, R. T. 1967. The significance of tumor-distinctive histocompatibility antigens, in J. J. Trentin (ed.), Cross-Reacting Antigens and Neoantigens, pp. 105. The Williams and Wilkins Co., Baltimore.

252. Prehn, R. T. 1971. Immunosurveillance, regeneration, and oncogenesis. Progr. Exp. Tumor Res. 14: 1–24.

253. Prehn, R. T. 1972. Immune involvement in oncogenesis, in Seventh National Cancer Conference Proceedings, pp. 401–404. J. B. Lippincott, Philadelphia.

254. Prehn, R. T. 1972. Role of tumor antigens in the biology of neoplasia, in A. Nowotny (ed.), Cellular Antigens, pp. 303–313. Springer-Verlag, New York.

255. Prehn, R. T. 1972. The immune reaction as a stimulator of tumor growth. Science 176: 170–171.

256. Prehn, R. T. 1974. Immunological surveillance: pro and con, in F. H. Bach and R. A. Good (eds.), Clinical Immunobiology, Vol. 2, pp. 191–203. Academic Press, New York.

257. Prehn, R. T. 1975. Nongenetic variability in susceptibility to oncogenesis. Science 190: 1095–1096.

258. Prehn, R. T., and Lappé, M. A. 1971. An immunostimulation theory of tumor development. Transplant. Rev. 7: 26–54.

259. Price, G. B., and Makinodan, T. 1972. Immunologic deficiencies in senescence. I. Characterization of intrinsic deficiencies. J. Immunol. 108: 403–417.

260. Proffitt, M. R., Hirsch, M. S., and Black, P. H. 1973. Murine leukemia: a virus-induced autoimmune disease? Science 182: 821–823.

261. Purtilo, D. T., and Pangi, C. 1975. Incidence of cancer in patients with leprosy. Cancer 35: 1259–1261.

262. Rafferty, K. A., Jr. 1973. Herpes viruses and cancer. Sci. Amer. 229: 26–33.

263. Rapp, F. 1973. Question: Do herpesviruses cause cancer? Answer: Of course they do! J. Natl. Cancer Inst. 50: 825–832.

264. Rauscher, F. J., and O'Connor, T. E. 1973. Virology, in J. F. Holland and E. Frei (eds.), Cancer Medicine, pp. 15–44. Lea and Febiger, Philadelphia.

264a. Reich, E., Rifkin, D., and Shaw, E. (eds.), 1975. Proteases and Biological Control, Cold Spring Harbor Conferences on Cell Proliferation, Vol. 2. Cold Spring Harbor Laboratory, Cold Spring Harbor, New York.

265. Reid, R. H., Pirofsky, B., and Dawson, P. J. 1972. The influence of immunosuppression and allografting on virus-induced lymphatic leukemia in mice. Transplantation 13: 61–65.

266. Reif, A. E. 1958. International cancer congress. Science 128: 1512–1522.

267. Reif, A. E. 1966. Immunity, cancer and chemotherapy. Science 154: 1475–1478.

268. Reif, A. E. 1975. Immune defenses against initiation of tumors, in A. E. Reif (ed.), Immunity and Cancer in Man: An Introduction, pp. 1–18. Marcel Dekker, New York.

269. Reif, A. E. 1976. Public information on smoking: an urgent responsibil-

ity for cancer research workers. *J. Natl. Cancer Inst.* 57: 1207–1210.

270. Richter, M. N. 1957. The spleen, lymph nodes, and reticuloendothelial system, in W. A. D. Anderson (ed.), *Pathology*, 3rd ed., p. 936. C. V. Mosby Co., St. Louis.

271. Riesz, T., Riskó, Z., Winkler, V., and Juhász, J. 1976. A clinico-pathological study on the correlation of immunosuppression and multiple primary malignant neoplasmas. *Neoplasma* 23: 409–420.

272. Roelants, G. E., Mayor, K. S., Hägg, L.-B., and Loor, F. 1975. T lineage lymphocytes in athymic mice, in M. Seligmann, J. L. Preud'homme and F. M. Kourilsky, (eds.), *Membrane Receptors of Lymphocytes*, pp. 361–362. American Elsevier Publishing Company, New York.

273. Roizman, B., and Kieff, E. D. 1975. Herpes simplex and Epstein-Barr viruses in human cells and tissues: a study in contrasts, in F. F. Becker (ed.), *Cancer*, Vol. 2, pp. 241–322. Plenum Press, New York.

274. Rose, N. R., and Bartholomew, W. R. 1976. Discussion paper: loss of cellular antigens during malignant transformation. *Ann. N.Y. Acad. Sci.* 276: 243–253.

275. Rosenberg, S. A., and Rogentine, Jr., G. N., 1972. Natural antibodies in human immune surveillance. *Surg. Forum* 23: 96–98.

276. Rosenberg, S. A., and Rogentine, Jr., G. N., 1972. Natural human antibodies to "hidden" membrane components. *Nature New Biol.* 239: 203–204.

277. Rushmer, R. F., Buettner, K. J. K., Short, J. M., and Odland, G. F. 1966. The skin. *Science* 154: 343–348.

278. Russell, E. S. 1966. Lifespan and aging patterns, in E. L. Green (ed.), *Biology of the Laboratory Mouse*, 2nd ed., pp. 511–519. McGraw-Hill Book Co., New York.

279. Rygaard, J., and Povlsen, C. O. 1974. Is immunological surveillance not a cell-mediated immune function? *Transplantation* 17: 135–136.

280. Ryser, H. J.-P. 1971. Chemical carcinogenesis. *N. Engl. J. Med.* 285: 721–734.

281. Ryser, H. J.-P. 1974. Special report: chemical carcinogenesis. *Ca.-A Cancer Journal for Clinicians* 24: 351–360.

282. Sampson, W. I. 1976. Cancer at insulin injection site. *JAMA* 235: 374.

283. Scheid, M. P., Goldstein, G., and Boyse, E. A. 1975. Differentiation of T cells in nude mice. *Science* 190: 1211–1213.

284. Schwartz, R. S. 1972. Immunoregulation, oncogenic viruses, and malignant lymphomas. *Lancet* 1: 1266–1269.

285. Schwartz, R. S. 1974. Immunosuppressive chemotherapy and malignancy. *Transplant. Proc.* 6: 45–48.

286. Schwartz, R. S. 1975. Another look at immunological surveillance. *N. Engl. J. Med.* 293: 181—184.

287. Schwartz, R., and Borel, Y. 1968. Principles of immunosuppressive drug action, in P. A. Miescher and H. J. Muller-Eberhard (eds.), *Textbook of Immunopathology*, Vol. I, pp. 227–235. Grune and Stratton, New York.

288. Segre, D., and Segre, M. 1976. Humoral immunity in aged mice. II. Increased suppressor T cell activity in immunologically deficient old mice. *J. Immunol.* 116: 735–738.

289. Seligmann, M., Preud'homme, J. L., and Kourilsky, F. M. (eds.). 1975. *Membrane Receptors of Lymphocytes*. American Elsevier Publishing Co., New York.

290. Selikoff, I. J., and Hammond, E. C. 1975. Multiple risk factors in Environmental cancer, *in* J. F. Fraumeni, Jr. (ed.), *Persons at High Risk of Cancer. An Approach to Cancer Etiology and Control*, pp. 467–483. Academic Press, New York.

291. Sendo, F., Aoki, T., Boyse, E. A., and Buafo, C. K. 1975. Natural occurrence of lymphocytes showing cytotoxic activity to BALB/c radiation-induced leukemia RL♂1 cells. *J. Natl. Cancer Inst.* 55: 603–609.

292. Sethi, K. K., and Brandis, H. 1972. *In vitro* cytotoxicity of normal serum factor(s) on neuraminidase-treated Ehrlich ascites tumor cells and murine leukemia L1210 cells. *Z. Immunitaets-Forsch. Exp. Klin. Immunol.* 143: 426–429.

293. Shearer, W. T., Philpott, G. W., and Parker, C. W. 1973. Stimulation of cells by antibody. *Science* 182: 1357–1359.

294. Sieber, S. M. 1975. Cancer chemotherapeutic agents and carcinogenesis. *Cancer Chemother. Rep.*, Part 1, 59: 915–918.

295. Siegler, R., and Rich, M. A. 1964. Comparative pathogenesis of murine viral lymphoma. *Cancer Res.* 24: 1406–1417.

296. Silverman, A. Y., Yagi, Y., Pressman, D., Ellison, R. R., and Tormey, D. C. 1973. Monoclonal IgA and IgM in the serum of a single patient (S C) III. Immunofluorescent identification of cells producing IgA and IgM. *J. Immunol.* 110: 350–353.

297. Slaga, T. J., and Scribner, J. D. 1973. Brief communication: Inhibition of tumor initiation and promotion by anti-inflammatory agents. *J. Natl. Cancer Inst.* 51: 1723–1725.

298. Smith, R. D. 1976. Checking out the fiber fad. *Sciences*, Mar./Apr: 25–29.

299. Smith, R. T. 1968. Tumor-specific immune mechanisms. *N. Engl. J. Med.* 278: 1207–1214.

300. Smith, R. T., and Landy, M. (eds.). 1970. *Immune Surveillance*. Academic Press, New York.

301. Smith, R. T., and Landy, M. (eds.). 1975. *Immunobiology of the Tumor-Host Relationship*. Academic Press, New York.

302. Snell, G. D., Dausset, J., and Nathenson, S. 1976. *Histocompatibility*. Academic Press, New York.

303. Snell, G. D., and Stimpfling, J. H. 1966. Genetics of tissue transplantation, *in* E. L. Green (ed.), *Biology of the Laboratory Mouse*, 2nd ed., pp. 457–491. McGraw-Hill Book Co., New York.

304. Southam, C. M. 1967. Cancer immunology in man, *in* M. Busch (ed.), *Methods in Cancer Research*, Vol. 2, pp. 1–43. Academic Press, New York.

305. Southam, C. M. 1967. Tumor resistance in cancer patients, *in* R. W. Wissler, T. L. Dao, and S. Wood, Jr. (eds.), *Endogenous Factors Influencing Host-Tumor Balance*, pp. 199–219. The University of Chicago Press, Chicago.

306. Southam, C. M. 1968. The immunologic status of patients with nonlymphomatous cancer. *Cancer Res.* 28: 1433–1440.

307. Southam, C. M., and Friedman, H. (eds.). 1976. *International Conference on Immunotherapy of Cancer. Ann. N.Y. Acad. Sci.* 277.

308. Spiegelberg, H. L. 1974. Biological activities of immunoglobulins of different classes and subclasses, in F. J. Dixon and H. G. Kunkel (eds.), *Advances in Immunology*, Vol. 19, pp. 259–294. Academic Press, New York.

309. Starzl, T. E., Penn, I., Putnam, C. W., Groth, C. G., and Halgrimson, C. G. 1971. Iatrogenic alterations of immunologic surveillance in man and their influence on malignancy. *Transplant. Rev.* 7: 112–145.

310. Steiner, P. E. 1954. *Cancer: Race and Geography*. The Williams and Wilkins Co., Baltimore.

311. Storer, J. B. 1975. Radiation carcinogenesis, in F. F. Becker (ed.), *Cancer*, Vol. 1, pp. 453–483. Plenum Press, New York.

312. Stutman, O. 1974. Tumor development after 3-methylcholanthrene in immunologically deficient athymic-nude mice. *Science* 183: 534–536.

313. Tax, A., and Manson, L. A. 1975. Antibody activity to a spontaneous mouse mammary adenocarcinoma in normal sera. *Fed. Proc.* 34: 1023.

314. Terasaki, P. I., Esail, M. L., Cannon, J. A., and Longmire, Jr., W. P., 1961. Destruction of lymphocytes in vitro by normal serum from common laboratory animals. *J. Immunol.* 87: 383–385.

315. Tevethia, S. S., and Tevethia, M. J. 1975. DNA virus (SV 40) induced antigens, in F. F. Becker (ed.), *Cancer*, Vol. 4, pp. 185–207. Plenum Press, New York.

316. Thomas, L. 1959. Discussion, in H. S. Lawrence (ed.), *Cellular and Humoral Aspects of the Hypersensitive States*, p. 529. Cassell, London.

317. Thompson, T. F. 1976. Diet and diseases of the colon. *JAMA* 235: 2815.

318. Tomasi, T. B. 1970. The concept of local immunity and the secretory system, in D. H. Dayton, P. A. Small, R. A. Chanock, H. E. Kaufman, and T. B. Tomasi (eds.), *The Secretory Immunologic System*, pp. 3–10. U.S. Govt. Printing Office, Washington, D.C.

319. Tomasi, T. B., Bull, D., Tourville, D., Montes, M., and Yurchak, A. 1970. Distribution and synthesis of human secretory components, in D. H. Dayton, P. A. Small, R. A. Chanock, H. E. Kaufman and T. B. Tomasi (eds.), *The Secretory Immunologic System*, pp. 41–53. U.S. Govt. Printing Office, Washington, D. C.

320. Townsend, C. M., Jr., Eilber, F. R., and Morton, D. L. 1976. Skeletal and soft tissue sarcomas. Treatment with adjuvant immunotherapy. *JAMA* 236: 2187–2189.

321. Trentin, J. J. 1976. Tumor immunotherapy in experimental animals: current status and prospectus. *Ann. N.Y. Acad. Sci.* 277: 716–721.

322. Treves, N., and Pack, G. T. 1930. The development of cancer in burn scars. *Surg. Gynec. Obstet.* 51: 749–782.

323. Twomey, P. L., Catalona, W. J., and Chretien, P. B. 1974. Cellular immunity in cured cancer patients. *Cancer* 33: 435–440.

324. Tyler, A. 1946. An auto-antibody concept of cell structure, growth, and differentiation. *Growth Suppl.* 10: 7–19.

325. Tyler, A. 1960. Clues to the etiology, pathology, and therapy of cancer provided by analogies with transplantation disease. *J. Natl. Cancer Inst.* 25: 1197–1229.

326. Tyler, A. 1962. A developmental immunogenetic analysis of cancer, in M. J. Brennan and W. L. Simpson (eds.), *Biological Interactions in Normal and*

Neoplastic Growth, pp. 533–571. Little, Brown and Co., Boston.

327. Uhr, J. W., and Scharff, M. 1969. Delayed hypersensitivity: The effect of X-irradiation on the development of delayed hypersensitivity and antibody formation. *J. Exp. Med.* 112: 65–76.

328. Upton, A. C. 1973. Radiation, *in* J. F. Holland and E. Frei (eds.), *Cancer Medicine*, pp. 90–101. Lea and Febiger, Philadelphia.

329. U.S. Dept. Health, Education and Welfare. 1968. *Vital Statistics of the United States*. Vol. 2. *Mortality*, pp. 1–150. U. S. Govt. Printing Office, Washington, D. C.

330. U.S. Dept. of Health, Education, and Welfare. 1973. *The Health Consequences of Smoking*. DHEW Publ. No. (HSM)73-9704. U.S. Govt. Printing Office. Washington, D.C.

331. Vaage, J. 1973. Humoral and cellular immune factors in the systemic control of artificially induced metastases in C3Hf mice. *Cancer Res.* 33: 1957–1965.

332. Vesselinovitch, S. D., Rao, K. V. N., Mihailovitch, N., Rice, J. M., and Lombard, L. S. 1974. Development of broad spectrum of tumors by ethylnitrosourea in mice and the modifying role of age, sex, and strain. *Cancer Res.* 34: 2530–2538.

333. Walburg, Jr., H. E., 1974. Experimental radiation carcinogenesis, *in* J. T. Lett, H. Adler and M. Zelle (eds.), *Advances in Radiation Biology*, Vol. 4, pp. 209–254. Academic Press, New York.

334. Walder, B. K., Robertson, M. R., and Jeremy, D. 1971. Skin cancer and immunosuppression. *Lancet* 2: 1282–1283.

335. Walsh, P. C. 1976. *Benign Prostatic Hyperplasia: Etiological Considerations*. Alan R. Liss, New York.

336. Walters, C. S., and Claman, H. N. 1975. Age-related changes in cell-mediated immunity in BALB/C mice. *J. Immunol.* 115: 1438–1443.

337. Watson, W. L. (ed.). 1968. *Lung Cancer*. C. V. Mosby Co., St. Louis.

338. Weigle, W. O., and Romball, C. G. 1975. Humoral and cell-mediated immunity in experimental progressive thyroiditis in rabbits. *Clin. Exp. Immunol.* 21: 351–361.

339. Weigle, W. O., Sieckmann, D. G., Doyle, M. V., and Chiller, J. M. 1975. Possible roles of suppressor cells in immunological tolerance. *Transplant. Rev.* 26: 186–205.

340. Weisburger, J. H. 1973. Chemical carcinogenesis, *in* J. F. Holland and E. Frei (eds.), *Cancer Medicine*, pp. 45–90. Lea and Febiger, Philadelphia.

341. Weiss, D. W. (ed.). 1974. *Immunological Parameters of Host-Tumor Relationships*, Vol. 3. Academic Press, New York.

342. Weiss, L. (ed.). 1976. *Fundamental Aspects of Metastasis. Papers from a Symposium*, Buffalo, N.Y., July 1975. Elsevier, New York.

343. Weiss, P. A., and Kavanau, J. L. 1957. A model of growth and growth control in mathematical terms. *J. Gen Physiol.* 41: 1–47.

344. Weissman, I. L. 1973. Tumor immunity *in vivo*: evidence that immune destruction of tumor leaves "bystander" cells intact. *J. Natl. Cancer Inst.* 51: 443–448.

345. Wigzell, H., and Stjernswärd, J. 1966. Age-dependent rise and fall of

immunological reactivity in the CBA mouse. *J. Natl. Cancer Inst.* 37: 513–517.

346. Wissler, R. W., Dao, T. L., and Wood, S., Jr. (eds.). 1967. *Endogenous Factors Influencing Host-Tumor Balance.* University of Chicago Press, Chicago.

347. Woodruff, M. F. A. 1964. Immunological aspects of cancer. *Lancet* 2: 265–269.

348. Wynder, E. L. 1975. The epidemiology of large bowel cancer. *Cancer Res.* 35: 3388–3394.

349. Wynder, E. L. 1976. Tobacco and tobacco smoke. *Seminars in Oncology* 3: 5–15.

350. Wynder, E. L., and Reddy, B. S. 1975. Dietary fat and colon cancer. *J. Natl. Cancer Inst.* 54: 7–10.

351. Yardley, J. H., and Keren, D. F. 1974. "Precancer" lesions in ulcerative colitis. A retrospective study of rectal biopsy and colectomy specimens. *Cancer* 34: 835–844.

352. Zarling, J. M., Nowinski, R. C., and Bach, F. H. 1975. Lysis of leukemia cells by spleen cells of normal mice. *Proc. Natl. Acad. Sci. USA* 72: 2780–2784.

CHAPTER 7

FUNCTIONS OF CELL SURFACE IMMUNO- GLOBULINS

John J. Marchalonis,
Gregory W. Warr,
Jane M. Moseley, and
Janet M. Decker

Laboratory of Molecular Immunology
The Walter and Eliza Hall Institute
of Medical Research, P.O.
Royal Melbourne Hospital
Victoria 3050, Australia
Present Address:
Basic Research Program
Frederick Cancer Research Center
Frederick, Maryland 21701

The current status of our knowledge about the types and function of immunoglobulins found on the surface of a variety of cells is presented. The immunoglobulins endogenously synthesized by thymus-derived (T) lymphocytes and bone-marrow-derived (B) lymphocytes are described, and their involvement in antigen recognition, lymphocyte activation, and cell collaboration is discussed. In addition, the passive adsorption of serum antibody on to the surface of various cell types (macrophages, granulocytes, mast cells, and lymphocytes) and the role of these cell types in the immune defenses of the body are discussed.

I. INTRODUCTION

Various cell types including lymphocytes, macrophages, mast cells, and polymorphonuclear leukocytes, can possess surface immunoglobulin. This immunoglobulin can, in principle, arise in two ways.

a) Lymphocytes, particularly bone-marrow-derived cells (B cells), synthesize and express readily detectable surface immunoglobulins. Thymus-derived lymphocytes (T cells), those cells active in cell-mediated processes such as allograft rejection, usually do not possess surface immunoglobulin detectable by relatively insensitive screening techniques which show B cell surface immunoglobulin (172). Although the existence and function of T cell immunoglobulin has been an issue of major controversy for the past five years (91), recent data indicate that these cells synthesize and express an immunoglobulin, T Ig,[1] which differs from B cell immunoglobulins in certain antigenic and functional properties (26, 151, 152, 207).

b) In addition to endogenously synthesized surface immunoglobulins, B cells and some T cells (55) possess receptors which bind the Fc fragment of exogenously produced antibodies, which are usually of the IgG class. The nonlymphoid cells listed above lack the capacity to synthesize immunoglobulin; but macrophages, granulocytes, and platelets can bind some serum immunoglobulins via Fc receptors, mast cells can bind IgE via a receptor for the Fc region of these molecules, and some tumor cells can be coated with antibodies directed against tumor antigens. Similarly, antibodies directed against self antigens can bind to tissues and cells in autoimmune conditions.

The endogenously produced surface immunoglobulin is implicated in three lymphocyte functions; namely, (1) recognition of antigen by B and T lymphocytes, (2) activation of lymphocytes (B and T cells), and (3) antigen-specific cooperation among B and T cells in an interaction requiring macrophages as accessory cells. Exogenously produced surface immunoglobulin is implicated or directly involved in a number of host reactions to immunization or infection which might be considered part of the inflammatory response. For example, the immunoglobulins passively displayed by macrophages act as opsonins in phagocytosis of foreign antigen by these cells and the binding of antigen to the passive IgE of mast cells initiates anaphylactic reactions. This chapter will discuss the nature of surface immunoglobulins, their interactions with the plasma membrane, and their involvement in specific and nonspecific immune phenomena.

II. PROPERTIES OF SERUM IMMUNOGLOBULINS

Prior to considering surface immunoglobulins, it is necessary to review briefly some of the properties of circulating antibodies which are germane to those of the membrane-associated receptor molecules. Immunoglobulin molecules have now been identified in representative species of all vertebrate classes (40, 153, 158), and the primary amino acid sequence of the polypeptide chains of immunoglobulins of man (59, 205), mouse (110), and guinea pig (215) have been elucidated (see 60, 81, 185). A high degree of conservation of immunoglobulin structure has been maintained throughout vertebrate evolution (147, 150, 153). All normally occurring immunoglobulins are glycoproteins consisting of a basic four-chain structure comprising two heavy and two light chains linked covalently by disulfide bonds, and also by noncovalent interactions. Each heavy chain (molecular weight, 50,000–77,000), plus one light (L) chain (molecular weight, 23,000) provides one binding site. Carbohydrate moieties are associated with the heavy chains and account for about 2% of γ chain mass and about 10% of μ chain mass. The basic four-chain unit may exist as the only unit, as in IgG, which can be written $(L\gamma)_2$, or as polymers, as in pentameric IgM, which has a structural formula that may be written $(L\mu)_{10}$ to emphasize that the molecule is a cyclic polymer having 10 combining sites. Additional chains may also occur, such as the "J" chain in polymeric IgM or the secretory component of IgA (38). Each immunoglobulin class or isotype is characterized by its heavy chain species and the number of basic units linked together. Subclasses exist within the major classes. All light chains fall into two classes, kappa (κ) and lambda (λ), and variable proportions of each are found in all vertebrate species. Both have an approximate molecular weight of 23,000 and their structural differences are reflected in antigenic differences. It should be noted that approximately 95% of murine light chains are kappa type, whereas κ and λ chains occur in roughly equal frequency in man.

The N-terminal 105–115 amino acid residues of both heavy and light chains show considerable variation in their sequence, and this domain is referred to as the variable (V) region. This variability occurs within a species and within individual animals and is believed to be responsible for the wide range of binding specificities for antigen. The remaining portion of the chains is highly conserved and thus constitutes the constant (C) region. This region defines the antigenic and structural properties of the class. Each constant region consists of domains which are each in turn specialized for a specific function (60, 81). The basic four-subunit structure of immunoglobulin is relatively stable chemically but can be broken by treatment with the enzyme papain into three parts of similar size, but having distinct properties.

1. Two Fab fragments containing the V region of both chains representing the antigen binding fragment.
2. One Fc fragment from the C region of the heavy chains.

These subunits will be referred to in the following pages. The model of IgG circulating antibody depicted in Figure 1 illustrates the domain structure of this molecule including its combining site (V_H–V_L), Fab fragment, and Fc region. The main immunoglobulin classes or isotypes pertinent to this discussion are IgG, IgM, and IgD because these have been definitely found on the surface of human B cells, with IgM and IgD constituting the major endogenously produced surface immunoglobulin. In addition, properties of certain IgA immunoglobulins will be discussed because these molecules show an organization that bears a number of similarities to that of T cell immunoglobulin.

IgG is the most abundant immunoglobulin of mammals (including man), to which it is unique (7), and has been studied in great detail. It has a heavy chain (γ) of molecular weight 50,000 and consists of a monomeric unit written $\kappa_2\gamma_2$ or $\lambda_2\gamma_2$. Serum IgM is characterized by a heavy chain (μ) of molecular weight 70,000 and exists as a pentamer $(\kappa_2\mu_2)_5$ or $(\lambda_2\mu_2)_5$ although monomeric forms exist in disease states (245) in man and are common among lower vertebrates (153, 161). IgM is the only immunoglobulin of many primitive vertebrates (41, 161, 162). In some species, notably sharks, both pentameric (19S) and monomeric (7S) forms of IgM occur in the serum, and dimeric, tetrameric, and hexameric forms of IgM have been reported in various other species (147). IgM immunoglobulins of all placoderm-derived species exist as polymers in which μ chains and light chains are linked covalently via disulfide bonds, but the IgM-like antibodies of cyclostomes such as the lamprey deviate from this pattern because the light and heavy chains are not covalently linked. IgA is found in mammals and birds, has a heavy chain of mass 55–65,000 daltons, and usually occurs as monomers of the form $(\kappa\ \alpha)_2$ or $(\lambda\ \alpha)_2$ but may also polymerize to form higher aggregates (145). It is interesting that mammalian IgA molecules bearing certain allotypes, IgA$_2$Am+ (123) in man, the BALB/c allotype in mice (1, 265), and IgA molecules found in chicken bile (254), form units in which the α heavy chains are joined via disulfide bonds, but are not covalently associated with light chains. The light chains can exist as dimers or monomers and dissociate from the heavy

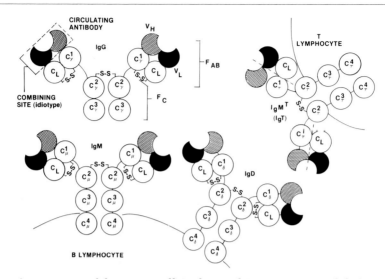

Fig. 1. The Structure of the Major Cell Surface and Serum Immunoglobulins. The domain structure of B cell surface IgM (monomeric) and IgD, T cell surface Ig (IgMT or TIg), and the major circulating antibody, IgG, are depicted diagrammatically. The number of domains in the heavy chains of the IgD and TIg molecules has been assigned on the basis of the apparent mass of these molecules. The heavy chain of the TIg molecule has been designated τ, on the assumption that it may represent a distinct class of immunoglobulin.

chains in the presence of denaturants such as urea or guanidine. IgD is considered a major class of human immunoglobulins although it occurs at relatively low levels in serum (0.003–0.4 mg/ml) and definitive evidence of its antibody function was difficult to obtain (241). It has now been conclusively shown to be a major B cell surface immunoglobulin (79, 223), as will be discussed below.

Classification of immunoglobulins would appear to be ill defined in the light of phylogenetic studies in recent years and comparison of the amino acid sequences of α, γ, and μ chains from various species indicate a closer evolutionary relationship between IgM and IgA than between IgM and IgG (261). The problem of homologous relationships among immunoglobulins of diverse species becomes acute in comparing other molecules with the IgD surface molecule of man, which is extremely similar to the monomeric subunit of human IgM in a number of physicochemical properties (76, 160, 163, 268). In contrast, the murine IgD analogue differs markedly from the IgM subunit, both in intact size and in properties of its heavy chain as analyzed by polyacrylamide gel electrophoresis in SDS-containing buffers (267); see Figure 2 as well.

III. ENDOGENOUSLY PRODUCED SURFACE IMMUNOGLOBULIN

A. Methods of Detection of Surface Immunoglobulin

The presence of immunoglobulin on the surface of lymphocytes has been demonstrated in many vertebrate species and the mass of evidence accumulated largely through the use of fluoresceinated or radio-iodinated antiglobulin reagents and by other indirect immunological techniques has been reviewed extensively by Warner (262) and Marchalonis (151, 152). Some difficulty was experienced with these methods applied to T cells, but immunoglobulin could be detected both with radioiodinated reagents and stringent autoradiographic conditions (10, 186) and by immunofluorescence (87, 226, 274). Use of chicken antisera to murine and human Ig also allowed ready detection of surface Ig on thymus lymphocytes (97, 128).

Direct techniques utilizing radio-iodination of cell surface proteins followed by extraction and isolation of immunoglobulin by precipitation with specific antisera (2, 3, 18, 131, 159) or the use of immunoadsorbents (105, 117, 267) have also been applied to membrane preparations or cell suspensions. This immunoglobulin can then be analyzed by polyacrylamide gel electrophoresis in sodium dodecylsulfate containing buffers, and in addition other chemical analyses such as cleavage with cyanogen bromide and analysis of labelled peptides can be performed. Some of the methods used in these sorts of investigations have been reviewed elsewhere (268).

These approaches have successfully led to the isolation of a monomeric IgM-like immunoglobulin from normal and neoplastic B lymphocytes of various species (76, 131, 157, 160, 239, 257). The IgM-like nature of B cell immunoglobulin has been confirmed chemically and antigenically, though other classes may be present. Notably, IgG may be present because of passive adsorption via Fc receptors, although a small proportion of B cells can clearly produce IgG surface molecules (190). T cell immunoglobulin, although similar to monomeric IgM, is probably not identical to this molecule (see below). A second class of B cell surface Ig molecules, IgD in man (79, 223) and a putative homologue in mice (3, 168, 258), has received considerable attention in recent months and will be considered in more detail below.

Since antibodies to immunoglobulin have been universally used in the detection and isolation of surface immunoglobulins reported to date, it is worthwhile commenting on the antigenic determinants with which "anti-immunoglobulin" reagents react. Figure 1 depicts the domain structure of circulating IgG antibody of a particular specificity, that is, a particular V_H–V_L combining site. Antisera produced to this molecule by animals of another species would usually react with determinants occurring within the constant region. Antisera specific for γ chain would bind determinants lying within the Fc region of the γ chain and analogous statements can be made for antisera specific for μ, α, δ, and ϵ chains. Often cross-reactions among various heavy chains can occur when antisera are directed against the F_D portion of the heavy chain, that is, that are present in the Fab piece. Since all usual immunoglobulins possess light chains as well as heavy chains, antisera to κ or λ chains would be expected to react with all immunoglobulin isotypes. For example, anti-light chain (chiefly anti-κ) precipitates both IgM and the IgD-like surface molecule of murine B cells whereas an antiserum directed against the Fc-region of μ chain precipitates only surface IgM, and an alloantiserum (made in the same species) to the delta-like chain precipitates only the IgD molecule (86, 268). Antibodies directed against the V region combining site for antigen can be made both in heterospecific or allogeneic combinations (35). These antisera can compete with antigen for the combining site and therefore are "antireceptor" antibodies. They can be directed against a determinant formed by V_H–V_L combination, or predominantly against V_H or V_L. This is a property of the particular antibody population under consideration. Since the combining site of a particular immunoglobulin, for example, that of a myeloma protein, was thought to be restricted to that molecule, these antisera were considered to be directed against "idiotypic" determinants and, therefore, were called anti-idiotypes (191). It has now been observed that antibodies to certain antigens can share idiotypic determinants of the combining site, even though they represent distinct isotypes (82).

B. B Cell Immunoglobulin

Immunoglobulin isolated from cell surfaces may be either synthesized endogenously or adsorbed cytophilically from exogenous sources. B cells have been demonstrated to bear receptors which will bind exogenous IgG (15) so the possibility exists that this immunoglobulin could be passively adsorbed from the surrounding milieu. There is, however, no question that membrane-bound IgM is actually synthesized endogenously (169), and the use of monoclonal cell lines cultured in vitro, and thus free of exogenous antibody contamination, has allowed clear confirmation of this (131, 144, 236). The apparent high density of immunoglobulin on B lymphocytes as detected by mammalian antisera is a characteristic feature of these cells and may be used as a B cell marker, since relatively insensitive techniques can readily detect it under conditions where T cells are virtually negative (93, 186). We would note, however, that workers using avian antisera to murine (97; Szenberg and Marchalonis, 282) and human (128) Ig-detected surface Ig on both T and B cells by immunofluorescence and autoradiography. It is well established that a major surface immuno-globulin of B cells is monomeric IgM, (Lμ)$_2$ consisting of typical μ chains and light chains (18, 94, 131, 157, 159, 257). Half-molecules have also been reported in the mouse (3) and rat (239), and occasionally free light chains (117) are also observed. Lower vertebrates possess only IgM serum immunoglobulins (153, 161), and the spleen cells of goldfish (266) and B cells of chicken (249) appear to express only that immunoglobulin class. IgG, on the other hand, has been found in addition to IgM on the B lymphocytes of the rat (137, 173, 239), mouse (157, 159) and guinea pig (76, 160), though it is present in much smaller amounts relative to the IgM, and may well be of cytophilic origin. A small proportion of murine B cells ($<$ 5%) bear surface IgG as their predominant membrane immuno-globulin (86, 108).

Figure 2 presents a diagram comparing the electrophoretic mobilities on SDS-polyacrylamide gel electrophoresis of surface immunoglobulins of B and T cells of man, mouse and guinea pig. Intact surface monomeric IgM has a mobility substantially slower than that of IgG (mass 150,000 daltons). Since the actual mass difference between monomeric IgM (180,000) and IgG (150,000) is not great, this differential migration in SDS gels is striking (131) and might reflect the aberrant mobility of heavily glycosylated proteins in this type of gel system (7, 230). Upon reduction, monomeric IgM is resolved into μ chains and light chains. γ and μ chains clearly separate, but once again the mobility of μ chain is abnormally slow by comparison of its mobility and known mass (70,000 daltons) with those of non-glycosylated standard proteins (7). Since gel electrophoresis in SDS is widely used to obtain molecular weights of surface proteins, we would emphasize that the method has high resolving power but suffers from the drawback that glycoproteins do not show true mobilities because they bind less detergent per mass unit than do pure polypeptides. There-fore, molecular weight estimates derived from SDS-polyacrylamide gel electrophoresis must, in the absence of measurement by independent techniques, be considered approximate or "nominal." (230).

Examination of the surface Ig from murine B lymphocytes isolated from the spleen of athymic (and normal) mice reveals an additional heavy chain with a mobility faster than μ (approximate molecular weight 60,000). Antigenically, the μ chain resembles serum μ, but the second peak is clearly distinct (3, 86, 117, 146, 168). Analogy has been drawn between this molecule and that of human IgD, which appears on human B lymphocytes together with IgM. However, double isotope mixing experi-ments show that the mouse δ-like chain migrates considerably faster than

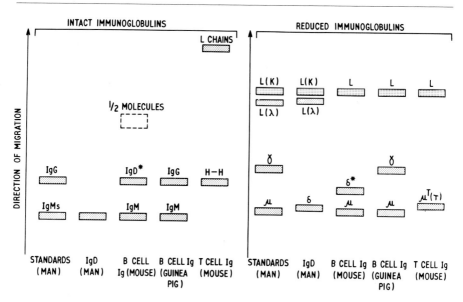

Fig. 2. An Analysis of Cell Surface Immunoglobulins and Their Constitutent Polypeptide Chains. The mobilities of the molecules on polyacrylamide gel electrophoresis in sodium dodecyl sulfate containing buffers are shown as stylized autoradiographs. The standard human immunoglobulins whose mobilities are shown are serum-derived IgG and IgD, and the monomeric ($\mu_2 L_2$) form of IgM (IgMs). The asterisk (*) marks the murine immunoglobulin class, apparently restricted to the B cell surface, which has been suggested to represent the murine homologue of human IgD.

that of human IgD in polyacrylamide gel electrophoresis (76, 160, 267). The intact murine IgD, moreover, has a mobility more similar to that of IgG rather than IgD or monomeric IgM. Human δ chain migrates only slightly faster than does human μ, and double isotope techniques on gels of high resolving power are required to show this difference (267). The murine IgM and IgD-like molecules can appear together on mouse cells and such "doubles" comprise approximately 85% of normal murine splenic B cells (85).

Complete homology between B cell surface immunoglobulins and their serum counterparts is not yet proven in mammals or lower vertebrates. Thus B cells of lower vertebrates bear only IgM while those of man and mouse possess two types of surface immunoglobulin consisting of antigenically distinct heavy chains; μ and δ in man (223) and μ and the product of the Ig5 locus in mouse (86). It is possible that species such as rat (173, 239), rabbit, and guinea pig (76, 160) possess surface Igs in

Table 1. Surface immunoglobulins of lymphocytes.

Immunoglobulin Isotype	Heavy Chain	Light Chain	Serum Form	Surface Form	Endogenously Synthesized by	Comments
IgM (all species)	μ (70,000)	K or λ (23,000)	$(K\mu)_{10}$ $(\lambda\mu)_{10}$	$(K\mu)_2$ $(\lambda\mu)_2$	B cells	H-L Disulfide bonded
IgD (man)	δ (approx.)	K or λ	$(K\delta)_2$ $(\lambda\delta)_2$	$(K\delta)_2$ $(\lambda\delta)_2$	B cells	SDS-PAGE extremely similar to IgM monomer: H-L disulphide bonds
IgD-like (mouse)	δ^a (approx. 60,000)	K or λ	Not detected	$(K\,\delta^a)_2$ $(\lambda\delta^a)_2$	B cells	Distinct from IgM; H-L disulfide bonded
IgG	γ (50,000)	K or λ	$(K\gamma)_2$ $(\lambda\gamma)_2$	$(K\gamma)_2$ $(\lambda\gamma)_2$	B cells (small percentage in man and mouse)	Major serum Ig H-L disulfide bonded
IgM^T (TIg)	μ^T (τ) (approx. 70,000)	K or λ K or λ	Not detected	$(K\tau)_2$ $(\lambda\tau)_2$	T cells	Distinct from IgM; H-L may not be covalently bonded

a. Murine immunoglobulin class, apparently restricted to the B cell surface, which has been suggested to represent the murine homologue of human IgD.

addition to IgM and IgG. If this is the case, however, the second surface Ig class must have a heavy chain with a mobility on SDS-polyacrylamide gels identical to that of μ chain. This surmise has been proven true in the case of the rat, where IgD has recently been reported to be present on the B cell surface (283).

Table 1 summarizes some of the salient properties of endogenously produced surface immunoglobulins.

C. T Cell Immunoglobulin

Certain routine B-cell immunoglobulin extraction procedures, notably use of the nonionic detergent Nonidet P-40 at concentrations higher than the critical micelle concentration, are unsuitable for extraction of surface Ig of normal and neoplastic mammalian T lymphocytes (43, 44, 46, 102, 104, 239). This phenomenon added to the controversy over the identification of immunoglobulin on T cells, and many negative reports emerged (93, 94, 146, 257). Moreover, it is of particular difficulty to obtain T cell preparations free of B cells and plasma cells, which could contribute to passive adsorption of exogenous immunoglobulin on to the T cell surface (115, 118, 201, 271). In addition, it must be borne in mind that thymus lymphocytes consist largely of immunologically unreactive cells which may possess very small amounts of immunoglobulin (91, 172). Thus, the use of antigen-specific activated cells (243, 259) or T cell populations of continuously cultured monoclonal T lymphoma cells (99) free of B cells can facilitate the study of T cell immunoglobulin (30, 99, 102, 104, 135). Indirect and direct evidence (151, 262) indicated that T cell surface immunoglobulin analyzed under non-dissociating conditions has a molecular weight of approximately 150,000 to 200,000 daltons (obtained by gel filtration in physiological buffer). The Ig consists of μ-like heavy chains, having an electrophoretic mobility slightly faster than μ (103, 104) and typical light chains. Without reduction of disulfide bonds, the molecule migrates slightly more slowly than IgG on SDS-PAGE. The light chains are usually κ type in the mouse. It has also been reported that IgA is present and synthesized on the surface of BALB/c thymocytes (177).

Much present evidence shows that T cell immunoglobulin exhibits functional and cytophilic properties distinct from those of B cell surface IgM or secreted IgM (45, 73, 246). In addition theta-positive monoclonal T lymphoma lines, free of exogenous contamination, have been demonstrated to synthesize immunoglobulin (99, 102, 135), and, although some T lymphoma cells bear an Fc receptor capable of binding exogenous IgG, the cells themselves synthesize IgM-like immunoglobulin (104). Other studies on monoclonal T lymphoma lines have provided much structural

(30) and functional (72, 246) data on the properties of murine T cell immunoglobulin.

Studies of thymocytes (putative T cells) of some lower vertebrates have also indicated that T cells make a unique type of surface immunoglobulin possibly analogous to that of mammals (266).

Recent studies suggest that the heavy and light chains comprising the T Ig molecule may not be covalently linked by disulfide bonds (44, 160, 176, 177, 178) and that under certain conditions it may be isolated as a heavy chain dimer with noncovalently associated light chains. There is an analogy here with the molecule isolated by Binz and Wigzell (26) from T cells by the use of antireceptor (anti-idiotype) reagents. This molecule has an intact molecular weight of 150,000 and consisted of only two chains of similar size. Whether T Ig and this idiotype-positive molecule are really identical awaits confirmation, but it is a reasonable surmise at the time of writing.

A hypothetical model illustrating similarities and differences between the major mammalian antibody isotype (IgG) and surface immunoglobulins of T and B lymphocytes is shown in Figure 1. The domain structures depicted are based upon the molecular weights of the respective chains. Based upon the use of anti-receptor (anti-idiotype) reagents, it has been shown (25, 167, 207), that circulating antibodies, and T and B cell surface receptors of the same specificity can bear the same idiotype even though they are distinct isotypes. The constant regions of γ, μ, δ, and μ (T) or τ differ from one another structurally and these differences probably condition distinct functional properties of each. Light chains of T Ig may not be covalently linked to the heavy chains and can be lost during fractionation. This diagram illustrates a modern restatement of Ehrlich's minimal hypothesis (61) that surface receptors which mimic circulating antibodies in specificity must be antibodies. This minimal hypothesis as applied to B and T cells can be stated that *surface receptor immunoglobulin possesses combining sites comprised of Ig variable regions but its constant regions are not necessarily identical to those of circulating antibodies.*

IV. FUNCTIONS OF LYMPHOCYTE SURFACE IMMUNOGLOBULIN

A. General Considerations

The proposal that membrane-bound antibody serves as a specific receptor for antigen on immunocompetent cells is a very old one (61), but the experimental evidence supporting this hypothesis is still of a rather indirect nature. Reasons for this state of affairs include, on the one hand, the complexity of cell types and humoral factors which have been implicated in the immune response, and on the other hand, the small numbers of lymphocytes in an unstimulated population which respond to a given antigen. The first of these conditions has meant that the requirements for triggering of one cell type must be deduced while satisfying the requirements of all the accessory cell types involved, while the second demands very sensitive biochemical and functional assays or the use of cell populations enriched for responsiveness to a given antigen.

In order to conclusively establish the function of membrane-bound Ig as antigen receptor and lymphocyte trigger, one would like to do the following: (1) isolate Ig from the surface of lymphocytes; (2) demonstrate antigen binding by isolated membrane Ig; (3) show that removing the membrane associated Ig from a cell or blocking its antigen-binding site results in failure of activation, whereas resynthesis of membrane Ig or reversing the block of antigen binding restores the ability of the cells to be stimulated by antigen; and (4) obtain a positive demonstration that binding of reagents specific for membrane Ig initiates immune differentiation. We have already discussed the molecular properties of the Ig molecules isolated from the surfaces of T and B lymphocytes. Following a brief presentation of the work on the antigen-binding properties of isolated membrane Ig, we will consider the evidence bearing on its function in lymphocyte activation.

B. Membrane Immunoglobulin Isolated from Lymphocytes Binds Antigen Specifically

Experiments have been performed with membrane Ig isolated from both T and B lymphocytes to demonstrate its binding specificity for antigen. In a typical protocol, Rolley and Marchalonis (221) isolated membrane Ig by metabolic release at 37°C from a murine splenocyte population which had been incubated with an ^{125}I-labeled antigen. Using a coprecipitation system, they showed that rabbit antibodies to Ig precipitated some of the labeled antigen, as well as surface Ig. With the converse experiment, it could be shown that antibody to the antigen precipitated some of the labeled membrane Ig as well as the antigen. These results indicated that a complex of membrane Ig and its specific antigen had been isolated. Further studies (154) showed that a subpopulation of both the monomeric IgM and the IgD-like molecules extracted by detergent from B cell surfaces bound to an antigen-immunoadsorbent. IgM was more reliably detected, however. Using "anti-receptor" antibodies directed against the idiotype of the phosphoryl choline-binding myeloma protein TEPC

Table 2. Binding specificity of surface immunoglobulin of BALB/c T cells activated to the syngeneic tumor line HPC 108[a]

[125]I-labeled cell Surface Proteins[b]	Radioactivity (cpm $\times 10^{-3}$) Binding to	
	HPC 108	MOPC 315 (control tumor)
Coprecipitated with a heterologous system, i.e., Ig present[c]	14.5 ± 1.0	0.6 ± 0.1
Coprecipitated with rabbit anti-mouse Ig + mouse Ig; i.e. Ig depleted	3.0 ± 1.5	1.0 ± 0.1

a. Data of Röllinghoff, Wagner, Cone and Marchalonis, Release of antigenspecific immunoglobulin from cytotoxic effector cells and syngeneic tumor immunity in vitro (222).

b. T cells were radioiodinated by a lactoperoxidase-catalyzed reaction and ^{125}I-labeled surface proteins obtained by metabolic release.

c. Chicken Ig+ rabbit antiserum to chicken Ig.

15, Strayer et al. (248) isolated cell surface Ig bearing this idiotype from spleen cells of immunized mice. Antigen binding by isolated T cell membrane Ig has been demonstrated with molecules isolated from T cell populations activated to histocompatibility antigens (48), syngeneic tumor-associated transplantation antigens (222), foreign erythrocytes (46) and foreign proteins (73). In all cases, the binding was specific for the activating antigen. Table 2 illustrates binding of surface Ig of BALB/c T cells activated against tumor antigens of the syngeneic plasmacytoma HPC 108 to the activating antigen, but not to a second syngeneic tumor MOPC 315. Depletion of Ig reduces specific binding by more than 80%. Thus, the second condition for establishing membrane Ig as antigen receptor has received experimental support.

C. Membrane Immunoglobulin of T Cells: A Possible Role in Cell Collaboration

Before we consider the function of membrane Ig directly in lymphocyte triggering, we will examine the capacity of T cell membrane Ig to suppress or enhance antibody production in systems dependent on T cell help. Cooperation between T and B cells is a complex process which requires the intervention of accessory cells such as macrophages (or "adherent" cells) and appears to involve antigen-specific factors, of which T cell Ig is the best characterized (73, 250), and various nonspecific factors. Moreover, it has been proposed that products of the major histocompatibility complex are implicated in antigen-recognition by T cells and in various phases of T/B cooperation (19, 20, 66, 130, 180). It is beyond the scope of this review to discuss the role of MHC products, notably Ia antigens, in T/B cooperation and the reader is referred to the above articles.

Evidence for a collaborative role for T cell surface Ig in T/B cooperation in a macrophage-dependent in vitro system was obtained largely by Feldmann and his collaborators (70, 73, 74). It was found that T cells and B cells could collaborate in a T-dependent immune response without direct cell-cell contact, and Feldmann et al. (73) obtained evidence that a monomeric Ig which contained μ-like heavy chains was responsible for antigen-specific T/B cooperation in this system. Taniguchi and Tada (250), working with an in vivo cooperative system in the rat, also obtained evidence supporting the capacity of monomeric IgM to act in T/B cooperation. Because the source of this collaborative Ig was open to some question, studies using Ig of T lymphoma cells might be considered easier to interpret in establishing a role for Ig produced by T cells. Stocker et al. (246) showed that culture supernatants from a thymoma (WEHI 22) suppressed an in vitro antibody response to a T-dependent but not a T-independent antigen. The factor responsible for the suppression could be adsorbed on a rabbit anti-mouse Ig immunoadsorbent. They proposed that T cell Ig of the thymoma competed with antigen-specific T cell Ig of helper cells for sites on the macrophage surface. Feldmann et al. (72) confirmed that Ig of T lymphoma cells could suppress T cell dependent IgM responses in vitro, but, perhaps surprisingly, enhance IgG responses. These effects could not be mimicked by a variety of myeloma proteins tested.

Based on these experiments and the finding that T cell membrane Ig is cytophilic for macrophages (45, 216), the following model for antigen-specific T/B cell collaboration can be proposed (Figure 3). Combination of antigen with T cell membrane Ig results in the release of antigen-membrane Ig complexes, which bind to macrophages and (possibly in combination with nonspecific T cell or macrophage products) trigger B cells to produce antibody. The absence of T cell membrane Ig release (for example, in the case of T cell tolerance) or a lack of macrophages at the time of antigen contact would result in either lack of stimulation or tolerization of the B cells. As with any data obtained from in vitro systems, one must be judicious in extrapolating to in vivo mechanisms; however, this model does suggest one mechanism by which membrane Ig might function as an antigen-specific collaborative factor, although alternative schemes have been proposed (see references cited above).

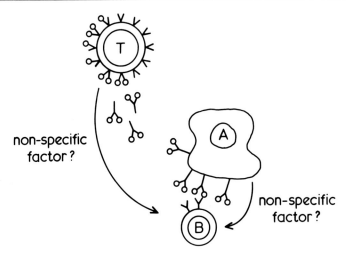

Fig. 3. Schematic diagram of a possible cooperation mechanism for T cells and B cells in antibody formation to thymus-dependent antigens. Macrophages (A for "adherent" cells) are included in this generalized interaction scheme. Released antigen-specific T cell receptor Ig (Y), bound to antigen (o), is concentrated on the macrophage surface. Ig receptors on B cells recognize antigen presented in this fashion and respond by differentiating into antibody-secreting cells. In addition, the macrophages and the T cells might give a nonspecific signal to the B cell.

D. Antibodies to Immunoglobulin Inhibit T and B Lymphocyte Function

The earliest experiments designed to demonstrate that lymphocyte membrane Ig was the receptor for antigen triggering involved the use of heterologous anti-Ig sera in attempts to block antigen binding and immune function. These studies have been extensively reviewed (51, 89, 140, 151, 152, 220, 262) and we will only give a general summary of the results here. The main caution we must bear in mind when interpreting these results and those with anti-idiotypic antibodies to be discussed later is that not all anti-Ig sera are equally effective, and that this irreproducibility can only partially be accounted for by their known combining site specificities.

1. Populations of antigen-binding lymphocytes have been shown to contain the precursors of immunocompetent T and B lymphocytes by depletion experiments utilizing antigen-coated adsorbents and sui-

cide with high specific activity radiolabelled antigen and by enrichment using the fluorescence-activated cell sorter.

2. Immunoglobulin can be detected easily on the surfaces of B lymphocytes and with more difficulty on the surfaces of T lymphocytes by the use of fluorochrome- or isotope-tagged anti-Ig sera.

3. Anti-Ig plus complement will kill some lymphocytes, presumably those with high levels of membrane Ig.

4. Pre-treatment of both B and T lymphocytes with anti-Ig blocks antigen binding, and antigen-binding B cells can be removed from a lymphocyte population by passage of the cells over anti-Ig immunoadsorbents.

5. Antigen and Ig appear to be associated on the membrane of antigen-binding cells because capping the Ig with antibody to Ig results in antigen redistribution and vice versa.

6. Pretreatment of lymphocytes with anti-Ig inhibits the ability of antigen to stimulate antibody production, graft-versus-host reactivity, delayed-type hypersensitivity, and T cell helper function, but not the generation of cytotoxic T cells against histocompatibility antigens.

7. Injection of antiserum directed against μ chain determinants or against specific Ig allotypes results in suppression of the synthesis of Ig generally or of the given allotype specifically. Anti-μ and in some cases anti-γ chain antisera will suppress secondary immune responses in vitro.

The simplest interpretation of these data is that the specific combination of lymphocyte membrane Ig with antigen results in lymphocyte triggering, and that this binding is inhibited by the binding of anti-Ig to the membrane Ig receptors. It does not follow that binding of antigen to membrane Ig is alone sufficient for triggering (see next section) or that the antigen receptor is identical to secreted Ig (see above), only that the receptor shows antigen-binding specificity and shares some antigenic determinants with secreted antibodies. Steric hindrance of antigen-binding to a non-Ig molecule, in close association with membrane Ig, is difficult to rule out completely. Moreover, since some groups have reported inhibition of T cell antigen-binding and antigen-specific "suicide" using antisera directed against histocompatibility (H-2) antigens (14, 96, 262), the possibility that H-2 antigens might be part of the antigen receptors on T cells has been a popular alternative to an Ig-like antigen receptor. The discovery of genetic loci (immune responsiveness or Ir genes) controlling the ability to respond to certain antigens (for example, synthetic polypeptides) and linked to the H-2 gene complex was additional evidence that the H-2 system was involved in antigen recognition, and it was suggested that Ir genes coded for the antigen-binding (V) region of an antigen receptor unique to T cells (180). However, more recent work forces us to question the interpretation of studies using alloantisera because Goding et al. (86) observed that alloantisera ostensibly specific for H-2 antigens contained antibodies directed against allotypic markers on the heavy chain of the murine IgD-like molecule. In addition, similar alloantisera have been shown to possess activity against a μ chain allotype (108, 263).

The model that we favour to reconcile both sets of data is that a second cell surface molecule, encoded by the Ir genes, may be involved in lymphocyte activation or cell collaboration, but that the antigen specificity of the receptors is coded for the same genes coding for the V regions of serum Ig and B cell antigen receptors.

E. Antibodies to Immunoglobulin Stimulate Lymphocyte Differentiation

It was hoped that the action of antigen on combination with its membrane receptor could be mimicked by the binding of anti-Ig to membrane Ig, so that anti-Ig would stimulate T accessory cell and B antibody-producing cell activities. The results of many such experiments have been variable, with success depending to some extent on the animal model chosen or the assay system used. We have divided these experiments into three groups: stimulation of blastogenic transformation by anti-Ig or anti-allotype sera, possible functions of membrane IgD, and stimulation of T and B cell functions by antibodies to Ig combining site determinants.

i. ANTI-Ig STIMULATION OF LYMPHOCYTE BLASTOGENE-SIS. Lymphocytes from humans, rabbits and chickens have been shown to undergo blastogenic transformation (usually measured by counting the percentage of blast cells, or the uptake of ^{3}H-thymidine) following incubation in vitro with anti-Ig sera (262, 272). Rabbit peripheral blood lymphocytes (PBL) are the most thoroughly studied cell type which can be stimulated by anti-Ig; both heterologous anti-Ig sera and alloantisera with specificity for heavy or light chain Ig allotypic markers will stimulate blast transformation (83, 232). Since a high percentage of rabbit PBL are transformed by anti-Ig, this reagent is presumed to stimulate cells with Ig of many different antigenic specificities. Most studies identify lymphocytes which respond in vitro to anti-Ig as B cells; i.e. cells which adhere to nylon wool and are resistant to killing with anti-T cell serum plus complement (34, 69, 235, 272). However, there does seem to be some overlap in the reactivity of T and B cell populations in the rabbit, which suggests that T cells may play some part in the response to anti-Ig (234, 235). ^{3}H-thymidine uptake by chicken T cells can be stimulated by turkey anti-

chicken Ig plus turkey antichicken thymocyte serum, although each anti-body alone has no effect as a lymphocyte activator (273). Stimulation of rabbit lymphocytes does not result in increased synthesis of immuno-globulin (233; Decker and Marchalonis, unpublished observations), and it is not clear what relationship blastogenic transformation may have to the differentiative events following antigenic stimulation of lymphocytes. However, Ig synthesis can be stimulated in rabbit spleen cells by incuba-tion with the mitogen concanavalin A, which also stimulates blas-togenesis (52). It has been shown for rabbit mesenteric lymph node cells that incubation with anti-Ig followed by a nonspecific soluble T cell factor (obtained from cultures of *Ascaris suum* primed lymph node cells plus *Ascaris* antigens) results in the synthesis of antibody specific for an anti-gen previously used to prime the rabbits (133). There are conflicting re-ports concerning the requirement for cross-linking of membrane Ig to stimulate rabbit PBL (68, 231). These diverse observations made in a va-riety of experimental systems make it difficult to draw any general con-clusions about the role of membrane Ig and its interactions with other membrane components during antigen-induced triggering of rabbit lym-phocytes.

In the mouse, anti-Ig will not trigger lymphocytes into either blas-

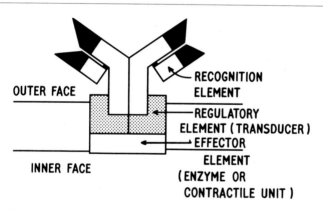

Fig. 4. Hypothetical model for an activation complex in lymphocyte plasma membranes. The recognition element consists of membrane-bound immunoglobu-lin, in particular the V-region combining site. Binding of antigen to the recogni-tion unit causes a signal to be transmitted through the membrane to the effector element, which might be adenylate or guanylate cyclase or contractile protein(s). Since the Fc portion of the membrane Ig probably does not span the membrane, a transducer or regulatory element which interacts with both membrane Ig and effector element is probably required; the nature of this component is unknown.

togenesis or Ig production, although the mitogens LPS (lipopolysac-charide from gram negative bacteria) and concanavalin A (in an insol-ubilized form) will induce both responses in murine B cells (89, 90). Since in most systems antigen alone is not a sufficient signal for B cell trigger-ing, it has been postulated that a second stimulus besides antigen-receptor contact is required (71, 155, 228, 229). It may be that membrane Ig on rabbit and human lymphocytes exists in an activation complex (Fig. 4) which will lead to blastogenic activation of the cells (but not necessar-ily differentiation into antibody-forming cells), while murine membrane Ig is separated from part of its triggering complex and a second signal is required for any sort of activation (152).

ii. IgD AND LYMPHOCYTE ACTIVATION.

With the discovery of an Ig molecule which comprised a large fraction of the detectable membrane Ig of mature B lymphocytes in the mouse but was undetectable in serum, a new candidate for the lymphocyte triggering receptor had appeared (258). There has so far been no proof that this murine cell-surface molecule is identical to human IgD, and, furthermore, the two molecules differ in some physicochemical properties (76, 267). However, certain similarities in distribution among B cell populations have led to the use of the nomenclature IgD and delta for the heavy chain when referring to the murine molecule (3, 168, 258). Since B lymphocytes in fetal mice and bone marrow lymphocytes (which are more immature B cells than those in the spleen) do not possess membrane IgD (256), Vitetta and Uhr (258) suggested that membrane IgD might be the "on" switch for lymphocytes; in their model, combination of antigen with IgD would result in activation, while antigen binding to only membrane IgM would lead to tolerance. IgD and IgM on the same cell have been shown to possess the same antigen-combining site in both mice (85) and men (80).

To date, experiments involving direct stimulation of murine lympho-cytes with hetero- or allo-antibodies specific for putative IgD have not resulted in blastogenic transformation, or shown any marked effect on immune responsiveness of cells (187, 197). However, there are very few anti-IgD sera available as yet, and based on the varied effects of different anti-IgM and anti-light chain sera on immune function (see previous sec-tion) it is too early to conclude that no anti-IgD serum will stimulate murine B lymphocytes. Although cells bearing membrane IgD will re-spond to lipopolysaccharide by ^{3}H-thymidine incorporation, it has been shown that murine B cells which synthesize Ig in response to lipopolysaccharide stimulation also have membrane IgM, either alone or together with membrane IgD (255).

It has been reported that, as with antibodies to IgM, anti-IgD will stimulate ^{3}H-thymidine uptake in human PBL (132). Anti-IgD has also been reported to enhance responses to the mitogen phytohemagglutinin by human PBL (132) and to stimulate *in vivo* synthesis of IgG in rhesus monkeys (200). The former response is marginal, however, and the latter is open to various interpretations. Based on these few experiments, the suggestion of a central role of membrane IgD in lymphocyte activation must for the present receive the verdict "not proven." Recent data (284) suggests that IgD in the mouse might be implicated in reducing the sensitivity of B cells to tolerance induction.

iii. ANTI-IDIOTYPIC ANTIBODIES STIMULATE BOTH B AND T CELL FUNCTIONS. The most direct and compelling evidence that membrane Ig on B and T lymphocytes acts as the antigen trigger comes from work in several laboratories with anti-idiotypic antibodies (for a recent review on the T helper cell receptor, see Ref. 207). These antibodies are usually (though not always) directed against determinants in the antigen-combining region of Ig molecules (35). Some anti-idiotype antisera were literally anti-receptor antibodies (165, 166, 212), but they have also been raised against serum antibodies (26, 35, 62, 167).

Anti-idiotypic antibody has been shown to have a variety of effects on immune responses, both *in vivo* and *in vitro*. These include (1) the suppression of antibody formation (27, 198, 224) and graft-versus-host reactions (24, 124, 166); (2) the specific priming of B and helper T cells (27, 65); and (3) the generation of suppressor T cells (63, 64). The ability of anti-idiotypic antibody to stimulate helper cells or suppressor cells seems to be related to its heavy chain class: IgG_1 antibodies stimulate helper cells and IgG_2 antibodies stimulate suppressor cells (63). It is not known whether this functional dichotomy is related to the complement-fixing capacity of IgG_2 but not IgG_1 antibodies. The capacity of anti-idiotypic antibody to specifically suppress immune responses has been suggested to be the basic mechanism for regulating the immune response (109, 122). Although much more experimental evidence is needed before such model systems can be proved to have any relationship to actual *in vivo* regulatory events, they are worth considering in our discussion of functions for membrane Ig since they propose regulatory as well as receptor capacities for Ig antigen receptors.

V. EXOGENOUSLY-DERIVED CELL SURFACE IMMUNOGLOBULIN

A. General Considerations

Immunoglobulin can bind to the surface of cells as the result of two major and distinct types of reaction. The first is the recognition of cell-bound antigenic structures by the antigen-binding site in the

N-terminal portion of the molecule (see above for an outline of the structure of the Ig molecule). The antigen-binding capacity of the Ig molecule can be localized to the Fab portion of the molecule, and is considered to reside specifically in the V region sequences of the constitutent light and heavy polypeptide chains (81). This classical, specific and generally aggressive recognition by antibody of foreign tissue, tumor, or autoantigens at the cell surface is more relevant to the function of the immune response directed against these antigens, rather than to the function of the cells bearing the recognized antigens. We therefore do not propose to consider this phenomenon further, but to concentrate on the second type of reaction which can result in the passive acquisition of immunoglobulin by cells. This reaction is entirely unrelated to the antigen specificity of the Ig molecule, and involves a site in the C terminal Fc portion of the molecule. The corresponding site on the cell surface which takes part in this binding

Table 3. Cytophilic antibodies.

Cell Type	Species	Class of Ig Cytophilically Bound	References
Macrophage	Man	IgG_1 and IgG_3	106
	Guinea pig	IgG_2	23
	Mouse	IgM and all IgG subclasses	42, 141, 251
Neutrophil	Man	IgA and all IgG subclasses	107
Basophils and mast cells	Man, Rat, Mouse Guinea pig Rabbit	IgE (and IgG)	58, 120, 204, 244, 281
Eosinophils	Man	IgE	114
Lymphocytes			
Thymocytes and T cells	Man, Mouse Rat	IgM and IgG	6, 16, 21, 32, 55, 56, 75, 78, 94, 99, 100, 118, 135, 136, 142, 175, 208, 240, 262, 264, 279
Bursa-equivalent derived (B cells)	Man, Mouse	IgM and IgG	6, 17, 42, 55, 57, 95, 139, 195, 210, 217, 240, 262

reaction has been termed the Fc receptor (195). A number of investigators have isolated from the lymphocyte membrane molecules which are possible candidates for the Fc receptor (103, 104, 203, 214). The Ig molecule bound to the Fc receptor of a cell still has its antigen-combining site free, and it is generally upon this passively acquired reactivity for antigen that a function for the cells bearing the Fc receptor has been postulated. Mammalian cell types which have been shown to possess Fc receptors for Ig include lymphocytes, platelets, macrophages, and granulocytes (see Table 3). A brief review of the data pertinent to the properties and postulated functions of the passively bound antibodies found on cells follows below.

Whatever the diversity of the Ig classes showing binding to cells, some progress in localizing the region of the molecule responsible for reaction with the cell-bound Fc receptor has been made. The site appears to be localized to the subterminal, or terminal domain in the constant region of the heavy chain (5, 39, 171, 189, 211, 253, 277, 278).

B. Exogenously Derived Lymphocyte Surface Immunoglobulin

That receptors for the Fc region of the Ig molecule exist on both T and B lymphocytes, or subpopulations thereof, is now undisputed (for reviews see references 55, 262). Most studies of this phenomenon have confined themselves to observing the reaction between lymphocytes and immunoglobulins using in vitro laboratory techniques. It is obviously very difficult to draw any conclusions as to function from these sorts of experiments, and it is of interest to ask whether lymphocytes in the whole animal bear passively adsorbed Ig. Some lymphocytes appear to do so, although it is extremely sensitive to washing off during subsequent procedures involving centrifugation and incubation (15). Other experiments demonstrating Ig passively bound to lymphocytes in the in vivo situation have been reported (115, 116, 118, 271). In the rabbit it appears that, in some situations, passively acquired Ig may be masking the phenomenon of allelic exclusion of the expressed cell surface Ig (126, 127). Whatever the problems involved in determining the function of Ig passively bound to the lymphocyte, it is proposed to first outline our knowledge of the lymphocyte Fc receptor, and then to discuss briefly some of its postulated functions.

The lymphocyte Fc receptor is generally detected by reacting cells in vitro with antigen/antibody complexes (6, 15, 54, 77, 276), aggregated immunoglobulin (55, 57), or immunoglobulin on an indicator cell (i.e., a cellular antigen/antibody complex). In the case of antigen/antibody complexes and aggregated Ig, radioisotopes or fluorochromes can be covalently linked to either the antigen or the antibody to provide a sensitive indication of reaction. In the case of the cellular antigen/antibody complex, reaction is observed when cells (usually erythrocytes) coated with specific antibody, adhere to the lymphocyte, giving rise to the characteristic "rosette" (42, 148, 279).

i. Fc RECEPTORS ON B CELLS.

There is clear evidence that B cells bind IgG (17, 42, 57, 195). Although there have been reports of IgM binding to B cells (17), there is some controversy on this point (6, 95, 139, 210, 217, 240). While some binding of IgE to human B cells has been reported (139), IgA and IgD do not appear to bind (17, 42, 139, 240).

Although there is evidence that all subclasses of IgG can bind to B cells, in man IgG_1 and IgG_3 appear to bind more strongly than IgG_2 and IgG_4 (139). In the mouse, there is disagreement in the literature as to which IgG subclass binds most strongly, either roughly equal binding of IgG_1, IgG_{2a}, and IgG_{2b} being reported (42), IgG_1 binding most strongly (17) or the IgG_2 subclasses binding most strongly (6, 95, 240). As pointed out by some authors (210), the efficiency of binding of the IgG subclasses is difficult to quantitate accurately because of the possible presence of IgG aggregates in a preparation. IgG aggregates bind much more efficiently than IgG monomers to the Fc receptor of B cells (210).

ii. Fc RECEPTORS ON T CELLS.

It has been clearly established that IgG can bind to T cells of mice and men (6, 21, 32, 56, 78, 94, 99, 100, 142, 208, 240, 279). There is evidence that IgG_1, IgG_{2a} and IgG_{2b} all bind to T lymphocytes, activated T cells, and T lymphoma cells, although there is some question as to which class binds most strongly (6, 16, 99, 135, 136, 142, 208, 240, 264).

The binding of IgM to T cells is more controversial. While some investigators have reported the presence of passively adsorbed IgM on T cells (188), a number of laboratories have reported negative results (78, 95, 99, 135, 136, 208, 217, 240, 247, 279). Moreover, it has been reported that human T lymphocytes can express a receptor for IgM only after a period of in vitro culture (175) and this has been interpreted by the authors to suggest that freshly isolated cells still have their receptor blocked by IgM adsorbed in vivo. It is of interest that only pentameric IgM, and not its monomeric subunit, bound to the human T cell Fc receptor (75). This passively adsorbed IgM should therefore be readily distinguishable from the monomeric Ig synthesized by T cells (vide supra). An additional complication arising from observations of IgM on T cells is that in certain experimental situations where the cells are stimulated by alloantigens, the IgM is bound not by its Fc receptor, but in combination with specifically recognized alloantigen already adsorbed on the cell surface (115, 181). The significance of these and other observations made in such highly artificial situations is obscure, and likely to remain so.

iii. POSSIBLE FUNCTIONS OF THE LYMPHOCYTE Fc RECEPTOR.

A number of possible functions for the Fc receptor of lymphocytes, some of which are discussed in detail in the review by Dickler (55), are listed below.

a. Regulation of Immune Responses.   It is known that specific antibody can regulate the level of an immune response (252) and that for some of these effects an intact Fc portion of the antibody molecule is required (37, 88, 129, 143, 238, 269). However, the evidence linking these observations with a functional role for the Fc receptor of lymphocytes is tenuous, and this is only one of a number of hypotheses which can explain the observed phenomena. The macrophage with very strong Fc receptors (see below) may be more attractive cells to invoke for the control of the immune response in antibody-mediated feedback.

b. Antibody-Mediated Cell Lysis.   Populations of nonimmune lymphocytes have been shown to be capable of lysing antibody-coated target cells (36, 174), and this function requires an intact Fc portion of the Ig molecule bound to the target (138, 149). This phenomenon of antibody-mediated cell lysis appears to be carried out by a poorly characterized lymphocyte-like cell (K cell), neither T nor B in type (92, 199, 213). This phenomenon may prove to be of importance as an effector mechanism in specific immunity, but since it appears at present to involve an uncharacterized cell type, it does not shed any light on the function of the Fc receptors on the more thoroughly studied T and B lymphocytes.

c. Receptor for Endogenously Synthesized Immunoglobulin.   It has been suggested (209) that the Fc receptor is the molecule to which endogenously synthesized membrane Ig is bound *in situ*. It is not yet possible to reach any conclusion about this hypothesis; observations that lymphocytes bear mostly endogenously produced IgM and IgD (see above), molecules which, by and large, do not bind strongly to Fc receptors, appear to militate against this possibility. Studies of lymphocyte activation initiated by binding of anti-Ig reagents suggest, however, that receptor IgM might be associated with other membrane components (*vide supra*).

d. Transport of Antigen.   Although a role for the Fc receptor in transporting antigen to the spleen may be postulated on the basis of experiments using aggregated Ig (31), the fact that complement plays a role in this localization (194) makes interpretation more difficult. It is hard to see why antigen-antibody complexes in the circulation should need any help from lymphocytes in actually reaching the spleen, although interaction with lymphocyte Fc or antigen receptors once there, would be a different matter.

The tentative conclusion which we would draw regarding the Fc receptor of lymphocytes is that, apart from antibody dependent cell lysis, a convincing role for this structure remains to be elucidated. In the meantime, it continues to provide intriguing questions and a useful cell marker for cellular immunologists.

C. Antibodies Cytophilic for Macrophages

i. GENERAL CONSIDERATIONS.   Although antibody has been detected in extracts of washed macrophages taken from the rabbit (84, 119), most demonstrations of cytophilia are carried out by exposing macrophages to antibody under controlled in vitro conditions. The cell bound antibodies can then be assayed by reaction of the "passively sensitized" macrophages with antigen. This antigen may be detected by means of a radioactive label (28) or in the case of particulate antigens (bacteria, tumor cells, erythrocytes), adherence of the particle to the sensitized macrophages may be monitored directly by light microscopy. The erythrocyte has proved a particularly popular test particle, the rosettes formed with sensitized cells providing an easy, and apparently very sensitive (182) test system. Erythrocytes can also be used as test particles with the antigen of interest (e.g., soluble proteins, haptens, carbohydrates) coupled to their surfaces (22, 125, 196).

It has been reported that reaction of the antigen with antibody prior to contact with the macrophage surface (generally termed the opsonic adherence test) provides a more sensitive system (22). There is reason however to question whether or not this method detects antibodies which would still be truly cytophilic in the absence of antigen (29). This is especially relevant in view of the fact that conformational changes have been postulated to take place in both IgG and IgM antibodies on combination with specific antigen (33, 101, 227), for such changes could alter the degree of exposure of the sites for cytophilic binding in the Fc region of the molecule. It appears, however, from the work of Philips-Quagliata et al. (202) that a conformational change in the Ig molecule is not necessary for binding to the Fc receptor to occur, and furthermore that the enhanced binding of aggregated Ig as compared to the monomeric form probably results from the effectively multivalent Fc regions possessed by such aggregates. However, there is in addition some evidence that in the mouse, the true cytophilic reaction detects different antibodies from the opsonic adherence system (196, 251). In some experiments (141, 251) both IgM and IgG showed cytophilic activity, whereas IgG alone was active in opsonic adherence (23, 251). The released monomeric IgM-like surface Ig of normal and activated murine T cells was observed to be cytophilic for macrophages both as free Ig (45) and as a complex with antigen (216). B cell surface Igs did not show this property. Rhodes (218), however, reported that the monomer produced by reduction of guinea-pig serum IgM bound to macrophages. The cytophilic properties of T cell Ig are consistent with its proposed role in one model of T/B collaboration (see above). Recent evidence derived from studies of an established cell line of murine macrophages (260) suggested that IgG_{2a} would only bind in aggregated form. In addition this report suggested that the receptors for IgG_{2a} and IgG_{2b} on this macrophage cell line were separate and distinct. Yet another functional test requiring recognition of antibody by the macrophage is opsonization, that is, the promotion of phagocytosis of bacteria or other particles by antibody present not on the macrophage, but on the particle being engulfed. Using this approach, it is clear that, in the mouse (53, 219, 225) IgM as well as IgG is an effective antibody for bacterial opsonization. Attempts to define the subclass of murine IgG in the mouse responsible for opsonic adherence have yielded conflicting results. While Cline et al. (42) suggested that IgG_{2a} might be the major subclass involved, Shevach et al. (237) have presented evidence that IgG_1 and IgG_{2b} might be more effective. Another unusual class of cytophilic antibodies in the mouse has been reported (112, 184). This poorly characterized molecule migrates electrophoretically like a fast $\alpha 1$-globulin, and has remained relatively unstudied since its original description.

In humans and guinea pigs the antibodies mediating opsonic adherence appear to be exclusively IgG, that is, IgG_2 in guinea pigs (22) and IgG_1 and IgG_3 in man (4, 106, 113). As might be expected from this differential effectiveness of different subclasses, the amount and nature of cytophilic antibody produced in an animal is highly dependent on a number of variables such as dose and route of antigen, use of adjuvant, etc. (182). Limited data on the nature of the macrophage Fc receptor are available. The receptor is sensitive to phospholipase A (50, 111, 134) and whereas the receptor for IgG on mouse macrophages is trypsin resistant, treatment with this enzyme can destroy the receptor for cytophilic IgM (141, 183, 251).

ii. POSSIBLE FUNCTIONAL SIGNIFICANCE OF IMMUNO-GLOBULIN ON MACROPHAGES.
Macrophages have been implicated in many important functions: phagocytosis and digestion of invading path-

ogenic microorganisms, and foreign particulate material; reactions against neoplastic cells; participation in the responses of delayed-type hypersensitivity and graft rejection; presentation of antigen to lymphocytes in the immune response; mediation of collaboration between T and B cells in the immune response (for review see reference 182).

Cell surface antibody would clearly be of advantage in facilitating the phagocytosis of microorganisms by macrophages, although direct evidence has proved difficult to obtain. While some investigators have postulated a role for cytophilic antibodies in defence against bacterial infection, it would seem that cytophilic antibodies would have no specific advantages over opsonic antibodies in this regard. First cytophilic antibodies must represent a heterogeneous population in terms of binding specificity for a given antigen, while on the other hand serum antibodies can bind specifically to a microorganism to present a high concentration of antibody Fc regions to the phagocytosing macrophage. In support of this view is the observation that Ig binds more efficiently to macrophages when complexed with polyvalent antigen. In addition, some opsonizing antibodies can also be expected to fix complement, in this manner facilitating phagocytosis (179).

Macrophages are virtually universal in their distribution in the animal kingdom, and phagocytose efficiently in animals which lack specific antibody responses. In some of these animals (121) they appear to utilize other less specific systems of recognition by serum proteins (opsonins?). It is not unlikely that the differences between cytophilia, opsonic adherence, and opsonization mediated by antibodies in vertebrates may have been enhanced by laboratory manipulation, and that it may be more fruitful to consider these phenomena as interacting, perhaps in some senses identical, aspects of a system designed to facilitate phagocytosis of microorganisms.

Similar arguments apply to cytophilic antibodies in delayed-type hypersensitivity, graft rejection, and tumor immunity. Clearly, refinements of the specific recognition system of the phagocytic cells might be expected to be advantageous. Definitive evidence for such a role of acquired antibody is lacking, although some reports involving reactions against alloantigens, and specific arming of macrophages for reaction against tumors (67, 182) are suggestive.

Whether Ig on the surface of macrophages mediates any of their interactions with lymphocytes in the immune response is a matter for debate. There is no clear evidence that the phagocytosis and processing of antigen by macrophages in the inductive stage of the immune response are mediated by passive antibody. The hypothesis that passively acquired T cell surface Ig on the membrane of the macrophage mediates lymphocyte collaboration in the antibody response has been dealt with above.

D. Antibody Cytophilic for Granulocytes

i. NEUTROPHILS. Receptors for Ig on neutrophils have been shown by (opsonic) promotion of bacterial phagocytosis (e.g., Ref. 206), by a rosetting technique (170), and by the release of intracellular lysosomal enzymes upon reaction with aggregated Ig (107, 242). Investigations using the latter approach suggested that all IgG and IgA subclasses in man could react with neutrophils, but that IgD, IgE and IgM were inactive. By the use of rosetting tests, it was suggested that only IgG_1 and IgG_3 were active. The studies utilizing opsonization of bacteria as a test for Ig receptors on neutrophils suggest that in man, IgG is the active class, although there is some dispute about the efficiency of IgA in this respect (206, 275). In sheep IgG_2 seems to be the active subclass (270) in promoting phagocytosis of bacteria by granulocytes.

It seems reasonable to suppose that the function of the receptors for Ig on the neutrophil membrane is to promote phagocytosis of invading microorganisms although, as for the macrophage, it is unclear whether or not the distinction between cytophilic and opsonic antibodies is a significant one in the normal physiology of the animal.

ii. BASOPHILS AND MAST CELLS. Immediate (Type 1; see Ref. 49) hypersensitivity reactions are mediated by serum antibodies passively bound to the membrane of basophils and mast cells. Upon reaction with the specific antigen, the cells then undergo degranulation, releasing their complement of pharmacologically active mediators (120). The antibodies mediating these reactions are cytophilic, as can be shown by their ability to fix in the skin of a nonsensitized recipient, and then mediate a reaction on subsequent challenge with antigen. These skin-fixing antibodies fall into two groups. One, which is heat labile, is present in low amounts in serum, remains fixed in the skin for long periods of time, and has been termed reaginic, has clearly been shown to be of the IgE class. Reaginic antibodies have been detected in the mouse (192, 204), rat (244), guinea-pig (58) and rabbit (281). A second class of skin-sensitizing antibody, belonging to the IgG class, has been described as heat stable and long-lived in the serum but with a short life fixed in the skin. In rats, mice and guinea pigs this Ig is of the IgG_1 (fast anodic mobility on electrophoresis) class (8, 193). Many classes of Ig which do not sensitize skin of an animal of the same species (i.e., are not homocytotropic) show the curious capacity to sensitize the skin of animals of other species (i.e., are heterocytotropic (see Ref. 242). One would probably be quite justified in regarding the phenomenon of heterocytotropic sensitization as an interesting laboratory demonstration with little relevance to normal function, either of antibodies or mast cells. In contrast to this, the immediate hypersensitivity reaction is very common (occurring perhaps as low in the phylogenetic scale as the teleosts) (9) and might, on teleological grounds, be expected to mediate some function of use to the animal. Although most of the manifestations of immediate hypersensitivity in man, as for example in atopic sensitivities leading to anaphylaxis, are more harmful than beneficial, a role, albeit controversial, has been claimed for these reactions in protection against parasites (188) and in tumor rejection (11).

iii. EOSINOPHILS.   Although levels of eosinophils in the blood of animals appear to be responsive to certain immunologically relevant events, such as immunization, especially with parasites (12, 13, 164, 280), the function of these cells remains an enigma. There is a report that in ragweed-pollen sensitive humans, both basophils and eosinophils bear passively adsorbed IgE antibody with specificity for the allergen (114), but the functional significance of this observation is unknown.

ACKNOWLEDGMENTS

Original work of the authors cited in this review was supported by grants from the American Heart Association (AHA 75-877) and the U.S.P.H.S. (AI-12565 and CA-20085). This is publication 2288 from The Walter and Eliza Hall Institute of Medical Research.

NOTE

1. Various investigators have used a number of designations for T cell immunoglobulin, e.g., IgM(T) or IgT (72, 250). We will use the terminology TIg.

REFERENCES

1. Abel, C. A., and Grey, H. M. 1968. Studies on the structure of mouse γA myeloma proteins. *Biochem.* 7: 2682–2688.

2. Abney, E. R., Hunter, I. R., and Parkhouse, R. M. E. 1976. Preparation and characterization of an antiserum to the mouse candidate for immunoglobulin D. *Nature* (*Lond.*) 259: 404–406.

3. Abney, E. R., and Parkhouse, R. M. E. 1974. Candidate for immunoglobulin D present on murine B lymphocytes. *Nature* (*Lond.*) 252: 600–602.

4. Abramson, N., Gelfand, E. W., Jandl, J. H., and Rosen, F. S. 1970. The interaction between human monocytes and red cells. Specificity for IgG subclasses and IgG fragments. *J. Exp. Med.* 132: 1207–1215.

5. Alexander, M. D., Leslie, R. G. Q., and Cohen, S. 1976. Cytophilic activity

of enzymatically derived fragments of guinea pigs IgG2. *Eur. J. Immunol.* 6: 101–107.

6. Anderson, C. L., and Grey, H. M. 1974. Receptors for aggregated IgG on mouse lymphocytes. Their presence on thymocytes, thymus-derived, and bone marrow-derived lymphocytes. *J. Exp. Med.* 139: 1175–1188.

7. Atwell, J. L., and Marchalonis, J. J. 1975. Phylogenetic emergence of immunoglobulin classes distinct from IgM. *J. Immunogenet.* 1: 367–391.

8. Bach, M. K., Bloch, K. J., and Austen, K. F. 1971. IgE and IgA antibody-mediated release of histamine from rat peritoneal cells. I. Optimum conditions for *in vitro* preparation of target cells with antibody and challenge with antigen. *J. Exp. Med.* 133: 752–771.

9. Baldo, B. A., and Fletcher, T. C. 1975. Phylogenetic aspects of hypersensitivity: intermediate hypersensitivity reactions in flat fish. *Adv. Exp. Med. Biol.* 64: 365–372.

10. Bankhurst, A. D., Warner, N. L., and Sprent, J. 1971. Surface immunoglobulins on thymus and thymus-derived lymphoid cells. *J. Exp. Med.* 134: 1005–1015.

11. Bartholomaeus, W. N., and Keast, D. 1972. Reaginic antibody to tumour and alloantigens in mice. *Nature (New Biol.)* 239: 206–207.

12. Basten, A., and Beeson, P. B. 1970. Mechanism of eosinophilia. II. Role of the lymphocyte. *J. Exp. Med.* 131: 1288–1305.

13. Basten, A., Boyer, M. H., and Beeson, P. B. 1970. Mechanism of eosinophilia. I. Factors affecting the eosinophil response of rats to *Trichinella spiralis*. *J. Exp. Med.* 131: 1271–1287.

14. Basten, A., Miller, J. F. A. P., and Abraham, R. 1975. Relationship between Fc receptors, antigen-binding sites on T and B cells, and H-2 complex-associated determinants. *J. Exp. Med.* 141: 547–560.

15. Basten, A., Miller, J. F. A. P., Sprent, J., and Pye, J. 1972. A receptor for antibody on B lymphocytes. I. A method of detection and functional significance. *J. Exp. Med.* 135: 610–626.

16. Basten, A., Miller, J. F. A. P., Warner, N. L., Abraham, R., Chia, E., and Gamble, J. 1975. A subpopulation of T cells bearing Fc receptors. *J. Immunol.* 115: 1159–1165.

17. Basten, A., Warner, N. L., and Mandel, T. 1972. A receptor for antibody on B lymphocytes. II. Immunochemical and electron microscopy characteristics. *J. Exp. Med.* 135: 627–642.

18. Baur, S., Vitetta, E. S., Sherr, C. J., Schenkein, I., and Uhr, J. W. 1971. Isolation of heavy and light chains of immunoglobulin from the surfaces of lymphoid cells. *J. Immunol.* 106: 1133–1135.

19. Benacerraf, B., and Katz, D. H. 1975. The histocompatibility-linked immune response genes. *Adv. Cancer Res.* 21: 121–173.

20. Benacerraf, G., and McDevitt, H. O. 1972. Histocompatibility-linked immune response genes. *Science* 175: 273–279.

21. Bentwich, Z., Douglas, S. D., Siegal, F. P., and Kunkel, H. G. 1973. Human lymphocyte-sheep erythrocyte rosette formation: some characteristics of the interaction. *Clin. Immunol. Immunopathol.* 1: 511–522.

22. Berken, A., and Benacerraf, B. 1966. Properties of antibodies cytophilic for macrophages. *J. Exp. Med.* 123: 119–144.

23. Berken, A., and Benacerraf, B. 1968. Sedimentation properties of antibody cytophilic for macrophages. *J. Immunol.* 100: 1219–1222.

24. Binz, H., Lindemann, J., and Wigzell, H. 1973. Inhibition of local graft-versus-host reaction by anti-alloantibodies. *Nature* 246: 146–148.

25. Binz, H., and Wigzell, H. 1975. Shared idiotypic determinants on B and T lymphocytes reactive against the same antigenic determinants. I. Demonstration of similar or identical idiotypes on IgG molecules and T-cell receptors with specificity for the same alloantigens. *J. Exp. Med.* 142: 197–211.

26. Binz, H., and Wigzell, H. 1976. Shared idiotypic determinants on B and T lymphocytes reactive against the same antigen determinants. V. Biochemical and serological characteristics of naturally occurring soluble antigen binding T lymphocyte-derived molecules. *Scand. J. Immunol.* 5: 559–571.

27. Black, S. J., Hämmerling, G. J., Berek, C., Rajewsky, K., and Eichmann, K. 1976. Idiotypic analysis of lymphocytes *in vitro*. I. Specificity and heterogeneity of B and T lymphocytes reactive with anti-idiotypic antibody. *J. Exp. Med.* 143: 846–860.

28. Blaskovec, A. A. 1966. A study of delayed hypersensitivity in guinea pigs injected with antigen-antibody complexes. *Int. Arch. Allergy Appl. Immunol.* 30: 482–496.

29. Boyden, S. V. 1963. Cytophilic Antibody, *in* B. Amos and H. Koprowski (eds.), *Cell Bound Antibodies*, pp. 7–17, Wistar Inst. Press, Philadelphia, Pa.

30. Boylston, A. W., and Mowbray, J. F. 1974. Surface immunoglobulin of a mouse T-cell lymphoma. *Immunol.* 27: 855–861.

31. Brown, J. C., De Jesus, D. G., Holborow, E. J., and Harris, G. 1970. Lymphocyte-mediated transport of aggregated human γ-globulin into germinal centre areas of normal mouse spleen. *Nature (Lond.)* 228: 367–369.

32. Brown, G., and Greaves, M. F. 1975. Cell surface markers for human T and B lymphocytes. *Eur. J. Immunol.* 4: 302–310.

33. Brown, J. C., and Koshland, M. E. 1975. Activation of antibody Fc function by antigen-induced conformational changes. *Proc. Natl. Acad. Sci. (USA)* 72: 5111–5115.

34. Calkins, C. E., Ozer, H., and Waksman, B. H. 1975. B cells in the appendix and other lymphoid organs of the rabbit: stimulation of DNA synthesis by anti-immunoglobulin. *Cell. Immunol.* 18: 187–198.

35. Capra, J. D., and Kehoe, J. M. 1975. Hypervariable regions, idiotypy and the antibody-combining site. *Adv. Immunol.* 20: 1–40.

36. Cerottini, J.-C., and Brunner, K. T. 1974. Cell-mediated cytotoxicity, allograft rejection and tumor immunity. *Adv. Immunol.* 18: 67–132.

37. Chan, P. L., and St. C. Sinclair, N. R. 1971. Regulation of the immune response. V. An analysis of the function of the Fc portion of antibody in suppression of an immune response with respect to interaction with components of the lymphoid system. *Immunology* 21: 967–981.

38. Chapuis, R. M., and Koshland, M. E. 1974. Mechanism of IgM polymerization. *Proc. Natl. Acad. Sci. (USA)* 71: 675–661.

39. Ciccimarra, F., Rosen, F. S., and Merler, E. 1975. Localization of the IgG

effector site for monocyte receptors. *Proc. Natl. Acad. Sci. (USA)* 72: 2081–2083.

40. Clem, L. W., and Leslie, G. A. 1969. Phylogeny of immunoglobulin structure and function, *in* M. Adinolfi (ed.), *Immunology and Development,* pp. 62–88. Spastics International Medical Publication, London.

41. Clem, L. W., and Small, P. A. 1967. Phylogeny of immunoglobulin structure and function. I. Immunoglobulins of the lemon shark. *J. Exp. Med.* 125: 893–920.

42. Cline, M. J., Sprent, J., Warner, N. L., and Harris, A. W. 1972. Receptor for immunoglobulin on B lymphocytes and cells of a cultured plasma cell tumor. *J. Immunol.* 108: 1126–1128.

43. Cone, R. E. 1976. Factors influencing the isolation of membrane immunoglobulins from T and B lymphocytes. I. Detergent effects and iodination conditions. *J. Immunol.* 116: 847–853.

44. Cone, R. E., and Brown, W. C. 1976. Isolation of membrane associated immunoglobulins from T lymphocytes by non-ionic detergents. *Immunochem.* 13: 571–580.

45. Cone, R. E., Feldmann, M., Marchalonis, J. J., and Nossal, G. J. V. 1974. Cytophilic properties of surface immunoglobulin of thymus-derived lymphocytes. *Immunology* 26: 49–60.

46. Cone, R. E., and Marchalonis, J. J. 1973. Antigen-binding specificity of cell surface immunoglobulin isolated from T helper cells. *Aust. J. Exp. Biol. Med. Sci.* 51: 689–700.

47. Cone, R. E., and Marchalonis, J. J. 1974. Surface proteins of thymus-derived lymphocytes and bone-marrow-derived lymphocytes. Selective isolation of immunoglobulin and the θ-antigen by non-ionic detergents. *Biochem. J.* 140: 345–354.

48. Cone, R. E., Sprent, J., and Marchalonis, J. J. 1972. Antigen-binding specificity of isolated cell-surface immunoglobulin from thymus cells activated to histocompatibility antigens. *Proc. Natl. Acad. Sci. USA* 69: 2556–2560.

49. Coombs, R. R. A., and Gell, P. G. H. 1975. Classification of allergic reactions responsible for clinical hypersensitivity and disease. *in* P. G. H. Gell, R. R. A. Coombs and P. J. Lachmann (eds.), *Clinical Aspects of Immunology,* 3rd ed., pp. 761–781. Blackwell, Oxford.

50. Davey, M. J., and Asherson, G. L. 1967. Cytophilic antibody. I. Nature of the macrophage receptor. *Immunology* 12: 13–20.

51. Davie, J. M., and Paul, W. E. 1974. Antigen-binding receptors on lymphocytes. *Contemp. Topics Immunobiol.* 3: 171–192.

52. Delamette, F., Hardt, N., and Panijel, J. 1975. *In vitro* induction of IgM synthesis and secretion in rabbit spleen cells by soluble concanavalin A. *Cell. Immunol.* 18: 41–48.

53. Del Guercio, P., Tolone, G., Andrade, F. B., Biozzi, G., and Binaghi, R. A. 1969. Opsonic, cytophilic and agglutinating activity of guinea-pig $\gamma 2$ and γM anti-*Salmonella* antibodies. *Immunology.* 16: 361–371.

54. Dickler, H. B. 1974. Studies of the human lymphocyte receptor for heat-aggregated or antigen-complexed immunoglobulin. *J. Exp. Med.* 140: 508–522.

55. Dickler, H. B. 1976. Lymphocyte receptors for immunoglobulin. *Adv. Immunol.* 24: 167–214.

56. Dickler, H. B., Adkinson, N. F., and Terry, W. D. 1974. Evidence for individual human peripheral blood lymphocytes bearing both B and T cell markers. *Nature (Lond.)* 247: 213–215.

57. Dickler, H. B., and Kunkel, H. G. 1972. Interaction of aggregated γ-globulin with B lymphocytes. *J. Exp. Med.* 136: 191–196.

58. Dobson, C., Rockey, J. H., and Soulsby, E. J. L. 1971. Immunoglobulin E antibodies in guinea pigs: characterization of monomeric and polymeric components. *J. Immunol.* 107: 1431–1439.

59. Edelman, G. M. 1970. The covalent structure of a human γG-immunoglobulin. XI. Functional implications. *Biochem.* 9: 3197–3205.

60. Edelman, G. M., and Gall, W. E. 1969. The antibody problem. *Ann. Rev. Biochem.* 38: 415–466.

61. Ehrlich, P. 1900. On immunity with special reference to cell life. *Proc. Roy. Soc.* 66: 424–448.

62. Eichmann, K. 1972. Idiotypic identity of antibodies to streptococcal carbohydrate in inbred mice. *Eur. J. Immunol.* 2: 301–307.

63. Eichmann, K. 1974. Idiotype suppression. I. Influence of the dose and of the effector functions of anti-idiotypic antibody on the production of an idiotype. *Eur. J. Immunol.* 4: 296–302.

64. Eichmann, K. 1975. Idiotype suppression. II. Amplification of a suppressor T cell with anti-idiotypic activity. *Eur. J. Immunol.* 5: 511–517.

65. Eichmann, K., and Rajewsky, K. 1975. Induction of T and B cell immunity by anti-idiotypic antibody. *Eur. J. Immunol.* 5: 661–666.

66. Erb, P., Meier, B., and Feldmann, M. 1976. Two-gene control of T-helper cell induction. *Nature (Lond.)* 263: 601–604.

67. Evans, R., and Alexander, P. 1972. Mechanism of immunologically specific killing of tumor cells by macrophages. *Nature (Lond.)* 236: 168–170.

68. Fanger, M. W., Hart, D. A., Wells, J. V., and Nisonoff, A. 1970. Requirement for cross-linkage in the stimulation of transformation of rabbit peripheral lymphocytes by antiglobulin reagents. *J. Immunol.* 105: 1484–1492.

69. Fanger, M. W., Pelley, R. P., and Reese, A. L. 1972. *In vitro* demonstration of two antigenically-distinct rabbit lymphocyte populations. *J. Immunol.* 109: 294–303.

70. Feldmann, M. 1972. Cell interactions in the immune response *in vitro*. V. Specific collaboration via complexes of antigen and thymus-derived cell immunoglobulin. *J. Exp. Med.* 136: 737–760.

71. Feldmann, M. 1977. Cell interactions in the immune response *in vitro*, in J. J. Marchalonis (ed.), *The Lymphocyte: Structure and Function*. Marcel Dekker, New York pp. 279–307.

72. Feldmann, M., Boylston, A., and Hogg, N. M. 1975. Immunological effects of IgT synthesized by theta-positive cell lines. *Eur. J. Immunol.* 5: 429–431.

73. Feldmann, M., Cone, R. E., and Marchalonis, J. J. 1973. Cell interactions in the immune response *in vitro*. VI Mediation by T cell surface monomeric IgM. *Cell. Immunol.* 9: 1–11.

74. Feldmann, M., and Nossal, G. J. V. 1972. Tolerance, enhancement and the regulation of interactions between T cells, B cells and macrophages. *Transplant. Rev.* 13: 3–34.

75. Ferrarini, M., Moretta, L., Mingari, M. C., Tonda, P., and Pernis, B. 1976. Human T cell receptor for IgM: specificity for the pentameric Fc fragment. *Eur. J. Immunol.* 6: 520–521.

76. Finkleman, F. D., Van Boxel, J. A., Asofsky, R., and Paul, W. E. 1976. Cell membrane IgD: Demonstration of IgD on human lymphocytes by enzyme catalised iodination and comparison with cell surface Ig of mouse, guinea pig and rabbit. *J. Immunol.* 116: 1173–1181.

77. Forni, L., and Pernis, B. 1975. Interactions between Fc receptors and membrane immunoglobulin on B lymphocytes, *in* M Seligmann, J. L., Preud'homme, and F. M. Kourilsky (eds.), pp. 193–201. North-Holland, Amsterdam.

78. Fridman, W. H., and Goldstein, P. 1974. Immunoglobulin-binding factor present on and produced by thymus-processed lymphocytes (T cells). *Cell. Immunol.* 11: 442–455.

79. Fu, S. M., Winchester, R. J., and Kunkel, H. G. 1974. Occurrence of surface IgM, IgD and free light chains on human lymphocytes. *J. Exp. Med.* 139: 451–456.

80. Fu, S. M., Winchester, R. J., and Kunkel, H. G. 1975. Similar idiotypic specificity for the membrane IgD and IgM of human B lymphocytes. *J. Immunol.* 114: 250–252.

81. Gally, J. A., and Edelman, G. M. 1972. The genetic control of immuno-globulin synthesis. *Ann. Rev. Med.* 6: 1–46.

82. Gehrhart, P. J., Sigal, N. H., and Klinman, N. R. 1975. Production of antibodies of identical idiotype but diverse immunoglobulin classes by cells derived from a single stimulated B cell. *Proc. Natl. Acad. Sci. (USA)* 72: 1707–1711.

83. Gell, P. G. H., and Sell, S. 1965. Studies on rabbit lymphocytes *in vitro.* II. Induction of blast transformation with antisera to six IgG allotypes and summation with mixtures of antisera to different allotypes. *J. Exp. Med.* 122: 813–821.

84. Girard, K. F., and Murray, E. G. D. 1954. The presence of antibody in macrophage extracts. *Canad. J. Biochem. Physiol.* 32: 14–19.

85. Goding, J. W., and Layton, J. E. 1976. Antigen-induced co-capping of IgM and IgD-like receptors on murine B cells. *J. Exp. Med.* 144: 852–857.

86. Goding, J. W., Warr, G. W., and Warner, N. L. 1976. Genetic polymorphism of IgD-like cell surface immunoglobulin in the mouse. *Proc. Natl. Acad. Sci. (USA).* 73: 1305–1309.

87. Goldschneider, L., and Cogen, R. B. 1973. Immunoglobulin molecules on the surface of activated T lymphocytes in the rat. *J. Exp. Med.* 138: 163–175.

88. Gordon, J., and Murgita, R. A. 1975. Suppression and augmentation of the primary *in vitro* immune response by different classes of antibodies. *Cell. Immunol.* 15: 392–402.

89. Greaves, M. F. 1970. Biological effects of anti-immunoglobulins. *Transplant. Rev.* 5: 45–75.

90. Greaves, M., Janossy, G., Feldmann, M., and Doenhoff, M. 1974. Poly-clonal mitogens and the nature of B lymphocyte activation mechanisms, *in* E. E. Sercarz, A. R. Williamson and C. F. Fox (eds.), *The Immune System: Genes, Receptors, Signals,* pp. 271–297. Academic Press, New York.

91. Greaves, M. F., Owen, J. J. T., and Raff, M. C. 1973. T and B lymphocytes: Origins, properties and roles in immune responses. Excerpta Medica, Amsterdam.

92. Greenberg, A. H., Hudson, L., Shen, L., and Roitt, I. M. 1973. Antibody-dependent cell-mediated cytotoxicity due to a "Null" lymphoid cell. *Nature New Biol.* 242: 111–113.

93. Grey, H. M., Colon, S., Campbell, P., and Rabellino, E. 1972: Immunoglobulins on the surface of lymphocytes. V. Quantitative studies on the question of whether immunoglobulins are associated with T cells in the mouse. *J. Immunol.* 109: 776–783.

94. Grey, H. M., Kubo, R. T., and Cerottini, J.-C. 1972. Thymus-derived (T) cell immunoglobulins, presence of a receptor site for IgG and absence of large amounts of "buried" Ig determinants on T cells. *J. Exp. Med.* 136: 1323–1328.

95. Gyöngyössy, M. I. C., Arnaiz-Villena, A., Soteriades-Vlachos, C., and Playfair, J. H. L. 1975. Rosette formation by mouse lymphocytes. IV. Fc and C3 receptors occurring together and separately on T cells and other leukocytes. *Clin. Exp. Immunol.* 19: 485–497.

96. Hämmerling, G. J., and McDevitt, H. O. 1974. Antigen binding T and B lymphocytes. II. Studies on the inhibition of antigen binding to T and B cells by anti-immunoglobulin and anti H-2 sera. *J. Immunol.* 112: 1734–1740.

97. Hämmerling, U., Mack, C., and Pickel, H. G. 1976. Immunofluorescence analysis of Ig determinants of mouse thymocytes and T cells. *Immunochem.* 13: 525–532.

98. Hämmerling, U., Pickel, H. G., Mack, C., and Masters, D. 1976. Immunochemical study of an immunoglobulin like molecule of murine thymocytes. *Immunochem.* 13: 533–538.

99. Harris, A. W., Bankhurst, A. D., Mason, S., and Warner, N. L. 1973. Differentiated functions expressed by cultured mouse lymphoma cells. II. θ antigen, surface immunoglobulin and a receptor for antibody on cells of a thymoma cell line. *J. Immunol.* 110: 431–438.

100. Hallberg, T., Gurner, B. W., and Coombs, R. R. A. 1973. Opsonic adherence of sensitized ox red cells to human lymphocytes as measured by rosette formation. *Int. Arch. Allergy. Appl. Immunol.* 44: 500–513.

101. Haustein, D. 1971. Untersuchungen zum Mechanismus der Hapten-Antikörper-Reaktion mit Hilfe eines solvatochromen Farbstoffs aus der Reihe der Pyridinium-N-(4-hydroxyphenyl)-betaine. Doctoral Dissertation, Albert-Ludwigs-Universität zu Freiburg im Bresgau.

102. Haustein, D. 1975. Effective radioiodination by lactoperoxidase and solubilisation of cell surface proteins of cultured murine T lymphoma cells. *J. Immunol. Methods* 7: 25–38.

103. Haustein, D., and Goding, J. W. 1975. Surface immunoglobulin heavy chains of murine splenocytes and thymocytes are different. *Biochem. Biophys. Res. Commun.* 65: 483–489.

104. Haustein, D., Marchalonis, J. J., and Harris, A. W. 1975. Immunoglobulin of T lymphoma cells. Biosynthesis, surface representation and partial characterization. *Biochemistry* 14: 1826–1834.

105. Haustein, D., and Warr, G. W. 1976. Use and abuse of Sepharose-conjugated antibodies for the isolation of lymphocyte-surface immunoglobulins. *J. Immunol. Methods.* 12: 323–336.

106. Hay, F. C., Torrigiani, G., and Roitt, I. M. 1972. The binding of human IgG subclasses to human monocytes. *Eur. J. Immunol.* 2: 257–261.

107. Henson, P. M., Johnson, H. B., and Spiegelberg, H. L. 1972. The release of granule enzymes from human neutrophils stimulated by aggregated immunoglobulins of different classes and subclasses. *J. Immunol.* 109: 1182–1192.

108. Herzenberg, L. A., Herzenberg, L. A., Black, S. J., Loken, M. R., Okumura, K., Van der Loo, W., Osborne, B. A., Hewgill, D., Goding, J. W., Gutman, G., and Warner, N. L. 1977. Surface markers and functional relationships of cells involved in murine B lymphocyte differentiation (including the description of IgM and IgD allotypes). *Cold Spring Harbor Symp. Quant. Biol.* 41:33–45.

109. Hoffmann, G. W. 1975. A theory of regulation and self-nonself discrimination in an immune network. *Eur. J. Immunol.* 5: 638–647.

110. Hood, L., Barstad, P., Loh, E., and Nottenburg, C. 1974. Antibody diversity: An assessment, in E. E. Sercarz, A. R. Williamson and C. F. Fox (eds.), *Genes, Receptors and Signals*, pp. 119–140. Academic Press, New York.

111. Howard, J. G., and Benacerraf, B. 1966. Properties of macrophage receptors for cytophilic antibodies. *Brit. J. Exp. Path.* 47: 193–200.

112. Hoy, W. E., and Nelson, D. S. 1967. Immunological responses to allografts in mice. *Proc. Australian Soc. Med. Res.* 2: 117 (abstract).

113. Huber, H., and Fudenberg, H. H. 1968. Receptor sites of human monocytes for IgG. *Int. Arch. Allergy Appl. Immunol.* 34: 18–31.

114. Hubscher, T., and Eisen, A. H. 1971. Allergen binding to human peripheral leukocytes. *Int. Arch. Allergy Appl. Immunol.* 41: 689–699.

115. Hudson, L., and Sprent, J. 1976. Specific adsorption of IgM antibody onto H-2-activated mouse T lymphocytes. *J. Exp. Med.* 143: 444–449.

116. Hudson, L., Sprent, J., Miller, J. F. A. P., and Playfair, J. H. L. 1974. B-cell-derived immunoglobulin on activated mouse T lymphocytes. *Nature (Lond.)* 251: 60–62.

117. Hunt, S. M., and Marchalonis, J. J. 1974. Radioiodinated lymphocyte surface glycoproteins. Concanavalin A binding proteins include surface immunoglobulin. *Biochem. Biophys. Res. Commun.* 61: 1227–1233.

118. Hunt, S. V., and Williams, A. F. 1974. The origin of cell surface immunoglobulin of marrow-derived and thymus-derived lymphocytes of the rat. *J. Exp. Med.* 139: 479–496.

119. Hunt, W. B., and Myrvik, Q. N. 1964. Demonstration of antibody in rabbit alveolar macrophages with failure to transfer antibody production. *J. Immunol.* 93: 677–681.

120. Ishizaka, K. 1970. Human reaginic antibodies. *Ann. Rev. Med.* 21: 187–200.

121. Jenkin, C. R., and Hardy, D. 1975. Recognition factors of the crayfish and the generation of diversity. *Adv. Exp. Med. Biol.* 64: 55–65.

122. Jerne, N. K. 1972. What precedes clonal selection? in *Ontogeny of Acquired Immunity.* pp. 1–15. Associated Scientific Publishers, Amsterdam.

123. Jerry, L. M., Kunkel, H. G., and Grey, H. M. 1970. Absence of disulfide bonds linking the heavy and light chains: a property of a genetic variant of γA2 globulins. *Proc. Natl. Acad. Sci. (USA)* 65: 557–563.

124. Joller, P. W. 1972. Graft-versus-host reactivity of lymphoid cells inhibited by anti-recognition structure serum. *Nature New Biol.* 240: 214–215.

125. Jonas, W. E., Gurner, B. W., Nelson, D. S., and Coombs, R. R. A. 1965. Passive sensitization of tissue cells. I. Passive sensitization of macrophages by guinea-pig cytophilic antibody. *Int. Arch. Allergy Appl. Immunol.* 28: 86–104.

126. Jones, P. P., Cebra, J. J., and Herzenberg, L. A. 1973. Immunoglobulin (Ig) allotype markers on rabbit lymphocytes: separation of cells bearing different allotypes and demonstration of the binding of Ig to lymphoid cell membranes. *J. Immunol.* 111: 1334–1348.

127. Jones, P. P., Tacier-Eugster, H., and Herzenberg, L. A. 1974. Lymphocyte commitment to Ig allotype and class. *Ann. Immunol. (Inst. Pasteur)* 125, C: 271–276.

128. Jones, V.E., Graves, H. F., and Orlans, E. 1976. The detection of F(ab')$_2$-related surface antigens on the thymocytes of children. *Immunol.* 30: 281–288.

129. Kappler, J. W., Van Der Hoven, A., Dharmarajan, U., and Hoffmann, M. 1973. Regulation of the immune response. IV. Antibody-mediated suppression of the immune response to haptens and heterologous erythrocyte antigens in vitro. *J. Immunol.* 111: 1228–1235.

130. Katz, D. H., and Benacerraf, B. 1975. The function and interrelationships of T-cell receptors, Ir genes and other histocompatibility gene products. *Transplant. Rev.* 22: 175–195.

131. Kennel, S. J., and Lerner, R. A. 1973. Isolation and characterisation of plasma membrane associated immunoglobulin from cultured human diploid lymphocytes. *J. Mol. Biol.* 76: 485–502.

132. Kermani-Arab, V., Leslie, G. A., and Burger, D. R. 1976. Anti-IgD activation of human lymphocytes and its enhancing effect on PHA responsiveness. *Fed. Proc.* 35: 822 (abstract).

133. Kishimoto, T., and Ishizaka, K. 1975. Regulation of antibody response in vitro. IX. Induction of secondary anti-hapten IgG antibody response by anti-immunoglobulin and enhancing soluble factor. *J. Immunol.* 114: 585–591.

134. Kossard, S., and Nelson, D. S. 1968. Studies on cytophilic antibodies. IV. The effects of proteolytic enzymes (trypsin and papain) on the attachment to macrophages of cytophilic antibodies. *Aust. J. Exp. Biol. Med. Sci.* 46: 63–71.

135. Krammer, P. H., Citronbaum, R., Read, S. E., Forni, L., and Lang, R. 1976. Murine thymic lymphomas as model tumors for T-cell studies. T-cell markers, immunoglobulins and Fc-receptors on AKR thymomas. *Cell. Immunol.* 21: 97–111.

136. Krammer, P. H., Hudson, L., and Sprent, J. 1975. Fc-receptors, Ia-antigens and immunoglobulin on normal and activated mouse T lymphocytes. *J. Exp. Med.* 142: 1403–1415.

137. Ladoulis, C. T., Misra, D. N., and Gill, T. J. III 1973. The isolation and characterization of rat lymphocyte plasma membranes, in H. Peeters (ed.), *Protides Biol. Fluids. Proc. Colloq. Bruges.* 21, pp. 67–71. Pergamon Press, Oxford.

138. Larsson, Å., and Perlmann, P. 1972. Study of Fab and F(ab')$_2$ from rabbit IgG for capacity to induce lymphocyte-mediated target cell destruction in vitro. *Int. Arch. Allergy Appl. Immunol.* 43: 80–88.

139. Lawrence, D. A., Weigle, W. O., and Spiegelberg, H. L. 1975. Immuno-

globulins cytophilic for human lymphocytes, monocytes and neutrophils. *J. Clin. Invest.* 55: 368–376.

140. Lawton, A. R., and Cooper, M. D. 1974. Modification of B lymphocyte differentiation by anti-immunoglobulins. *Contemp. Topics Immunobiol.* 3: 193–225.

141. Lay, W. H., and Nussenzweig, V. 1969. Ca^{++}-dependent binding of antigen 19S antibody complexes to macrophages. *J. Immunol.* 102: 1172–1178.

142. Lee, S.-T., and Paraskevas, F. 1972. Cell surface-associated gamma globulins in lymphocytes. IV. Lack of detection of surface γ globulin on B-cells and acquisition of surface γ_G globulin by T-cells during primary response. *J. Immunol.* 109: 1262–1271.

143. Lees, R. K., and St. C. Sinclair, N. R. 1973. Regulation of the immune response. VII. In vitro immunosuppression by $F(ab')_2$ or intact IgG antibodies. *Immunol.* 24: 735–750.

144. Lerner, R. A., McConahey, P. J., and Dixon, F. J. 1971. Quantitative aspects of plasma membrane-associated immunoglobulin in clones of diploid human lymphocytes. *Science* 173: 60–62.

145. Leslie, G. A., and Martin, L. N. 1973. Studies on the secretory immunologic system of fowl. III. Serum and secretory IgA of the chicken. *J. Immunol.* 110: 1–9.

146. Lisowska-Bernstein, B., Rinuy, A., and Vassalli, P. 1973. Absence of detectable IgM in enzymatically or biosynthetically labelled thymus-derived lymphocytes. *Proc. Natl. Acad. Sci. (USA)* 70: 2879–2883.

147. Litman, G. W. 1976. Physical properties of immunoglobulins of lower species: A comparison with immunoglobulins of mammals, in J. J. Marchalonis (ed.), *Comparative Immunology* pp. 239–275. Blackwell, Oxford.

148. LoBuglio, A. F., Cotran, R. S., and Jandl, J. H. 1967. Red cells coated with immunoglobulin G: Binding and sphering by mononuclear cells in man. *Science* 158: 1582–1585.

149. MacLennan, I. C. M., Connell, G. E., and Gotch, F. M. 1974. Effector activating determinants on IgG. II. Differentiation of the combining sites for C1q from those for cytotoxic K cells and neutrophils by plasmin digestion of rabbit IgG. *Immunol.* 26: 303–310.

150. Marchalonis, J. J. 1972. Conservation in the evolution of immunoglobulin. *Nature New Biol.* 236: 84–86.

151. Marchalonis, J. J. 1975. Lymphocyte surface immunoglobulins *Science* 190: 20–29.

152. Marchalonis, J. J. 1976. Surface immunoglobulins of B and T lymphocytes: molecular properties, association with cell membrane, and a unified model of antigen recognition. *Contemp. Topics Mol. Immunol.* 5:125–160.

153. Marchalonis, J. J. 1976. *Immunity in Evolution.* Harvard University Press (in press).

154. Marchalonis, J. J. 1976. Isolated DNP-binding B cell surface immunoglobulins. *Immunochem.* 13: 667–670.

155. Marchalonis, J. J. 1976. Cell cooperation in immune responses, in *Basic and Clinical Immunology*, eds. H. H. Fudenberg, D. P. Stites, J. L. Caldwell and J. V. Wells. Lange Med. Pub., Los Altos, pp. 88–96.

156. Marchalonis, J. J., Atwell, J. L., and Haustein, D. 1974. Molecular properties of isolated surface immunoglobulins of human chronic lymphocytic leukaemia cells. Biochem. Biophys. Acta. 351: 99–112.

157. Marchalonis, J. J., and Cone, R. E. 1973. Biochemical and biological characteristics of lymphocyte surface immunoglobulin. Transplant. Rev. 14: 3–49.

158. Marchalonis, J. J., and Cone, R. E. 1973. The phylogenetic emergence of vertebrate immunity. Aust. J. Exp. Biol. Med. Sci. 51: 461–488.

159. Marchalonis, J. J., Cone, R. E., and Atwell, J. L. 1972. Isolation and partial characterization of lymphocyte surface immunoglobulin. J. Exp. Med. 135: 956–971.

160. Marchalonis, J. J., Decker, J. M., DeLuca, D., Moseley, J. M., Smith, P. M., and Warr, G. W. 1977. Lymphocyte surface immunoglobulins: Evolutionary origins and involvement in activation. Cold Spring Harbor Symp. Quant. Biol., 41:261–273.

161. Marchalonis, J. J., and Edelman, G. M. 1965. Phylogenetic origins of antibody structure. I. Multichain structure of immunoglobulins in the smooth dogfish (Mustelus canis). J. Exp. Med. 122: 610–618.

162. Marchalonis, J. J., and Edelman, G. M. 1968. Phylogenetic origins of antibody structure. III. Antibodies in the primary immune response of the sea lamprey, Petromyzon marinus. J. Exp. Med. 127: 891–914.

163. Martin, L. N., Leslie, G. A., and Hindes, R. 1976. Lymphocyte surface IgD and IgM in non-human primates. Int. Arch. Allergy. Appl. Immunol. 51: 320–329.

164. McGarry, M. P., Speirs, R. S., Jenkins, V. K., and Trentin, J. J. 1971. Lymphoid cell dependence of eosinophil response to antigen. J. Exp. Med. 134: 801–814.

165. McKearn, T. J. 1974. Anti-receptor antiserum causes specific inhibition of reactivity to rat histocompatibility antigens. Science 183: 94–96.

166. McKearn, T. J., Hamada, H., Stuart, F. P., and Fitch, F. W. 1974. Anti-receptor antibody and resistance to graft-versus-host disease. Nature (Lond.) 251: 648–650.

167. McKearn, T. J., Stuart, F. P., and Fitch, F. W. 1974. Anti-idiotypic antibody in rat transplantation immunity. I. Production of anti-idiotypic antibody in animals repeatedly immunized with alloantigens. J. Immunol. 113: 1874–1882.

168. Melcher, U., Vitetta, E. S., McWilliams, M., Lamm, M. E., Philips-Quagliata, J. M., and Uhr, J. W. 1974. Cell surface immunoglobulin. X. Identification of an IgD-like molecule on the surface of murine splenocytes. J. Exp. Med. 140: 1427–1431.

169. Melchers, F., and Anderson, J. 1973. Synthesis, surface deposition and secretion of immunoglobulin M in bone marrow derived lymphocytes before and after mitogenic stimulation. Transplant. Rev. 14: 76–130.

170. Messner, R. P., and Jelineck, J. 1970. Receptors for human γG globulin on human neutrophils. J. Clin. Invest. 49: 2165–2171.

171. Michaelsen, T. E., Wisløff, F., and Natvig, J. B. 1975. Structural requirements in the Fc region of rabbit IgG antibodies necessary to induce cytotoxicity by human lymphocytes. Scand. J. Immunol. 4: 71–78.

172. Miller, J. F. A. P. 1972. Lymphocyte interactions in antibody responses. *Int. Rev. Cytol.* 33: 77–130.

173. Misra, D. N., Ladoulis, C. T., Gill, T. J., III, and Bazin, H. 1976. Lymphocyte plasma membranes. V. Immunoglobulins on isolated plasma membranes of the thymic and splenic lymphocytes of the rat. *Immunochem.* 13: 613–622.

174. Möller, E. 1965. Contact-induced cytotoxicity by lymphoid cells containing foreign isoantigens. *Science* 147: 873–879.

175. Moretta, L., Ferrarini, M., Durante, M. L., and Mingari, M. C. 1975. Expression of a receptor for IgM by human T cell *in vitro*. *Eur. J. Immunol.* 5: 565–569.

176. Moroz, C., and Hahn, J. 1973. Cell surface immunoglobulin of human thymus cells and its *in vitro* biosynthesis. *Proc. Nat. Acad. Sci. (USA)* 70: 3716–3720.

177. Moroz, C., and Lahat, N. 1974. *In vitro* biosynthesis and molecular arrangement of surface immunoglobulin of mouse thymus cells, *in* E. E. Sercarz, A. R. Williamson and C. F. Fox (eds.). *The Immune System, Genes, Receptor, Signals.* Academic Press. New York, pp. 233–246.

178. Moseley, J. M., Marchalonis, J. J., Harris, A., and Pye, J. 1977. Molecular properties of T lymphoma immunoglobulin I. Serological and general physicochemical properties. *J. Immunogenetics* 4:233–248.

179. Müller-Eberhard, H. J. 1975. Complement and phagocytosis, *in The Phagocytic Cell in Host Resistance.* J. A. Bellanti and D. H. Dayton (eds.), pp. 87–99. Raven Press, New York.

180. Munro, A. J., and Taussig, M. J. 1975. Two genes in the major histocompatibility complex control immune response. *Nature (Lond.)* 256: 103–106.

181. Nagy, Z., Elliott, B. E., Nabholz, M., Krammer, P. H., and Pernis, B. 1976. Specific binding of alloantigens to T cells activated in the mixed lymphocyte reaction. *J. Exp. Med.* 143: 648–659.

182. Nelson, D. S. 1969. Macrophages and immunity. North-Holland, Amsterdam.

183. Nelson, D. S., and Boyden, S. V. 1967. Macrophage cytophilic antibodies and delayed hypersensitivity. *Brit. Med. Bull.* 23: 15–20.

184. Nelson, D. S., Kossard, S., and Cox, P. E. 1967. Heterogeneity of macrophage cytophilic antibodies in immunized mice. *Experientia* 23: 490–491.

185. Nisonoff, A., Hopper, J. E., and Spring, S. B. 1975. *The Antibody Molecule,* Academic Press, New York.

186. Nossal, G. J. V., Warner, N. L., Lewis, H., and Sprent, J. 1972. Quantitative features of a sandwich radioimmunolabelling technique for lymphocyte surface receptors. *J. Exp. Med.* 135: 405–428.

187. Nossal, G. J. V., Pike, B. L., Stocker, J. W., Layton, J. E., and Goding, J. W. 1977. Hapten-specific B lymphocytes: Enrichment cloning, receptor analysis and tolerance induction. *Cold Spring Harbor Symp. Quant. Biol.* 41:237–243.

188. Ogilvie, B. M., and Jones, V. E. 1973. Immunity in the parasitic relationship between helminths and hosts. *Prog. Allergy.* 17: 93–144.

189. Okafor, G. O., Turner, M. W., and Hay, F. C. 1974. Localization of monocyte binding site of human immunoglobulin G. *Nature (Lond.)* 248: 228–230.

190. Okumura, K., Julius, M. H., Tsu, T., Herzenberg, L. A., and Herzenberg, L. A. 1976. Demonstration that IgG memory is carried by IgG-bearing cells. *Eur. J. Immunol.* 6: 467–472.

191. Oudin, J., and Michel, M. 1963. A new allotype form of rabbit serum γ-globulins, apparently associated with antibody function and specificity. *C.R. Acad. Sci. (Paris)* 257: 805–808.

192. Ovary, Z., Barth, W. F., and Fahey, J. L. 1965. The immunoglobulins of mice. III. Skin-sensitizing activity of mouse immunoglobulins. *J. Immunol.* 94: 410–415.

193. Ovary, Z., Benacerraf, B., and Bloch, K. J. 1963. Properties of guinea pig 7S antibodies. II. Identification of antibodies involved in passive cutaneous and systemic anaphylaxis. *J. Exp. Med.* 117: 951–964.

194. Papamichael, M., Gutierrez, C., Embling, P., Johnson, P., Holborow, E. J., and Pepys, M. B. 1975. Complement dependence of localization of aggregated IgG in germinal centres. *Scand. J. Immunol.* 4: 343–347.

195. Paraskevas, F., Lees, S. T., Orr, K. B., and Israels, L. G. 1972. A receptor for F_c on mouse B-lymphocytes. *J. Immunol.* 108: 1319–1327.

196. Parish, W. E. 1965. Differentiation between cytophilic antibody and opsonin by a macrophage phagocytic system. *Nature (Lond.)* 208: 594–595.

197. Parkhouse, R. M. E., Abney, E. R., Bourgois, A., and Wilcox, H. N. A. 1977. Functional and structural characterization of immunoglobulins on murine B lymphocytes. *Cold Spring Harbor Symp. Quant. Biol.* 41:193–200.

198. Pawlak, L. L., Hart, D. A., and Nisonoff, A. 1973. Requirements for prolonged suppression of an idiotypic specificity in adult mice. *J. Exp. Med.* 137: 1442–1458.

199. Perlmann, P., Biberfeld, P., Larsson, Å., Perlmann, H., and Wåhlin, B. 1975. Surface markers of antibody dependent lymphocytic effector cells (K-cells) in human blood. In *Membrane receptors of lymphocytes.* M. Seligmann, J. L. Preud'homme and F. M. Kourilsky, (eds.), pp. 161–169, North-Holland, Amsterdam.

200. Pernis, B. 1975. The effect of anti-IgD antiserum on antibody production in Rhesus monkeys, in *Membrane Receptors of Lymphocytes.* M. Seligmann, J. L. Preud'homme and M. F. Kourilsky (eds.), pp. 25–26. North-Holland, Amsterdam.

201. Pernis, B., Miller, J. F. A. P., Forni, L., and Sprent, J. 1974. Immunoglobulins on activated T-cells detected by indirect immunofluorescence. *Cell. Immunol.* 10: 476–482.

202. Philips-Quagliata, J. M., Levine, B. B., Quagliata, F., and Uhr, J. W. 1971. Mechanisms underlying binding of immune complexes to macrophages. *J. Exp. Med.* 133: 589–601.

203. Premkumar, E., Potter, M., Singer, P. A., and Sklar, M. D. 1975. Synthesis, surface deposition and secretion of immunoglobulins by Abelson Virus—transformed lymphosarcoma cell lines. *Cell* 6: 149–159.

204. Prouvost-Danon, A., Silva-Lima, M., and Queiroz-Javierre, M. 1966. Active anaphylactic reaction in mouse peritoneal mast cells *in vitro. Life Sci.* 5: 289–297.

205. Putnam, F. W., Florent, G., Paul, C., Shinoda, T., and Shimizu, A. 1973.

Complete amino acid sequence of the mu heavy chain of a human IgM immunoglobulin. *Science.* 182: 287–291.

206. Quie, P. G., Messner, R. P., and Williams, R. C. 1968. Phagocytosis in subacute bacterial endocarditis, localization of the primary opsomic site to Fc fragment. *J. Exp. Med.* 128: 553–570.

207. Rajewsky, K., and Eichmann, K. 1977. Antigen receptors of T helper cells. *Contemp. Topics in Immunobiology.* 7: 69–112.

208. Ramasamy, R., and Munro, A. J. 1974. Surface T- and B-cell markers on murine lymphomas and plasmacytomas. *Immunology* 26: 563–570.

209. Ramasamy, R., Munro, A., and Milstein, C. 1974. Possible role for the Fc receptor on B lymphocytes. *Nature (Lond.)* 249: 573–574.

210. Ramasamy, R., Richardson, N. E., and Feinstein, A. 1976. The specificity of the Fc receptor on murine lymphocytes for immunoglobulins of IgG and IgM classes. *Immunol.* 30: 851–858.

211. Ramasamy, R., Secher, D. S., and Adetugbo, K. 1975. C_H3 domain of IgG as binding site to F_c receptor on mouse lymphocytes. *Nature (Lond.)* 253: 656.

212. Ramseier, H., and Lindenmann, J. 1972. Allotypic antibodies. *Transpl. Rev.* 10: 57–96.

213. Ramshaw, I. A., and Parish, C. R. 1976. Surface properties of cells involved in antibody-dependent cytotoxicity. *Cell. Immunol.* 21: 226–235.

214. Rask, L., Klareskog, L., Östberg, L., and Peterson, P. A. 1975. Isolation and properties of a murine spleen cell F_c receptor. *Nature (Lond.)* 257: 231–233.

215. Ray, A., and Cebra, J. J. 1972. Localization of affinity-labeled residues in the primary structure of anti-dinitrophenyl antibody raised in strain 13 guinea pigs. *Biochem.:* 11: 3647–3657.

216. Rieber, E. P., and Riethmüller, G. 1974. Surface immunoglobulin on thymus cells. II. Release of heterologous anti-Ig-antibodies from thymus cells as an immunogenic complex. *Z. Immun.-Forsch.* 147: 276–290.

217. Revillard, J. P., Samarut, C., Cordier, G., and Brochier, J. 1975. Characterization of human lymphocytes bearing F_c receptors with special reference to cytotoxic (K) cells, *in* M. Seligmann, J. L. Preud'homme and F. M. Kourilsky, (eds.), *Membrane Receptors of Lymphocytes,* pp. 171–184, North-Holland, Amsterdam.

218. Rhodes, J. 1973. Receptor for monomeric IgM on guinea-pig splenic macrophages. *Nature (Lond.)* 243: 527–528.

219. Robbins, J. B., Kenny, K., and Suter, E. 1965. The isolation and biological activities of rabbit γM- and γG- anti-*Salmonella Typhimurium* antibodies. *J. Exp. Med.* 122: 385–402.

220. Roelants, G. E. 1975. Recognition of antigen by T lymphocytes, *in* M. Seligmann, J. L. Preud'homme and F. M. Kourilsky, (eds.), *Membrane Receptors of Lymphocytes,* pp. 65–78. North-Holland, Amsterdam.

221. Rolley, R. T., and Marchalonis, J. J. 1972. Release and assay of antigen-binding immunoglobulin from the surfaces of lymphocytes of unsensitised mice. *Transplant.* 14: 734–741.

222. Rollinghoff, M., Wagner, H., Cone, R. E., and Marchalonis, J. J. 1973. Release of antigen-specific immunoglobulin from cytotoxic effector cells and

syngeneic tumor immunity *in vitro*. *Nature New Biol.* 243: 21–23.

223. Rowe, D. S., Hug, K., Forni, L., and Pernis, B. 1973. Immunoglobulin D as a membrane receptor. *J. Exp. Med.* 138: 965–972.

224. Rowley, D. A., Köhler, H., Schreiber, H., Kaye, S. T., and Lorbach, I. 1976. Suppression by autogenous complementary idiotypes: the priority of the first response. *J. Exp. Med.* 144: 946–959.

225. Rowley, D., and Turner, K. J. 1966. Number of molecules of antibody required to promote phagocytosis of one bacterium. *Nature (Lond.)* 210: 496–498.

226. Santana, V., Wedderburn, N., and Turk, J. L. 1974. Demonstration of immunoglobulin on the surface of thymus lymphocytes. *Immunol.*. 27: 65–73.

227. Schlessinger, J., Steinberg, I. Z., Givol, D., Hochman, J., and Pecht, I. 1975. Antigen-induced conformational changes in antibodies and their Fab fragments studied by circular polarization of fluorescence. *Proc. Natl. Acad. Sci. (USA)* 72: 2775–2779.

228. Schrader, J. W. 1973. Specific activation of the bone marrow derived lymphocyte by antigen presented in a non-multivalent form. *J. Exp. Med.* 137: 844–849.

229. Schrader, J. W. 1973. Mechanism of activation of the bone marrow derived lymphocyte. III. A distinction between a macrophage produced triggering signal and the amplifying effect on triggered B lymphocytes of allogeneic interactions. *J. Exp. Med.* 138: 1464–1480.

230. Segrest, J. P., Jackson, R. L., Andrews, E. P., and Marchesi, V. T. 1971. Human erythrocyte membrane glycoprotein. A revaluation of the molecular weight as determined by S.D.S. polyacrylamide gel electrophoresis. *Biochem. Biophys. Res. Commun.* 44: 390–395.

231. Sell, S. 1967. Studies on rabbit lymphocytes *in vitro*. VII. The induction of blast transformation with the F(ab′)₂ and Fab fragments of sheep antibody to rabbit IgG. *J. Immunol.* 98: 786–791.

232. Sell, S., and Gell, P. G. H. 1965. Studies on rabbit lymphocytes *in vitro*. I. Stimulation of blast transformation with anti-allotype serum. *J. Exp. Med.* 122: 423–439.

233. Sell, S., Rowe, D. S., and Gell, P. G. H. 1965. Studies on rabbit lymphocytes *in vitro*. III. Protein RNA and DNA synthesis by lymphocyte cultures after stimulation with phytohemagglutinin, staphylococcal filtrate, antiallotype serum and heterologous antiserum to rabbit whole serum. *J. Exp. Med.* 122: 823–839.

234. Sell, S., and Sheppard, H. W., Jr. 1973. Rabbit blood lymphocytes may be T cells with surface immunoglobulins. *Science* 182: 586–587.

235. Sheppard, H. W., Jr., and Redelman, D. 1976. Mitogen responses of rabbit T and B cells. *Fed. Proc.* 35: 822 (abstract).

236. Sherr, C. J., Baurs, S., Grundke, I., Zeligs, J., Zeligs, B., and Uhr, J. W. 1972. Cell surface immunoglobulin. III. Isolation and characterization of immunoglobulin from nonsecretory human lymphoid cells. *J. Exp. Med.* 135: 1392–1405.

237. Shevach, E., Herberman, R., Lieberman, R., Frank, M. M., and Green, I. 1972. Receptors for immunoglobulin and complement on mouse leukemias and lymphomas. *J. Immunol.* 108: 325–328.

238. Sinclair, N. R. St.C. 1969. Regulation of the immune response. I. Reduction in ability of specific antibody to inhibit long-lasting IgG immunological priming after removal of the F_c fragment. J. Exp. Med. 129: 1183–1201.

239. Smith, W. I., Ladoulis, C. T., Misra, D. N., Gill, T. J., III, and Bazin, H. 1975. Lymphocyte plasma membranes. III. Composition of lymphocyte plasma membranes of normal and immunized rats. Biochim. Biophys. Acta. 382: 506–525.

240. Soteriades-Vlachos, C., Gyöngyössy, M. I. C., and Playfair, J. H. L. 1974. Rosette formation by mouse lymphocytes. III. Receptors for immunoglobulin on normal and activated T cells. Clin. Exp. Immunol. 18: 187–192.

241. Spiegelberg, H. 1972. γD immunoglobulin. Contemp. Top. Mol. Immunol. 1: 165–180.

242. Spiegelberg, H. L. 1974. Biological activities of immunoglobulins of different classes and subclasses. Adv. Immunol. 19: 259–294.

243. Sprent, J., and Miller, J. F. A. P. 1971. Activation of thymus cells by histocompatibility antigens. Nature New Biol. 234: 195–198.

244. Stechschulte, D. J., Orange, R. P., and Austen, K. F. 1970. Immunochemical and biologic properties of rat IgE. I. Immunochemical identification of rat IgE. J. Immunol. 105: 1082–1086.

245. Stobo, J. D., and Tomasi, T. B. 1967. A low molecular weight immunoglobulin antigenically related to 19S IgM. J. Clin. Invest. 46: 1329–1337.

246. Stocker, J. W., Marchalonis, J. J., and Harris, A. W. 1974. Inhibition of a T-cell dependent immune response in vitro by thymoma cell immunoglobulins. J. Exp. Med. 139: 785–790.

247. Stout, R. D., and Herzenberg, L. A. 1975. The F_c receptor on thymus-derived lymphocytes. I. Detection of a subpopulation of murine T lymphocytes bearing the F_c receptor. J. Exp. Med. 142: 611–621.

248. Strayer, D. S., Vitetta, E. S., and Köhler, H. 1975. Anti-receptor antibody. I. Isolation and characterization of the immunoglobulin receptor for phosphorylcholine. J. Immunol. 114: 722–727.

249. Szenberg, A., Cone, R. E., and Marchalonis, J. J. 1974. Isolation of surface immunoglobulins from lymphocytes of chicken thymus and bursa. Nature (Lond.) 250: 418–420.

250. Taniguchi, M., and Tada, T. 1974. Regulation of homocytotropic antibody formation in the rat. X. IgT-like molecule for the induction of homocytotropic antibody response. J. Immunol. 113: 1757–1769.

251. Tizard, I. R. 1969. Macrophage cytophilic antibody in mice. Differentiation between antigen adherence due to these antibodies and opsonic adherence. Int. Arch. Allergy. Appl. Immunol. 36: 332–346.

252. Uhr, J. W., and Möller, G. 1968. Regulatory effect of antibody on the immune response. Adv. Immunol. 8: 81–127.

253. Utsumi, S. 1969. Stepwise cleavage of rabbit immunoglobulin G by papain and isolation of four types of biologically active Fc fragments. Biochem. J. 112: 343–355.

254. Vaerman, J. P., Lebacq-Verheyden, A. M., and Heremans, J. F. 1974. Absence of disulfide bridges between heavy and light chains in IgA from chicken bile. Immunol. Commun. 3: 239–247.

255. Vitetta, E. S., Forman, J., and Kettman, J. R. 1976. Cell surface immunoglobulin. XVIII. Functional differences of B lymphocytes bearing different immunoglobulin isotypes. *J. Exp. Med.* 143: 1055–1066.

256. Vitetta, E. S., Melcher, U., McWilliams, M., Lamm, M., Philips-Quagliata, J. M., and Uhr, J. W. 1975. Cell-surface immunoglobulins. XI. The appearance of an IgD-like molecule on murine lymphoid cells during ontogeny. *J. Exp. Med.* 141: 206–215.

257. Vitetta, E. S., and Uhr, J. W. 1973. Synthesis, transport, dynamics and fate of cell surface Ig and alloantigens in murine lymphocytes. *Transplant. Rev.* 14: 50–57.

258. Vitetta, E. S., and Uhr, J. W. 1975. Immunoglobulin receptors revisited. *Science* 189: 964–969.

259. Wagner, H., and Feldmann, M. 1972. Cell mediated immune system *in vitro*. I. A new *in vitro* system for the generation of cell-mediated cytotoxic activity. *Cell. Immunol.* 3: 405–420.

260. Walker, W. S. 1976. Separate Fc-receptors for immunoglobulins IgG2a and IgG2b on an established cell line of mouse macrophages. *J. Immunol.* 116: 911–914.

261. Wang, A.-C., and Fudenberg, H. H. 1974. IgA and Evolution of Immunoglobulins. *J. Immunogen.* 1: 3–31.

262. Warner, N. L. 1974. Membrane immunoglobulins and antigen receptors on B and T lymphocytes. *Adv. Immunol.* 19: 67–216.

263. Warner, N. L., Goding, J. W., Gutman, G. A., Warr, G. W., Herzenberg, L. A., Black, S. J., Van Der Loo, W., and Loken, M. R. 1977. Allotypes of mouse IgM immunoglobulin. *Nature* 265: 447–449.

264. Warner, N. L., Harris, A. W., and Gutman, G. A. 1975. Membrane immunoglobulin and Fc receptors of murine T and B cell lymphomas, in M. Seligmann, J. L. Preud'homme, and F. M. Kourilsky (eds.), *Membrane Receptors of Lymphocytes*, pp. 203–216. North-Holland, Amsterdam.

265. Warner, N. L., and Marchalonis, J. J. 1972. Structural differences in mouse IgA myeloma proteins of different allotypes. *J. Immunol.* 109: 657–661.

266. Warr, G. W., DeLuca, D., and Marchalonis, J. J. 1976. Phylogenetic origins of immune recognition: lymphocyte surface immunoglobulins in the goldfish. *Carassius auratus. Proc. Natl. Acad. Sci. (USA)* 73: 2476–2480.

267. Warr, G. W., and Marchalonis, J. J. 1976. Heavy chains of murine splenocyte membrane immunoglobulins: a comparison with the heavy chains of human and toad serum immunoglobulins. *J. Immunogen.* 3: 221–227.

268. Warr, G. W., and Marchalonis, J. J. 1977. Lymphocyte surface immunoglobulins: Detection, characterization and occurrence in diseases of the lymphoid system. *C.R.C. Crit. Rev. Clin. Lab. Sci.* 7: 185–226.

269. Wason, W. M., and Fitch, F. W. 1973. Suppression of the antibody response to SRBC with F(ab')₂ and IgG in vitro. *J. Immunol.* 110: 1427–1429.

270. Watson, D. L. 1976. The effect of cytophilic IgG2 on phagocytosis by ovine polymorphonuclear leucocytes. *Immunol.* 31: 159–165.

271. Webb, S. R., and Cooper, M. D. 1973. T cells can bind antigen via cytophilic IgM antibody made by B cells. *J. Immunol.* 111: 275–277.

272. Weber, W. T. 1975. Avian B lymphocyte subpopulations: origins and functional capacities. *Transpl. Rev.* 24: 113–158.

273. Weber, W. T. 1976. Induction of T cell proliferation following sequential exposure to anti-T cell and anti-immunoglobulin serum. *Fed. Proc.* 35: 819 (abstract).

274. Whiteside, T. L., and Rabin, B. S. 1976. Surface immunoglobulin on activated human peripheral blood thymus-derived cells. *J. Clin. Invest.* 57: 762–771.

275. Wilson, I. D. 1972. Studies on the opsonic activity of human secretory IgA using an *in vitro* phagocytosis system. *J. Immunol.* 108: 726–730.

276. Winchester, R. J., Fu, S. M., Wernet, P., Kunkel, H. G., Dupont, B., and Jersild, C. 1975. Recognition by pregnancy serums of non-HL-A alloantigens selectively expressed on B lymphocytes. *J. Exp. Med.* 141: 924–929.

277. Wisløff, F., Michaelsen, T. E., and Froland, S. S. 1974. Inhibition of antibody-dependent human lymphocyte mediated cytotoxicity by immunoglobulin classes, IgG subclasses, and IgG fragments. *Scand. J. Immunol.* 3: 29–38.

278. Yasmeen, D., Ellerson, J. R., Dorrington, K. J., and Painter, R. H. 1973. Evidence for the domain hypothesis: Location of the site of cytophilic activity toward guinea pig macrophages in the C_H3 homology region of human immunoglobulin G. *J. Immunol.* 110: 1706–1709.

279. Yoshida, T. O., and Andersson, B. 1972. Evidence for a receptor recognizing antigen complexed immunoglobulin on the surface of activated mouse thymus lymphocytes. *Scand. J. Immunol.* 1: 401–408.

280. Zucker-Franklin, D. 1974. Eosinophil function and disorders. *Adv. Intern. Med.* 19: 1–25.

281. Zvaifler, N. J., and Robinson, J. O. 1969. Rabbit homocytotropic antibody. A unique immunoglobulin analogous to human IgE. *J. Exp. Med.* 130: 907–929.

282. Szenberg, A., Marchalonis, J. J., and Warner, N. L. 1977. Direct demonstration of marine thymus-dependent all surface endogenous immunoglobulin. *Proc. Natl. Acad. Sci.* (U.S.A.) 74: 2113–2117.

283. Ruddick, J. H., and Leslie, G. A. 1977. Structure and biologic functions of human IgD. XI. Identification and ontogeny of rat lymphocyte immunoglobulin having antigenic cross-reactivity with IgD. *J. Immunol.* 118: 1025–1031.

284. Scott, D. W., Layton, J. E., and Nossal, G. J. V. 1977. Role of IgD in the immune response I. Anti-δ pretreatment facilitates tolerance induction in adult B cells in vitro. *J. Exp. Med.* 146: 1473–1483.

CHAPTER 8

IMMUNITY AND METASTASIS

L. Weiss and D. Glaves

Department of Experimental Pathology
Roswell Park Memorial Institute
Buffalo, New York 14263

Immune responses may facilitate the initial step in metastasis. In cancer patients, although there is little general evidence for cytotoxic antibodies that destroy circulating cancer cells, there is substantial evidence for the presence of cytophilic, "blocking" factors which may protect them from hemodynamic trauma. In sensitized animals, the arrest pattern of circulating cancer cells is changed by immunospecific factors. The immune defense system may influence the overlapping steps of the metastatic cascade, but this influence may not be to the benefit of the patient.

Introduction

Of those patients dying with solid tumors, large numbers will succumb to metastases as distinct from their primary lesion. The metastatic process is extremely complex (62) and is therefore usually compartmentalized for purposes of study. However, although we can describe the process in sequential "steps," it should be emphasized that they are continuous rather than discrete, and that the whole process is additionally complicated by the metastasis of metastases (7, 34).

In man, some 270 different histologic types of cancer are recognized, which cover a whole spectrum of metastatic behavior; there is also considerable variation between patients with histologically similar tumors. Therefore, our following comments, which are of necessity based largely on in vitro and in vivo experiments with comparatively few types of animal tumors, must be considered speculative and are given only as tentative suggestions of feasible mechanisms of interactions between the host defense systems and cancer as they affect metastasis, rather than as dogmatic generalizations.

A number of the interactions of metastases or potential metastases with the host defense system are not unique, but appear similar to corresponding interactions involving primary cancers. The reader is referred to other sections of this volume for details of the latter, more general interactions, and use these as a base for evaluation of not only the importance of "immunity" in human cancer, but also whether "defense system" is a more appropriate term than "immune system."

THE METASTATIC CASCADE

The low overall efficiency of the metastatic cascade may be gauged in a quasi-quantitative manner from many observations indicating that in experimental animals, tens of thousands of cancer cells from solid tumors must be injected intravenously, to produce relatively few hematogenous "metastases" (26). It is difficult to arrive at assessments of the efficiency of the metastatic process in man where clinical measurements of tumor size and growth-rate do not usually permit discrimination between loss of tumor by liberation of live cancer cells and loss by cell death (52), and where detection and enumeration of subclinical "micrometastases" is not feasible. However, in spite of the lack of numeric data, the general feeling is that the establishment of metastases is statistically an uncommon or even rare event in the natural history of individual tumors, and that each viable secondary deposit is the monument to very many unsuccessful attempts. The fact that metastases are present in the majority of patients with cancer after the elapse of time (68), may simply indicate the cumulative results of many cancer cells continuously entering each step of the metastatic process. In this connection, Butler and Gullino's (9) work on the liberation of adonocarcinoma cells from solid cancers in experimental animals may be highly relevant, and shows release of more than 10^6 cells per gram of solid cancer per 24 hours. The viable parts of a solid tumor may contain between 10^8 to 10^9 cells per cm^3.

The precariousness of the metastatic process, in that the "success" of any one step depends on the comparatively few survivors from the preceeding one, emphasizes that studies of individual steps may not have prognostic value in determining whether metastases will occur or not *in vivo*. However, this interdependence of the progressive steps suggests that therapy aimed at interrupting any one step in the metastatic cascade may be beneficial to the patient.

With these various limitations in mind, we propose to discuss the progressive parts of the metastatic cascade in a stepwise manner.

The Primary Tumor

Solid cancers are heterogeneous populations of malignant and non-malignant cells which are in a highly dynamic state with respect to each other and their host environment. Different parts of the same tumor are often histologically distinct, and exhibit a whole spectrum of activities associated with cell proliferation on the one hand, to cell death on the other.

It is important to appreciate that at different stages in the natural history of a primary cancer, not only may the cancer cell population undergo changes but so may the host and these changes may well reflect in metastatic phenomena. Greene (25) studied the heterotransplantation of human tumor fragments into the anterior chamber of the guinea pig eye, and obtained a general correlation between transplantability and clinical deterioration associated with overt metastasis. Foulds (20) has also postulated progressive changes manifest in different facets of tumor cell behavior with time, which he regards as occurring in irreversible steps towards increased malignancy and associated metastasis.

Thus, regardless of detailed mechanisms, the concept has been advanced that selection for metastasis-associated and other changes can occur in an evolving tumor cell population. Evidence supportive of metastatic variants comes from the work of Yamada et al (69) showing that in a variety of human tumors, the karyotype of metastatic cells differed in general from that of their primary cancer.

Other work relating to the selection within cancer cell lines for metastatic variants comes from Fidler's (16) studies on the B16 melanoma in mice. Pulmonary tumor nodules growing in mice which had received intravenous injections of B16 cells were excised, maintained in vitro and reinjected into fresh animals. On repeating this process, the numbers of lung tumors developing after I. V. injections increased. This was associated with a higher retention of tumor cells in the lungs. These selected lines of cells were stable with respect to their arrest patterns after repeated subculture. Nicolson et al. (43), by use of similar techniques, have also selected variants of B16 populations showing specific organ arrest patterns. Specificity in organ arrest is not evident in karyotypic studies on human material, as Sandberg et al. (48) report no difference in the karyotype of metastases in different organs.

The possibility of metastatic sublines of cancer cells developing during the course of disease, focusses attention on appropriate selection mechanisms. On the basis of work on mouse tumors, immunoselection as evidenced by karyotypic change, is known to be associated with change in virulence (28). However, evidence for immunoselection in the human situation is lacking, and it must be borne in mind that other selective pressures not primarily based on immunologic mechanisms undoubtedly exist. In addition, it is important not to confuse selection resulting in change of immunologic expression, with selection caused by it.

CELL RELEASE AND MOVEMENT

By means of growth, and/or active locomotory and/or passive movements, cancer cells invade "solid" tissues, blood or lymphatic channels, and disseminate to other regions of the same organ and/or other organs. Loss of contiguity is by definition an essential part of metastasis, and therefore the detachment of cancer cells individually or en masse, is an essential component of the metastatic cascade (60).

The mode of cell detachment from a primary cancer may be complex (58), and its timing in relation to the whole metastatic process may be variable. Thus, detachment may occur as a preliminary to active infiltration or, alternatively, by expansive processes a solid cancer may invade blood-vessels prior to cell detachment, and cancer cells may separate from the main tumor mass in response to blood-flow, tissue movements, or surgical handling etc.

The pioneering work of Coman (14) and his colleagues was interpreted to indicate that inherent defects in cancer cell membranes made them less adherent to each other than was the case for normal cells, and that this was the key to the whole metastatic process. However, in common with so many other behavioral characteristics of cancer cells which are dependent on their peripheral properties, cell detachment is not a specific cancer-dependent property but rather reflects a general cellular response to processes associated with growth, damage and/or degeneration (60, 61). Various enzymes, among many other factors, promote cell detachment.

An important area of interaction between the immune system and cell detachment is through the agency of lysosomal activation. It has been shown in vitro that in the presence of complement, antisera induce the activation of lysosomes with the consequent enzyme activity in the pericellular region, which both degrades intercellular matrix (15) and promotes cell detachment (57).

The facilitated release of cells from solid mammary carcinomas of the mouse was also shown to be increased following exposure to either extrinsic lysosomal hydrolases or to excess vitamin A which is a lysosomal labilizer (65). The release of lysosomal enzymes from cells, which modify their own peripheral properties without killing them was termed "sublethal autolysis" (57). Interaction of sensitized lymphocytes with target cells and subsequent target cell lysis is accompanied by release of intracellular contents, thus exposing surviving cells to lysosomal components. In addition to direct interactions between the immune system and malignant cells facilitating the release of the latter, it should also be appreciated that lymphokines produced upon interaction of sensitized lymphocytes and antigen are capable of inducing lysosomal release from macrophages (44) which are frequently found in neoplastic tissues.

Malignant cell release from tumors could also result indirectly from interaction of immune complexes with non-malignant macrophages and leukocytes in or near tumors, leading to release of lysosome contents (10, 66).

Immune complexes in the form of soluble tumor antigen in combination with antibody have been detected in the circulation of experimental animals (2, 6, 54) and there is suggestive evidence for their occurrence in cancer patients (50). It would appear, therefore, that the immune response elicited to defend the host may actually facilitate the detachment of tumor cells by initiating the production of "extrinsic" enzymes potentially capable of acting upon the tumor cells which survive immunologic attack.

Another mode of expression of effects of "immune" factors on cell detachment is in connection with active cell movement which may occur in infiltration of normal tissues by cancer cells, or in the infiltration of cancers by non-malignant cells such as macrophages.

In order for a cell to actively move through tissues it must first adhere to the tissue in question to obtain a hand- or foothold against which it can "push" or "pull"; it must also generate locomotor energy to provide the "push" or "pull." Finally, as cells are not infinitely extensible, the actively moving cell must break regions of adhesion with the tissues in order to continue progressive movements.

It therefore follows that factors inhibiting cell detachment are also expected to inhibit cell movement. Weiss and Glaves (63) have attempted to define and quantitate the detachment-dependent arm of locomotion in macrophages with respect to mediators of the immune response. Supernatants from antigen-stimulated spleen cells, derived from mice injected with BCG, specifically inhibited both the migration of normal mouse peritoneal macrophages, and their detachment from protein-coated glass surfaces. Both macrophage migration- and detachment-inhibitory activities were thermostable, but were abrogated by neuraminidase- and chymotrypsin-treatment, indicating that migration and detachment are causally related, and that at least one mediator of the immune response, migration inhibitory factor (MIF), affects both parameters of cell behavior. These experiments yield no information on the effects of MIF on either macrophage adhesion or locomotor forces which are also expected to partially regulate locomotion.

Arrest

The next part of the metastatic cascade is concerned with the arrest of free or circulating cancer cells. Unless such circulating cells are arrested within a short period of time, they perish; this is partly due to haemodynamic damage related to the resistance of the cells to deform when passing through small blood-vessels (49) and partly to various cytotoxic humoral factors, including antitumor antibodies (8, 19, 42), lymphocyte-dependent antitumor antibody (1, 27) and peripheral blood lymphocytes (29, 31). In contrast, circulating tumor cells may be protected from direct immune cytotoxic attack by other factors associated with immune responses to tumors, including "blocking factors." In vitro studies have shown that blocking factors in the form of soluble tumor antigen shed by cancer cells, alone or in combination with antibody, are capable of binding to the receptors of sensitized lymphocytes and also tumor cell surfaces when antibody is present. These factors do not induce a cytotoxic effect but prevent subsequent lymphocyte recognition and destruction of target cells (6, 29, 54).

The presence of blocking factors could potentially increase the numbers of tumor cells which survive in the circulation to be subsequently arrested at sites distant from the primary tumor.

All mammalian cells so far examined carry a net negative charge at their surfaces, thus circulating cancer cells are expected to be electrostatically repelled from any by the vascular endothelium (59). Boundary "layers," which are inherently due to plasma viscosity, consist of relatively immobile plasma near to vessel walls, and are also a major factor in provonting circulating cancer cells from making contact with the vascular endothelium (23). The magnitude of the combined hemodynamic and electrostatic forces makes direct collisions between tumor emboli and the vessel walls infrequent events, and plays an important part in directing arrest to the smaller blood vessels. It is emphasized that only a small proportion of cells initially arrested in a vascular bed remain there and, that of those remaining, only a small proportion give rise to metastases (17). Thus, direct correlation between the numbers of cells arrested in organs with the amount of metastatic growth developing subsequently may be technically difficult or impossible, particularly if population selection manifest in arrest occurs. For these reasons, it is extremely difficult to comment on the specific immunodependent mechanisms involved in observations of the type reported by Wexler (67), in which differences in the occurrence of tumors were noted following the injection of cancer cells into sensitized or nonsensitized animals.

The organ-arrest pattern of potential metastasis-forming cells has been traditionally followed in experimental animals by injecting them with radiolabeled cells and then making organ-counts. Previous work by others have usually involved the injection of such cells into non-tumor-bearing animals. These experiments are in many respects an unrealistic model of the clinical situation, where circulating cancer cells arise in tumor-bearing patients in whom immune status and other tumor-associated factors must be considered. We have therefore been investigating (64, 22) the early arrest patterns of tumor cells injected into the systemic circulation of mice, in normal, tumor-bearing and tumor sensitized animals. In the case of the two syngeneic tumor-host systems examined by us, a 3-methycholanthrene-induced fibrosarcoma and the estradiol-induced Gardner lymphosarcoma, differences in the initial distribution of ^{125}IUdR-labeled cells were observed in sensitized animals as shown in Tables 1 and 2.

Inflammatory reactions of various types are often associated with the conditions giving rise to immune responses, and it is thus often difficult to discriminate between the two. We have therefore made experiments to determine the specificity of the altered arrest patterns.

Mice bearing, and sensitized to, the 3-methylcholanthrene-induced

Table 1 In vivo localization of ^{125}IUdR-labeled fibrosarcoma cells (% Total Activity Recovered [+ SE].)

Recipient	Blood	Lymph[a] nodes	Spleen	Kidney	Liver	Lung
Ascites bearer	0.79 (± 0.18)[b]	0.18 (± 0.05)[b]	0.40 (± 0.09)	0.51 (± 0.10)	8.03 (± 1.05)[b]	88.97 (± 3.35)
Normal	0.16 (± 0.07)	0.05 (± 0.03)	0.13 (± 0.06)	0.23 (± 0.03)	1.71 (± 0.13)	100.11 (± 2.18)
Subcutaneous tumor bearer	0.60 (± 0.06)	0.36 (± 0.03)	1.23 (± 0.11)[b]	1.00 (± 0.12)[b]	15.90 (± 1.57)[b]	53.46 (± 3.62)[b]
Normal	0.35 (± 0.08)	0.21 (± 0.02)	0.35 (± 0.05)	0.29 (± 0.03)	2.22 (± 0.28)	90.55 (± 2.33)
Hyperimmunized	0.39 (±0.13)[b]	0.16 (± 0.07)	1.26 (± 0.32)	0.76 (± 0.21)[b]	14.59 (± 1.99)	69.07 (± 9.84)[b]
Normal	0.05 (± 0.03)	0.14 (± 0.08)	0.24 (± 0.12)	0.30 (± 0.09)	2.48 (± 0.36)	105.09 (± 3.13)

a. Cervical, axial, and mesenteric.
b. $P < 0.05$.

Table 2 In vivo localization of ^{125}IUdR-labeled lymphosarcoma cells. (% Total Activity Recovered [± SE]).

Recipient	Blood	Lymph nodes[a]	Spleen	Kidney	Liver	Lung
Ascites bearer	0.40 (± 0.08)	0.20 (± 0.06)	3.06 (± 0.45)	2.19 (± 0.45)	19.36 (± 2.14)	27.63 (± 2.4)
Normal	0.68 (± 0.07)	0.25 (± 0.04)	3.25 (± 0.46)	2.68 (± 0.44)	14.31 (± 1.55)	24.88 (± 3.02)
Subcutaenous tumor bearer	1.40 (± 0.20)[b]	0.55 (± 0.06)	4.23 (± 0.51)	1.93 (± 0.21)	20.45 (± 1.55)	27.80 (± 1.98)
Normal	2.02 (± 0.22)	0.76 (± 0.12)	2.78 (± 0.20)	1.58 (± 0.10)	22.30 (± 1.95)	19.22 (± 3.37)
Hyperimmunized	0.48 (± 0.04)[b]	0.27 (± 0.04)[b]	2.14 (± 0.19)	1.19 (± 0.07)[b]	17.82 (± 1.07)[b]	48.07 (± 4.37)[b]
Normal	0.84 (± 0.07)	0.47 (± 0.04)	3.03 (± 0.28)	1.69 (± 0.23)	20.39 (± 0.77)	32.86 (± 2.33)

a. Cervical, axial and mesenteric.
b. $P < 0.05$.

fibrosarcoma were injected with radiolabelled Gardner lymphosarcoma cells and vice versa. Analysis of the arrest patterns showed that sensitization to one tumor did not influence the distribution pattern of the unrelated tumor subsequently injected. These results indicate that pharmacological factors which potentially play a role in tumor cell arrest are different from those associated with the tumor-specific immune response.

Although the change in initial arrest patterns in the cases examined by us appear to be associated with specific immunity, the actual mechanisms of arrest are not known at present. It may be relevant in this respect to consider the role of clotting mechanisms in tumor cell arrest, particularly since many patients with cancer exhibit altered blood coagulation (41, 47). In the present context, it is of considerable interest that immunologic factors do interact with platelets, particularly through the agency of antibody/antigen complexes (36, 45), and other compartments of the thrombogenic system (5, 13, 30, 35). As previously mentioned, circulating complexes of tumor antigen and antibody do occur, and binding of non-lytic antibody to antigenic sites on liberated tumor cells could also elicit thrombogenic reactions.

It is a common observation that arrested tumor emboli are commonly associated with fibrin-containing thrombus and platelets; the ultrastructure of such associations has been carefully documented by Warren (55). Thus, the role of thrombogenic interactions in *initiating* tumor cell arrest has been stressed, and attempts have been made to prevent such arrest by treating patients with anticoagulants, without striking success (61). A different time relationship has been stressed by others, including Chew *et al.* (12), who shift the main tumor cell/platelet interactions to the period following cell arrest. Either, or both, time relationships may be appropriate for different types of cancer, since in general, carcinomas are often associated with thrombogenesis (e.g., thrombophlebitis migrans, particularly with pancreatic adenocarcinomas), whereas sarcomas are not, and may indeed even be associated with fibrinolysis.

In an unusually extensive study of platelet-tumor cell interactions in mice, Gasic *et al.* (21) observed that in a number of cases, thrombocytopenia reduced the number of metastases produced by a variety of tumors. In addition, some tumors aggregated platelets *in vitro* and produced a thrombocytopenia *in vivo* which was associated with platelet accumulation in the lungs. It was demonstrated that tumors with *in vitro* platelet-aggregating activity usually gave rise to lung metastases, while those not possessing these activities tended to produce more widespread metastases, although no immunologic factors were implicated.

Among other products released from platelets by antigen/antibody complexes are histamine and 5-hydroxytryptamine. The former, which is predominant in mast cells, is also released by the action of basic polypeptides and proteins including protamine, polylysine, histones and lysosomal proteins which are themselves expressions of cell damage. Histamine produces local dilation of capillaries, terminal arterioles and venules, which tends to slow down the microcirculation, and is coupled with increased permeability in the post-capillary venules due to endothelial cell contraction, might well promote both the arrest of cancer emboli and the escape of cells from them. These effects are not expected to be confined to the regions of vessels involved but may be widespread due to local axon reflex mechanisms. In man, 10% of the 5-hydroxytryptamine is found in platelets, and on release it acts directly on the smooth muscle of the vasculature-producing vasoconstriction (24). Therefore circulating antigen/antibody complexes, acting through platelets, mast and other cells by causing the release of vasoactive materials could conceivably alter patterns of cell arrest in metastasis.

The interactions between the immune and clotting systems may also affect other aspects of metastasis. Thus, among other factors, immune responses resulting in tissue damage can lead to released thromboplastic activity; such activity is not unique to cancer cells but is also exhibited by damaged non-malignant cells (33). In addition to catalyzing the conversion of fibrinogen to fibrin, the thrombin generated by tissue thromboplastins, together with activators from both malignant and normal cells converts plasminogen to plasmin. Thrombin and plasmin, by virtue of their proteolytic activities can induce sublethal autolysis in the region of the tumor cell periphery which, as discussed earlier, may well result in the increased liberation of cells from the primary tumor.

The Extravasation of Cancer Cells

There are basically two mechanisms by which arrested tumor cells can escape from blood vessels. The first is by active migration, in a manner similar to the egress of leukocytes which push through the potential spaces between the endothelial cells (37). In some vessels, histamine or agents associated with inflammatory change, may widen these spaces, and Gasic et al. (21) have speculated that materials released from platelets, directly and/or indirectly increase cancer cell locomotory movements and create gaps in the vascular endothelium through which they can crawl

The second mode of egress of arrested emboli is by destruction of the surrounding blood-vessel; first the endothelium and then the basement membrane. Cell processes invade the surrounding tissues through the gaps created in the basement membrane. As cell multiplication is continuous throughout this process, it is difficult to assess the relative importance of tumor invasion by expansive growth and invasion by active movements. The egress of tumor cells by destructive processes is well-documented and reviewed by Chew et al. (12), who present a good case for this mode of escape in many solid tumors.

Having escaped from blood vessels, or from lymphatic channels, the cancer cells are faced with the problem of establishing themselves in their new environment. An important factor is the establishment of an adequate blood-supply, since Thomlinson and Gray (53), among others, have calculated that in solid tumors, oxygen will only diffuse out approximately 150 μm from capillaries, and at distances exceeding this, tumor necrosis is observed. Electron microscopic observations of melanomas by Warren and Shubik (56) indicated that the tumors stimulated vascular endothelial proliferation in the nonmalignant adjacent tissues, and resulted in neovascularization of the tumor. Angiogenic factors have been isolated from tumors (18), and have prompted the suggestion that interference with their activity could form the basis of therapy. If the factor has antigenic specificity, immunotherapy is a possibility. Other host defense mechanisms may interfere with tumor blood flow, and Cater et al. (11) have shown that mediators of the inflammatory response, such as 5-hydroxytryptamine, act in this manner and reduce oxygen tension.

From the immunologic viewpoint, the further development of metastases is subject to the same general considerations as a primary tumor, and represents an increase in tumor load for the patient. However, there is some suggestion that metastases may exhibit different sensitivity to the host defense system than the primary tumor.

Potential differences between cell populations of primary and secondary cancers were referred to earlier with reference to arrest patterns, and these cellular variations together with site differences are reflected in variations in susceptibility to environmental factors. Thus, Slack and Bross' (51) analyses of the response to chemotherapy of primary and secondary cancers revealed marked differences between metastases in various anatomic sites, compared with statistically nonsignificant variations in response of primary lesions at different sites. It is possible that in an analogous manner, a metastatic lesion developed from a selected population, particularly by a process of immunoselection, could exhibit different interactions with the various humoral and cellular arms of the immune system, to the benefit or detriment of the host.

Immunotherapy of Metastasis

It is clear from examination of this volume that the role of immunity in human cancer is ill-defined, and its role in metastasis is largely speculative. Against this uncertain background, it is difficult to comment on the immunotherapy of metastasis; however two examples may help to clarify the situation, namely: use of the agents BCG and dinitrochloroben- zene (DNCB).

BCG may be administered systemically to patients, when it evokes a generalized, non-specific stimulation of the reticuloendothelial system. It may be injected directly into an accessible tumor, where it produces a local delayed hypersensitivity response to the BCG which may result in the partial or complete destruction of the tumor and immediate lymph nodes. BCG has been injected into either accessible tumor nodules to- gether with previously removed tumor, in the hope that it will act as an adjuvant, and produces heightened tumor-specific immunity-causing tumor destruction. This would indeed be the generalized type of im- munotherapy which is needed to combat widespread, non-accessible or unrecognized metastases, and has been the goal of very many im- munotherapists (40). However, recent work (4) on mice bearing a leukemia has shown that doses of BCG and tumor cells which produced local suppression of tumor growth did not induce detectable tumor im- munity, and doses inducing tumor immunity were relatively ineffectual in suppressing tumor growth. Several studies (3, 39, 46) also show that, in experimental animal tumor systems, the dose, route and timing of BCG administration, together with tumor load, are critical, and the balance between effective therapy and no effect, or even tumor growth potentia- tion, is extremely delicate.

DNCB has proved dramatically successful in the treatment of cutane- ous primary and secondary tumors. Some days after application of DNCB to the patient's skin, it is applied in very low dosage directly over the tumor(s), where a delayed hypersensitivity reaction occurs. Thymus- derived lymphocytes react with the DNCB (or a DNCB complex) locally, producing lymphokines which attract and activate macrophages, which in turn attack and destroy the tumor cells (32). Thus, as with BCG, this is not generalized immunotherapy, and tumors not accessible to the direct application of DNCB cannot be treated in this manner.

At present, with the possible exception of scattered case reports (38), there is little direct evidence that any other administered antigenic mate- rial has ever produced a generalized (adjuvant) immunotherapeutic effect in man. In assessing the therapeutic value of local destruction of accessi- ble tumors by delayed hypersensitivity, one has to compare this type of local therapy with local excision, X-irradiation, chemotherapy, etc. which are also highly successful. In the case of multiple primary lesions of the skin, hypersensitivity-therapy is often preferable. In the case of multiple metastases in the skin, where wide-spread dissemination to other organs is a near certainty, any form of local therapy will simply be palliative.

Apparently immunologic defense mechanisms, alone or in concert with immunologically initiated secondary defense mechanisms, potentially participate in many phases of the metastatic cascade. It would seem ironic that factors elicited to eradicate cancer cells could also play a role in facilitating metastasis; by increasing release of cells from primary tumors, by "protecting" circulating cells, by involvement in tumor cell arrest and finally by interacting to abrogate effective control of metastatic deposits.

REFERENCES

1. Avis, F., Avis, I., Hindsley, J. P., and Haughton, G. 1976. Interactions of cancer cells with antibodies and other humoral factors, in L. Weiss (ed.), *Fundamental Aspects of Metastasis*, pp. 191–204. North-Holland, Amsterdam.

2. Baldwin, R. W., Bowen, J. G., and Price, M. R. 1973. Detection of circulating hepatoma D23 antigen and immune complexes in tumour bearer serum. *Brit. J. Cancer* 28: 16–24.

3. Bansal, S. C., and Sjogren, H. O. 1973. Effects of BCG on various facets of the immune response against polyoma tumors in rats. *Int. J. Cancer* 11: 162–171.

4. Bartlett, G. L., Purnell, D. M., and Kreider, J. W. 1976. BCG inhibition of murine leukemia: local suppression and systemic tumor immunity require different doses. *Science* 191: 299–300.

5. Beneviste, J., Henson, P. M., and Cochrane, C. G. 1972. Leukocyte-dependent histamine release from rabbit platelets. *J. Exp. Med.* 136: 1356–1377.

6. Bowen, J. G., Robins, R. A., and Baldwin, R. W. 1975. Serum factors modifying cell mediated immunity to rat hepatoma D23 correlated with tumor growth. *Int. J. Cancer* 15: 640–650.

7. Bross, I. D. J., and Blumenson, L. E. 1976. Metastatic sites that produced generalized cancer: Identification and kinetics of generalizing sites, in L. Weiss (ed.), *Fundamental Aspects of Metastasis*, pp. 359–375. North-Holland, Amsterdam.

8. Bubenik, J., Perlmann, P., Helmstein, K., and Moberger, G. 1970. Cellular and humoral responses to human urinary bladder carcinomas. *Int. J. Cancer* 5: 310–319.

9. Butler, T. P., and Gullino, P. M. 1975. Quantitation of cell shedding into efferent blood of mammary adenocarcinoma. *Cancer Res.* 35: 512–516.

10. Cardella, C. J., Davies, P., and Allison, A. C. 1974. Immune complexes induce selective release of lysosomal hydrolases from macrophages. *Nature* 247: 46–48.

11. Cater, D. B., Adair, H. M., and Grove, C. A. 1966. Effects of vasomotor drugs and "Mediators" of the inflammatory reaction upon the oxygen tension of tumours and tumour blood-flow. *Brit. J. Cancer* 20: 504–516.

12. Chew, E. C., Josephson, R. L., and Wallace, A. C. 1976. Morphologic aspects of the arrest of circulating cancer cells, in L. Weiss (ed.), *Fundamental Aspects of Metastasis*, pp. 121–150. North-Holland, Amsterdam.

13. Colvin, R. B., Johnson, R. A., Mihm, M. C., and Dvorak, H. F. 1973. Role of the clotting system in cell-mediated hypersensitivity. *J. Exp. Med.* 138: 686–698.

14. Coman, D. R. 1953. Mechanisms responsible for the origin and distribution of blood-borne tumor metastases. *Cancer Res.* 13: 397–404.

15. Fell, H. B., and Weiss, L. 1965. The effect of antiserum, alone and with hydrocortisone, on foetal mouse bones in culture. *J. Exp. Med.* 121: 551–560.

16. Fidler, I. J. 1975. Biological behavior of malignant melanoma cells correlated to their survival *in vivo*. *Cancer Res.* 35: 218–224.

17. Fidler, I. J. 1976. Patterns of tumor cell arrest and development, in L. Weiss (ed.), *Fundamental Aspects of Metastasis*, pp. 275–290. North-Holland, Amsterdam.

18. Folkman, J., Merler, E., Abernathy, C., and Williams, G. 1970. Isolation of a tumor factor responsible for angiogenesis. *J. Exp. Med.* 133: 275–288.

19. Fossati, G., Colnaghi, M. I., Della Porta, G., Balnarzi, G. P., and Veronesi, U. 1971. Cellular immunity to human malignant melanoma. *Int. J. Cancer* 8: 344–350.

20. Foulds, L. 1969. *Neoplastic Development*. Academic Press, London.

21. Gasic, G. J., Gasic, T. B., Galanti, N., Johnson, T., and Murphy, S. 1973. Platelet-tumor cell interactions in mice. The role of platelets in the spread of malignant disease. *Int. J. Cancer* 11: 704–718.

22. Glaves, D., and Weiss, L. 1976. Initial arrest patterns of circulating cancer cells: effects of host sensitization and anticoagulation, in L. Weiss (ed.), *Fundamental Aspects of Metastasis*, pp. 263–273. North-Holland, Amsterdam.

23. Goldsmith, H. L. 1976. Collision of circulating cells with the vascular endothelium, in L. Weiss (ed.), *Fundamental Aspects of Metastasis*, pp. 99–120. North-Holland, Amsterdam.

24. Goodman, L. S., and Gilman, A. 1973. *The Pharmacological Basis of Therapeutics*, 5th ed., MacMillan, New York.

25. Greene, H. S. N. 1952. The significance of the heterologous transplantability of human cancer. *Cancer* 5: 24–44.

26. Griffiths, J. D., and Salsbury, A. J. 1965. *Circulating Cancer Cells*, p. 109 et seq. C.C. Thomas, Springfield.

27. Hakala, T. R., and Lange, P. H. 1974. Serum induced lymphoid cell-mediated cytotoxicity to human transitional cell carcinomas of the genitourinary tract. *Science* 184: 795–797.

28. Hauschka, T. S., Kvedar, B. J., Grinnell, S. T., and Amos, D. B. 1956. Immunoselection of polyploids from predominantly diploid cell populations. *Ann. N.Y. Acad. Sci.* 63: 683–705.

29. Hellström, K. E., and Hellström, I. 1974. Lymphocyte-mediated cytotoxicity and serum blocking activity to tumour antigens. *Advan. Immunol.* 18: 209–277.

30. Henson, P. M. 1970. Release of vasoactive amines from rabbit platelets induced by sensitized mononuclear leukocytes and antigen. *J. Exp. Med.* 131: 287–306.

31. Herberman, R. B. 1974. Cell-mediated immunity to tumor cells. *Advan. Cancer Res.* 19: 207–263.

32. Holtermann, O. A., Klein, E., Djfraffi, I., Bernhard, J. D., and Parmett, S.

1976. Immunotherapeutic approaches to tumors involving the skin, in D. S. Nelson (ed.), *Immunobiology of the Macrophage*, Academic Press, New York.

33. Holyoke, E. D., Frank, A. L., and Weiss, L. 1972. Tumor thromboplastin activity in vitro. *Int. J. Cancer* 9: 258–263.

34. Hoover, H. C., and Ketcham, A. S. 1975. Metastasis of metastases. *Amer. J. Surg.* 130: 405–411.

35. Lavelle, K. J., Ransdell, B. A., and Trygstad, C. W. 1975. Identification of a new platelet aggregating factor released by sensitized leukocytes. *Clin. Immunol. Immunopath.* 3: 492–502.

36. Lüscher, E. F. 1970. Induction of platelet aggregation by immune complexes. *Series Hematol.* 3: 121–129.

37. Marchesi, V. T., and Florey, H. W. 1961. Electron microscopic observations on the emigration of leukocytes. *Quart. J. Exp. Physiol.* 45: 343–348.

38. Mastrangelo, M. J., Bellet, R. E., Berkelhammer, J., and Clark, W. H. 1975. Regression of pulmonary metastatic disease associated with intralesional BCG therapy of intracutaneous melanoma metastases. *Cancer* 36: 1305–1308.

39. Mathé, G., Kamel, M., Dezfulian, M., Hallepannenko, O., and Bourut, C. 1973. An experimental screening for "systemic adjuvants of immunity" applicable in cancer immunotherapy. *Cancer Res.* 33: 1987–1997.

40. McKhann, C. F., and Gunnarson, A. 1974. Approaches to immunotherapy. *Cancer* 34: 1521–1531.

41. Merskey, C. 1974. Pathogenesis and treatment of altered blood coagulability in patients with malignant tumors. *Ann. N.Y. Acad. Sci.* 230: 289–293.

42. Nairn, R. C., Nind, A. P. P., Guli, E. P. G., Muller, H. K., Rolland, J. M., and Minty, C. C. J. 1971. Specific immune response in human skin carcinoma. *Brit. Med. J.* 4: 701–705.

43. Nicolson, G. L., Winkelhake, J. L., and Nussey, A. C. 1976. An approach to studying the cellular properties associated with metastasis: some in vitro properties of tumor variants selected in vivo for enhanced metastasis, in L. Weiss (ed.), *Fundamental Aspects of Metastasis*, pp. 291–303. American Elsevier, New York.

44. Pantalone, R. M., and Page, R. C. 1975. Lymphokine-induced production and release of lysosomal enzymes by macrophages. *Proc. Natl. Acad. Sci.* 72: 2091–2094.

45. Pfueller, S. L., and Lüscher, E. F. 1974. Studies on the mechanisms of human platelet release reaction induced by immunologic stimuli. *J. Immunol.* 112: 1201–1210.

46. Proctor, J. W., Auclair, B. G., and Lewis, M. G. 1976. The effect of BCG on B16 mouse melanoma: a comparison of routes of administration on tumour growth at different anatomical sites. *Eur. J. Cancer* 12: 203–210.

47. Samaha, R. J., Bruns, T. N. C., and Ross, G. J. 1973. Chronic intravascular coagulation in metastatic prostate cancer. *Arch. Surg.* 106: 295–298.

48. Sandberg, A. A., Yamada, K., Kikuchi, Y., and Takagi, N. 1967. Chromosomes and causation of human cancer and leukemia. III. Karyotypes of cancerous effusions. *Cancer* 20: 1099–1116.

49. Sato, H., and Suzuki, M. 1976. Deformability and viability of tumor cells by transcapillary passage, with reference to organ affinity of metastasis in cancer,

in L. Weiss (ed.), *Fundamental Aspects of Metastasis*, pp. 311–317. North-Holland, Amsterdam.

50. Sjögren, H. O., Hellström, I., Bansal, S. C., Warner, G. A., and Hellström, K. E. 1971. Suggestive evidence that the "blocking antibodies" of tumor bearing individuals may be antigen-antibody complexes. *Proc. Natl. Acad. Sci.* 68: 1372–1375.

51. Slack, N. H., and Bross, I. D. J. 1975. The influence of site of metastasis on tumour growth and response to chemotherapy. *Brit. J. Cancer* 32: 78–86.

52. Steel, G. G. 1960. Cell loss from experimental tumours. *Cell Tissue Kinet.* 1: 193–207.

53. Thomlinson, R. H., and Gray, L. H. 1955. The histological structure of some human lung cancers and the possible implications for radiotherapy. *Brit. J. Cancer* 9: 539–549.

54. Thompson, D. M. P., Eccles, S., and Alexander, P. 1973. Antibodies and soluble tumour-specific antigens in blood and lymph of rats with chemically induced sarcomata. *Brit. J. Cancer* 28: 6–15.

55. Warren, B. A. 1970. The ultrastructure of platelet pseudopodia and the adhesion of homologous platelets to tumour cells. *Brit. J. Exp. Path.* 51: 570–580.

56. Warren, B. A., and Shubik, P. 1966. The growth of the blood supply to melanoma transplants in the hamster cheek pouch. *Lab. Invest.* 15: 464–478.

57. Weiss, L. 1965. Studies on cell adhesion in tissue-culture. VIII. Some effects of antisera on cell detachment. *Exp. Cell Res.* 37: 540–551.

58. Weiss, L. 1967. *The Cell Periphery, Metastasis and Other Contact Phenomena*, North-Holland, Amsterdam/Wiley, New York.

59. Weiss, L. 1971. Biophysical aspects of initial cell interactions with solid surfaces. *Fed. Proc.* 30: 1649–1657.

60. Weiss, L. 1976a. Cell detachment and metastasis. *Gann Monogr. Cancer Res.* 20:25–35.

61. Weiss, L. 1976b. A pathobiologic overview of metastasis. *Seminars in Oncol.* 4: 5–17.

62. Weiss, L. (ed.) *Fundamental Aspects of Metastasis*, 1976. North-Holland, Amsterdam.

63. Weiss, L., and Glaves, D. 1975. Effects of migration inhibiting factor(s) on the *in vitro* detachment of macrophages. *J. Immunol.* 115: 1362–1365.

64. Weiss, L., Glaves, D., and Waite, D. A. 1974. The influence of host immunity on the arrest of circulating cancer cells and its modification by neuraminidase. *Int. J. Cancer* 13: 850–862.

65. Weiss, L., and Holyoke, E. D. 1969. Some effects of hypervitaminosis A on metastasis of spontaneous breast cancer in mice. *J. Natl. Cancer Inst.* 43: 1045–1054.

66. Weissmann, G., Zurier, R. B., Spieler, P. J., and Goldstein, I. M. 1971. Mechanisms of lysosomal enzyme release from leukocytes exposed to immune complexes and other particles. *J. Exp. Med.* 134: 149–165.

67. Wexler, H., Chretien, P. B., and Ketcham, A. S. 1972. Effect of tumor immunity on production of lung tumors after intravenous inoculation of antigenically identical tumor cells. *J. Natl. Cancer Inst.* 48: 657–663.

68. Willis, R. A. 1952. *The Spread of Tumours in the Human Body,* Butterworth, London.

69. Yamada, K., Takagi, N., and Sandberg, A. A. 1966. The chromosomes and causation of human cancer and leukemia. II. Karyotypes of human solid tumors. *Cancer* 19: 1879–1890.

CHAPTER 9

RADIATION, CELL-MEDIATED IMMUNITY, AND CANCER

Kong-oo Goh

Medical Oncology Unit
Monroe Community Hospital and
Department of Medicine
University of Rochester School
of Medicine and Dentistry
Rochester, New York 14603

This chapter reviews some clinical and experimental data obtained from studying the radiation effects supporting the hypothesis that cancer is the final phenotypical expression of mutant cells. It discusses the development of B and T cell classifications and demonstrates examples of an association between radiation and cancer, radiation-caused mutations in somatic cells, and radiation alterations of cell-mediated immunity. It raises the possibility that the cell-mediated immunosuppressive effects of radiation may result in T cell mutations.

I. INTRODUCTION*

The cause of cancer has been postulated to be a result of events such as the aging process, radiation, chemical agents or viruses. Many of these can produce mutant cells which may be detected with cytogenetic techniques in the form of chromosomal breakages or morphologically abnormal chromosomes. There are, however, occasional chromosomal abnormalities in "normal" persons (29). If mutant cells lead to cancer as proposed by Boveri (6), why do so many people not have the disease? Also, how can a mutant cell develop into cancer? To answer these questions, explanation in addition to the mutant-cell theory is necessary. Self-recognition and self-defense are important in maintaining homeostasis. When self-recognition (autoimmune) or self-defense (cancer) is impaired, phenotypical disease is produced (29). In cancer, the basic abnormality that leads to the phenotypical expression of cancer may be due to the rate of mutant cell-production exceeding the ability of the natural self-defense mechanism. Alternatively, there is an impairment of the self-defense mechanism. This chapter will review the available clinical and experimental data obtained from irradiation to support this hypothesis.

II. RADIATION

A. General

Radiation may be defined as the energy moving through space as waves or invisible particles. It can be divided into two major categories—ionizing and nonionizing radiation. The ionizing radiation includes: (1) photons (x-ray and gamma rays) which have the ability to strip electrons from atoms that create ions which are electrically charged, (2) uncharged particles (neutrons), and (3) charged particles (electrons or beta particles and helium, nuclei or alpha particles). Nonionizing radiation does not create ions and includes as an area of major interest the microwaves emitted by radar equipment and microwave ovens.

Ionizing radiation is measured in roentgens (R). A roentgen is the quantity of ionizing radiation that will produce in 1 ml (0.001295 gm) of dry air at 0°C and 760 mm Hg pressure, ions carrying 1 electrostatic unit of

*See page 329 for glossary of terms used in this chapter.

electricity of either sign. The biological radiation dose is measured in rads, which is defined as the quantity of radiation that deposits 100 ergs per gm of tissue.

B. Biological Effects

The biological effect of microwaves is most likely through their heat production, while that of ionizing radiation is more complex. Extensive investigations have been carried out in studying these effects since the end of World War II because of their potential military and medical uses. It has been found that the biological effect of ionizing radiation increases with increased ion pair density along the path of the radiation beam. Also, different tissues appear to have different sensitivities to radiation. The former finding has led to considerable interest in using neutron radiation as a possible therapeutic agent. If the biological effect of radiation depends on the energy liberated in a tissue mass (rads), it follows that the greater the density of the ionizing rays, the greater the biological effects produced.

The biological effects of ionizing radiation can be characterized by their induced somatic or genetic changes. The genetic effects of radiation may involve gene damage in the reproductive cells which may not be expressed clinically in their offspring until several years have elapsed. This unknown radiation effect upon future mankind has created great concern among many individuals regarding the use of nuclear energy. The acute and long-term mutation effects of ionizing radiation upon somatic cells will be reviewed in the following.

C. Radiation Mutation

In 1927, Muller found that there was an increase of about 150× mutation rate in the eggs and sperms of *Drosophila* radiated with high doses of X-ray. He also found that lethal mutations greatly outnumbered phenotypic mutants and that there were frequent chromosomal breakages and rearrangements in the treated insects. This important discovery of induced mutation opened a new field in experimental genetics. Muller's finding of radiation-induced mutation in the fruit fly was immediately confirmed by the independent work of Stadler from the University of Missouri with barley and corn treated with X-ray and radium. Since then radiation-induced mutation has been confirmed from bacteria to mammals.

Although radiation can affect cells in various ways, its more permanent and urgent effects are the changes in chromosomes, either demonstrated as gene mutation by pedigree studies or by analyzing chromosomal changes in cells exposed to either in vivo or in vitro radiation. It is possible the visible chromosomal changes may not be a major component of the mutation induced by radiation. But it is much simpler and easier to study the radiation effects upon somatic cells with this technique. In fact it was because of technical reasons that most of the radiation-induced chromosomal aberration research was done in animals other than man until recently. Man has a relatively large number of chromosomes, and the chromosomes are relatively small. These made an accurate study more difficult. However, in the late 1950s, simpler and more reliable techniques for cytogenetic studies were introduced for clinical and experimental studies in man (24).

D. Radiation and Human Chromosomes

Bender (1) showed that X-radiation affected chromosomes of human epitheloid and fibroblast cells in vitro. This observation was complemented by a report by Tough et al. (68) that chromosomal aberration can be seen in man after X-ray exposure. These observations have been confirmed and extended to include patients who were exposed to accidental, diagnostic, and therapeutic radiation. Although abnormal chromosomes can be seen in patients as soon as 30 minutes after radiation, the most remarkable and significant is the observation that the radiation-induced chromosomal abnormalities can be seen long after exposure for the treatment of ankylosing spondylitis (10) and the atomic bomb (42).

In 1958 a group of eight men at Oak Ridge, Tennessee, were accidentally exposed to total-body irradiation from fast neutrons and gamma rays with an exposure range of 22.8 to 365 rads. Abnormal chromosomes were found in these men 2 1/2 and 3 1/2 years after the accident. Six of the original eight men continued to participate in our studies of the long-term radiation effects. Chromosomal abnormalities were found in these men, 7 (25, 27, 30), 8, and 10 1/2 (34) years after the accident in the phytohemagglutinin (PHA)-stimulated peripheral blood leukocyte cultures (25, 27, 34), direct bone marrow preparations (25, 27) and bone marrow cultures (30, 34). The abnormal chromosomes found in cells at mitosis in the PHA-stimulated peripheral blood leukocyte cultures were thought to be lymphocytes. Therefore, our observation confirmed other reports that radiation can cause chromosomal breaks in human peripheral blood lymphocytes and has a long-lasting effect. In addition, we found chromosomal aberrations in the metaphases obtained from the direct bone marrow preparations (25, 27). Information obtained from direct bone marrow studies in patients with chronic myelocytic leukemia (CML) suggested that the metaphases obtained in these preparations were probably myeloid cells that differentiated to myelocytes, erythrocytes, and possibly megakaryocytes (28). Assuming that the same types of metaphases were seen in our direct bone marrow preparations of these irradiated patients, one may conclude that radiation also injures the human myeloid cells, and its effect is also long-lasting. The abnormalities found in these patients were independent of the level of radiation exposure.

We found a small G chromosome, morphologically resembling the Philadelphia (Ph[1]) chromosome seen in patients with CML. Similar morphological abnormal chromosomes were also found in a group of Japanese fishermen who were 90 miles away from the atomic bomb explosion on March 1, 1954. These fishermen received an external exposure dose estimated to range from 200 to 600 rads (43).

In the few cases reported in which Ph[1] chromosomes were found in patients after radiation therapy (21, 23), the patients had clinical evidence of CML at the time of the cytogenetic studies. Kamada (46) did not find any cytogenetic differences between the radiation-exposed and the nonradiation-exposed CML patients with one exception (Case 4), a 51-year-old woman was exposed to atomic radiation in 1945. In 1962 she was found to be in an early stage of CML. At that time only 62% of the metaphases obtained from a direct bone marrow preparation had a Ph[1] chromosome. The frequency of Ph[1] chromosome increased to 100% when her disease became more typical in 1964. In our patients, however, we found the frequencies of the small G chromosomes were between 1.4% to 3.0%, and the patients did not have clinical leukemia 10½ years after accidental irradiation.

III. CANCER AND RADIATION

Because of the latent period between the radiation exposure and the development of cancer, it has been very difficult to prove the direct cancer-causing effect of ionizing radiation in man. Furthermore, victims of high dose exposure usually die from more acute radiation effects than secondary consequences of radiation. But there is much indirect evidence linking ionizing radiation and cancer. The following are some of the cancers that have been found in association with radiation exposure.

A. Skin

Skin cancer was the first type of cancer found in high frequencies in irradiated subjects, prominently in the hands, forearms, and faces of radiologists and technicians who were chronically exposed to radiation. The cancer usually develops in skin that has had previous radiation dermatitis. The latent period of the skin tumors varies between 6 and 56 years with an average of about 13 to 26 years (41, 71). Abnormal chromosomes have been found in the dermal connective tissue cultures from patients who had received conventional radiation treatment from 6 months to 60 years previously. However, the skin neoplasms which developed after irradiation were predominantly squamous cell or basal cell carcinoma. Fibrosarcoma of the skin after irradiation is uncommon, despite the persistent cytogenetic damage (55).

B. Thyroid

The thyroid gland has been classified as a radioresistant organ based on the fact that large doses are needed to suppress the secretory function of the gland and produce histological evidence of tissue damage. External irradiation as a treatment for an enlarged thymus has been used since 1907. This treatment for the enlarged thymus gland was commonplace in this country from 1930 to 1945 (62). In 1950, Duffy and Fitzgerald (19) reported that 9 of 28 children who were treated with irradiation for thymus enlargement had thyroid cancer. The radiation that the thyroid glands received was not all due to scattered radiation as previously thought, but because of the size of the child the thyroid glands were sometimes in the primary beams of radiation (39). Studies of the late radiation effects indicate that under certain conditions, neoplastic transformation of the gland can be produced by radiation doses much lower than those formerly considered to be damaging to the tissue. The greater awareness of the relation between thyroid cancer and radiation for benign diseases has resulted in decreased use of this type of treatment. Consequently, the incidence of thyroid cancer in children has decreased, but there still is an increased occurrence of radiation-associated thyroid neoplasms in adults who were exposed to irradiation during infancy (54).

The histological findings in these thyroid tumors have included hyperplasia, adenoma, and carcinoma. Doida et al. (18) found that there were chromosomal aberrations in the metaphases obtained from cultured neoplastic and nonneoplastic cells of the thyroid gland after irradiation, some as long as 37 years after exposure. This indicates that lasting radiation-induced cellular damage has occurred. There is a latent period of 10–20 years between the radiation exposure and the development of neoplasms. The minimum latent period was 5 years for thyroid cancer and 10 years for benign tumors (40). Although Hempelmann and associates did not find a direct relation between the thyroid dose and the latent period, they found many benign tumors developed in the low-dose categories. This suggested that there was a longer latent period after the smaller dose exposure to develop benign nodular thyroid lesions (40).

Besides the increased incidence of thyroid cancer in the group of patients who were exposed to external irradiation, radioiodine (^{131}I) has been suspected to have tumorigenic effects in adolescents or adults who were treated with ^{131}I for thyrotoxicosis (60). On March 1, 1954, 64 people on Rongelap Island, about 100 miles from Bikini Island, were exposed to radiation from the fallout of fission products from a nuclear test on nearby Eniwetok Island. Following this accidental fallout exposure, many thyroid lesions occurred (12).

C. Leukemia

Since the first report of leukemia developed in radiological workers some years ago (69), there has been abundant evidence of the capacity of ionizing radiation to produce leukemia. March (50) analyzed the obituary notices of *JAMA* from 1929 to 1943 and found that leukemic deaths among the radiologists was 10× more frequent than other physicians. Similar results were also found between 1935–1944 (51). These findings support the earlier suspicions by investigators (75).

The epidemiological studies from 24,000 individuals in Japan who were exposed to 10 or more rads of equal rate radiation have made a significant contribution in association with radiation and leukemia (44). Leukemia was diagnosed first in 1948 among the atomic bomb survivors who had received large doses of radiation (8). This indicated that there was a latent period of at least two years before the expression of clinical leukemia in this population. Although the leukemic death rate is still significantly elevated among those who had received more than 100 rads (56), the peak incidence reached in 1951–1952 has been declining ever since. The majority (two-thirds) of the leukemias diagnosed in the survivors of the atomic bomb were acute leukemias, and the remainder CML.

In addition to the high incidence of leukemia developed in the atomic bomb exposed population, Court-Brown and Doll (14, 15) followed 14,000 ankylosing spondylitis patients between 5–25 years and found that the number of deaths from leukemia was nearly 10×, and the number of aplastic anemia, nearly 30× more frequent than as expected for the controls. They found that the latent periods in this group of patients were similar to those seen in the atomic bomb survivors, with the mortality from leukemia reaching a peak 3 to 5 years after irradiation. This then declined slowly. Again 80% of the leukemia in this population was acute leukemia and the remainder, CML.

D. Bone

Seventy-one presumably radiation-induced tumors have been identified among 780 former radium dial painters (70). Fifty-one of these tumors were osteogenic sarcomas, and the others were carcinomas of the paranasal sinus and mastoid. The tumors developed in persons who were exposed to accumulated radiation doses that exceeded 700 rads.

E. Breast

Mammary cancer can be produced in mice after long exposure to total-body irradiation. In rats Schellabarger and Schmidt (61) demonstrated that mammary neoplasia can develop in the transplanted mammary glands that were irradiated with 500r *in vitro*. In man it has been seen following the use of thorium dioxide in mammography. MacKenzie (49) found 13 breast cancers among 271 women who underwent multiple fluoroscopic examinations during the treatment of pulmonary tuberculosis by closed pneumothorax. In contrast they found only 1 among 510 tuberculosis patients who were not treated with artificial pneumothorax. Myrden and Hiltz (57) found that 22 of the 300 women exposed to multiple fluoroscopic examinations for the same treatment had developed breast cancer, an incidence of 7.3% as compared to 0.83% among 483 women who were not treated with pneumothorax. Because breast cancer is the leading cause of cancer death among American women, these reports aroused great interest regarding the hazards of diagnostic irradiation exposure, particularly, the recent popular mammography examination. Analyzing the statistics on the incidence of breast cancer among women who survived the atomic bombs of Hiroshima and Nagasaki (22) and the fluoroscopic examinations among the tuberculosis patients, a recent committee endorsed a recommendation that routine mammography for women under age 50 be discontinued because of the small but definite risk in developing cancer with this technique (17).

F. Comments

The two most interesting observations from the reports cited above are: (a) there is no morphological difference between cancers developed spontaneously and those thought to be associated with radiation, and (b) there is a latent period between the radiation exposure and the detection of the tumor.

There is no question from these studies that cancer is found in association with previous radiation exposure, especially in those exposed to a high dose. But our major concern should be whether radiation is hazardous to a larger population who were exposed to a small dose of radiation. There are data to suggest that the incidence of cancer is also high among populations with lower dose exposure (17). Although some of these exposures can be prevented by a complete eradication of the use of any kind of radiation, the more realistic approach would be that radiation be used only by skilled personnel, and more importantly, only for a specific potentially serious clinical indication.

G. Genotype (abnormal cells) and Phenotype (cancer or leukemia)

There is an increased incidence of cancer and leukemia among populations exposed to radiation, and radiation can produce chromosomal abnormalities as discussed in the preceding section. It is tempting to conclude that it is through the chromosomal aberration produced by the ionizing radiation that some of the irradiated patients develop cancer and leukemia. But there is a gap between the incidence of chromosomal abnormalities in the connective tissue culture of the skin and the frequency of the patients who developed skin cancer after irradiation and the frequency of small G chromosome in the total-body irradiated patients who do not have CML and the patients that do have CML. Also, there is a long latent period between the radiation and the development of cancer. Therefore, it seems that the development of cancer or leukemia (phenotype) must depend, not only on the presence of abnormal cells (genotype) but also on factors that allow these abnormal cells to continue to proliferate. This could result from an impairment of the defense mechanism (27, 28, 29, 31, 34). Alternatively, it may be due to a special advantage of the mutant cells whereby the rate of its production exceeds the ability of the natural defense mechanisms.

IV. CELL-MEDIATED IMMUNITY

A. General

One of the major natural defense mechanisms is through immunity. There are two types of immunity; namely, cellular and humoral. The humoral immune response is the type of immunity that can be transferred from a sensitized donor to a recipient by the serum. This usually involves a specific immunoglobulin (antibody). When an immune response that can *only* be transferred through the sensitized donor's cells to a recipient, it is called cell-mediated immunity. Both these immune responses are mediated either directly or indirectly through lymphocytes.

Previously, lymphocytes were classified according to their morphological appearance, for example, small, medium and large lymphocytes. In recent years it was found that there are at least two major subpopulations of morphologically similar lymphocytes, namely, T cells (thymus-dependent lymphocytes) and B cells (bursal-equivalent or thymus-independent lymphocytes). The T cells can be identified by their ability to form spontaneous rosettes with sheep erythrocytes, and B cells have surface immunoglobulins (Ig) detectable with fluorescent anti-Ig serum. There is another subpopulation of lymphocytes in the peripheral blood which is neither T nor B cells. This population of lymphocytes is called "Null" cells. The frequency of the "Null" cells is determined by subtracting the sum of the percentages of T and B cells from 100. The T and B cells have several roles in the immune system. The T cells function mainly in the cellular immune system. This involves delayed hypersensitivity, graft rejection, graft-versus-host reaction (GVHR) and cellular resistance to infections, notably viral, mycobacterial and fungal. B cells are the precursors of the plasma cells which produce specific antibodies. Although T and B cells have their own major function, they also function interdependently and interact with each other.

B. B Cells

In 1952 Bruton showed absence of gammaglobulin in the serum of a boy with repeated infections. The infections could be prevented by injections of gammaglobulin (9). Good (37) and Craig et al. (16) found no plasma cells or reactive lymphoid follicles in the lymph node cortex in agammaglobulinemic patients. Subsequently, Coons and associates (13) using fluorescent antibody demonstrated gammaglobulin in plasma cells. These observations indicated that at least some of the lymphocytes are involved in the production of immunoglobulins. This subpopulation of lymphocytes is derived from the bone marrow stem cells and has been shown to be dependent on the presence of bursa of Fabricius for their differentiation in birds. In mammals no organ equivalent to the bursa of Fabricius has been identified. Because of their dependence to the bursa in birds, this population of lymphocytes is called B cells or B lymphocytes.

C. T Cells

Thymus is the major lymphoid organ in the perinatal mouse at the time when the animal has not yet acquired the capacity to respond immunologically to antigenic stimuli. Therefore, thymectomy of the neonate will affect the maturation of immunological faculty. Miller (53) found no differences in the body weight of (AK × T$_6$)F$_1$ mice, either thymectomized or sham-thymectomized at birth during the first 4 months following the procedure. He found the mortality was high in the neonatal thymectomized mice after 2 months of age. The clinical condition before the death of these animals showed progressive wasting. This was rarely seen in mice who were thymectomized between 1 and 3 weeks old and not seen in mice thymectomized after 3 weeks old. Miller also found that 6-week-old healthy neonatal thymectomized mice had lower white blood cell counts than their sham-thymectomized littermates. The decrease in the white blood cells in these animals was entirely due to lymphopenia. The thymectomized mice showed involution of their lymphoid organs as indicated by a reduction in weight of their spleen and lymph nodes. Histologically, the spleen showed ill-defined, inactive follicles with slight basophilia and few mitoses as compared to the sham-operated mice.

These neonatal thymectomized mice have a long survival of allogenic or heterogenic skin grafts. If the neonatal thymectomized mice were grafted with whole intact thymuses from other neonatal mice between 7 and 14 days of age, the skin grafts were promptly rejected. These neonatal thymectomized mice with thymus grafts have well developed spleens, Peyer's Patches, and lymph nodes with active mitotic figures. Chromosomal analyses of cells obtained from the spleens of the thymus grafted, neonatal thymectomized mice showed 15–20% of the cells at metaphase were of donor origin. These observations are consistent with the hypothesis that cells differentiating in the thymus during embryonic or early postnatal life are progenitors of immunologically competent cells, a specific thymic lymphocyte (now called T cells). The majority of the cells found in the lymphoid organs were of the recipient rather than donor origin. This suggested that there must be another function of the thymus gland, possibly a humoral factor that can influence the progenitors of immunologically competent cells. This question was postulated by Metcalf (52) when he isolated a factor from the thymus which can produce temporary lymphocytosis in the peripheral blood when injected into newborn mice.

In order to test the hypothesis that there is a humoral factor from the thymus that can influence the lymphocytes, Osoba and Miller (58), ingeniously designed experiments in which neonatal thymectomized mice were implanted intraperitoneally with neonatal thymus enclosed inside a "Millipore" diffusion chamber. Animals with these implants partially restored their lymphopoiesis and promptly rejected their skin homografts while no rejection of homograft was seen in neonatal thymectomized mice implanted with an empty "Millipore" diffusion chamber. The lymphocyte population of neonatal thymectomized mice bearing thymus tissue inside a diffusion chamber was not significantly different from the control thymectomized mice. These experiments suggested that: (a) embryonic or neonatal thymus tissue elaborates in the diffusion chamber a humoral factor which is capable of homograft rejection, and (b) the capacity of mice to reject homografts is not necessarily dependent on the quantity of lymphocytes present in the animals.

D. Origin and Characteristics of B and T Cells

Injection of bone marrow cells with sex chromosome markers into lethally irradiated hosts showed that the proliferating cells in the thymus, as well as in other lymphoid structures, were of donor origin. Injection of lymph nodes, thymus or thoracic-duct lymphocytes resulted in repopulation only of the spleen and the lymph nodes, but not thymus. These indicated that the precursors of the T lymphocytes and the immunoglobulin-producing B lymphocytes are bone marrow cells.

Progenitors of T cells from the bone-marrow stem cells apparently enter the thymus via circulating blood, and within the thymus these cells divide and differentiate. During this procedure, the cells migrate from the cortex to the medulla as they become mature T cells. Although B cells in mammals also originate from the bone-marrow stem cells, there is no organ similar to thymus to produce mature B cells from their precursors. In chickens the bursa of Fabricius, a primary lymphoid organ adjacent to the cloaca, probably serves this function. Recently, Brand and associates (7) reported a bursal extract which could be the counterpart of thymosin of the thymus gland. This extract can induce differentiation of both B and T cells. At a low concentration, this extract produces a greater B cell differentiation than T cells. Therefore, it is possible there is also a humoral factor that can induce B cell differentiation as thymopoietin in the T cells. This bursal extract factor has been named bursopoietin (7).

The differences of B and T cells are summarized in Table 1.

V. RADIATION AND CELL-MEDIATED IMMUNITY

Since cell-mediated immunity depends largely on the subpopulation of lymphocytes that are dependent on the thymus gland, radiation effect on lymphocytes or thymus glands will result in an alternation of cell-mediated immunity.

A. Radiation of Lymphocytes

It has been shown experimentally that a decrease in lymphocyte counts in the peripheral blood occurs after an acute exposure to total-body irradiation. This can be seen as early as 15–30 minutes. The maximum depletion usually occurs with 48 to 72 hours. The cause of the lymphopenia found in irradiated subjects has been thought to be the result of a direct destruction of the cells by the radiation. After irradiation the lymphoid organs usually show the following sequence of events: a decrease of mitosis with congestion and edema; degeneration and necrosis of lymphocytes; phagocytosis of debris; aplasia and atrophy of the germinal centers; and recovery by regeneration of the germinal centers. The earliest morphological change in the lymphocytes after irradiation is clumping of the nuclear chromatin. This is followed by pyknotic degeneration of the nucleus and finally the disintegration of the cytoplasm and the disappearance of the cells when the nuclear degeneration is far advanced. Although it is difficult to determine when the lymphocytes die after radiation, it seems reasonable to assume that death occurs about 1–2 hours following the irradiation and the morphological nuclear degeneration process occurs in 2–6 hours as a result of autolysis of the cells.

B. Radiation of Thymus

Carter, Cronkite, and Bond found a decrease in the weight of the thymus and peripheral blood lymphocytes in animals after exposure to radiation, either from the nuclear devices or X-radiation (11). They considered the weight loss of the thymus gland as due to the loss of the lymphoid cells in the organs and the decrease in the peripheral lymphocytes as the result of the loss of the precursor cells from the lymphopoietic centers and the decrease of the total small lymphocyte masses of the animals. They found the biological effects of the neutron radiation in the thymus was twice those seen in the peripheral blood lymphocytes.

Morphologically, the thymus gland became nearly completely involuted following a large dose of irradiation. Two hours after irradiation, almost all the thymic lymphocytes became pyknotic with disintegrated nuclei. These nuclei contained agglutinated chromatin which appeared as homogenous round drops of various sizes. The disintegrated nuclei disappeared within 3–5 days. In low-dose X-irradiation, regeneration usually begins between 5–10 days after acute irradiation. Complete regeneration is a very slow process. Takada et al. (65) found that at 400 R of whole-body irradiation, the kinetics of thymic regeneration follows a

Table 1.   Summaries of T and B lymphocytes.

Characteristics	T	B
Origin	Bone marrow	Bone marrow
Dependency	Thymus	Bursa in birds or its equivalent in mammals
Life span	Long (months to years)	Short (days to weeks)
Recirculating	Majority	Minority
Cell surface (scanning electron microscope)	Smooth	Contains microvilli
Electrophoretic mobility	Fast	Slow
Adhesiveness (glass or nylon)	Less	More
Spontaneous rosette(s) formation with sheep erythrocytes	+	−
Fluorescence anti-human Ig or antibody C_3 receptor by sheep erythrocytes coated with human complement	−	+
Mitogenic Responses		
Phytohemagglutinin (PHA)	+	−
Concanavalin A (con A)	+	−
Lentil	+	−

biphasic pattern as measured by the change of thymic weight and the mitotic index. They showed that there was a precipitous drop in the weight of the thymus gland following irradiation. The weight of the gland recovered almost fully within 5–12 days after irradiation. This early recovery period, however, was followed by another drop in weight which persisted until about the 25th day.

The thymic lymphocytes are very radiosensitive; thus at higher doses

Table 1.   (Continued)

Characteristics	T	B
Waxbean	+	?
Pokeweed mitogen (PWM)	+	+
Insoluble fraction of PHA, con A, PWM	+	+
Bacterial lipo-polysaccharide (LPS)	−	+
Staphylococcal entero-toxin B	+	+
Allogeneic leukocytes	+	−
Distributions (%)		
Thymus	95–100	0
Thoracic duct	80–90	10–15
Peripheral blood	60–85	20–40
Lymph node	55–80	30–35
Spleen	23–32	18–30
Peyer's patches	20–40	60–75
Functions		
Cell-mediated immunity	Yes	?
Humoral production		
Induction	Yes	Yes
Antibody synthesis	No	Yes
Memory	Yes	Yes

of irradiation, the restoration of the thymic lymphocytes has to depend upon a migration of the bone-marrow-derived stem cells (20). This is indicated by: (a) a striking morphological similarity of the regenerating adult thymus following irradiation and the neonatal thymus, and (b) the recovery of the glands when the adult irradiated animals were given bone marrow cells. More definitive evidence regarding the migration of the bone marrow cells as stem cells to repopulate the thymus gland in adults after a high dose of total-body irradiation was reported by Takada and Takada (66). These investigators injected either bone marrow or thymus and bone marrow cells to recipient mice 1–2 hours after the animals were exposed to 800 R of total-body irradiation. The donor cells can be identified by their chromosomal pattern. The recipient mice were killed at various intervals, and slides from the bone marrow, spleen, thymus and lymph node cells were made. Takada and Takada (66) found the donor's bone marrow cells reached the host bone marrow and spleen and lymph nodes immediately after transplantation, and proliferation started in these organs 5–8 days later. However, the donor cells did not start to proliferate in the host thymus until 10 days after the bone marrow transplantation and did not reach 100% until after 30 days. They also showed that the donor's thymic cells did not proliferate in the host bone marrow or spleen but did proliferate in the lymph nodes and thymus of the irradiated animals.

More recently, Kadish and Basch (45) showed that there is a significant pool of radioresistant stem cells which are capable of partially restoring the thymus of heavily irradiated mice. This conclusion was based on their observations that there is no effect upon the thymic regeneration as measured by the incorporation of ^{3}H-thymidine in the whole-body and the lower-body shielded (bone marrow and spleen protected) irradiated mice during the first 12 days following the irradiation. During this period, they found that there was no difference in the incorporation of ^{3}H-thymidine in the glands of animals, either receiving syngeneic bone marrow or not. The observation of Kadish and Basch (45) complements and supports the report of Takada et al. (65) as they found that although the second weight loss of the thymus gland could be prevented when syngeneic bone marrow was given at the time of irradiation, the syngeneic bone marrow has no effect upon the initial thymus weight drop. Furthermore, they found that the first regeneration of the thymus following irradiation, as measured by weight, could be eliminated if the animals were irradiated with a dose higher than 500 R. This suggested that these two recovery phases were from different cell pools.

A transit cell pool is being proposed to define these more radiation resistant cells that cause the early phase of thymic regeneration (45). These cells may not continuously maintain themselves but are precommitted to undergo substantial expansion into a differentiated cell compartment: the thymic lymphocyte. The exact anatomical location of the radioresistant transit cell pool has not been established. But since shielding the lower half of the animal or transfer of a large dose of exogenous bone marrow cells does not influence the size of this pool, Kadish and Basch (45) concluded that this pool of cells is probably located in the thymus itself.

VI. RADIATION EFFECTS ON B AND T CELLS IN MAN

A. Cancer of Breast

Stjernsward et al. (64) presented the results of an investigation designed to detect shifts in the ratio between the two subpopulations of circulating small lymphocytes in 34 women with breast cancer who were treated with radiation. They also studied 19 patients with breast cancer treated with either preoperative or postoperative radiation to the breast or chest wall. Their controls included healthy, age-matched staff members, nine patients with primary brain tumors, before and after irradiation, and seven patients with chronic shoulder or knee diseases. The T cells were determined with spontaneous rosette formation with sheep erythrocytes and the B cells with EAC-binding lymphocytes. They found radiation produced a significant lymphopenia in spite of the fact that the patients received only a very limited area in the parasternal and supraclavicular regions. The lymphopenia was still seen in these patients one year after irradiation. They did not find lymphopenia in patients with brain tumors treated with radiation. In addition, Stjernsward et al. found that the proportion of peripheral blood B cells increased from 35% to 56%, and the T cells decreased from 55% to 50% after radiotherapy. These results suggest that it was the T cells that were specifically eliminated in radiated patients.

A rapid decrease in peripheral lymphocytes could be explained by irradiation of lymphocytes flowing through the large vessels within the radiation site. The long duration of the lymphopenia could be interpreted to be due to selective elimination of long-lived lymphocytes. Since half of the thymus gland was included in the radiation field, it is possible that radiation injured the thymus gland resulting in its failure to maintain the T cells. Recently, Lewis and Paterson (48) found that the irradiation of the mediastinum may be more crucial in producing leukopenia than the extent of bone marrow irradiation. Regrettably, they did not study the frequencies of B and T lymphocytes in the peripheral blood or the type of cells that resulted in producing the leukopenia in their patients.

Blomgren et al. (4) and Wood et al. (74), using various techniques to determine T and B lymphocytes in two groups of post-irradiated lymphopenia breast cancer patients, found no significant changes in the frequencies of B and T lymphocytes. Blomgren et al. (4) interpreted the discrepancy between their observation and those reported by Stjernsward et al. (64) as being caused by a technical difference in lymphocyte preparation. They routinely passed the leukocytes through a nylon column which would remove any cells that might adhere to the nylon. This step was not done in Stjernsward's lymphocyte preparations (64).

B. Cancer of Lung

Thomas et al. (67) investigated the ability of the peripheral blood lymphocytes to respond to PHA in a group of patients with advanced lung cancer who were treated with ^{60}Co-irradiation to the chest. The doses received by these patients were between 2950 and 5750 rads. The degree of response to PHA was measured by ^{3}H-thymidine uptake. These investigators found that there was a marked decrease in the responsiveness of the lymphocytes to PHA in all irradiation doses. This reached a low at the end of the third week with a slight improvement at the fourth week after irradiation. In addition, they showed that there was a significantly lower mean lymphocyte response to PHA in a group of patients, most of whom had received irradiation for carcinoma of the lung and had survived for a number of years. Since a decreased capacity of the lymphocytes to transform following stimulation with PHA is frequently associated with a decrease in an individual's general immunological response, these findings suggest an impairment of the immunological response after radiation.

Stefani et al. (63) evaluated the immunological competence of 29 male lung cancer patients who were referred to their service for radiation treatment. The patients ranged in age from 34 to 70 years. These patients were treated either with 6000 rads to the primary tumor and regional lymph nodes over a period of 6 weeks or 3000–4000 rads to the distant metastases in 2–4 weeks. The immunological evaluation included: (a) skin-test antigen response with dermatophytin; dermatophytin-O; streptokinase-streptodornase; mumps and intermediate strength tuberculin antigens, (b) dinitrochlorobenzene (DNCB) reactivity, and (c) rosette-forming cells assays. These investigators found an increased response to the skin-test antigens and to DNCB in patients following radiotherapy. They attributed this observation to patient selection, for example, the nonresponders had either died or were too sick to return for further testing.

No difference in the frequencies of skin reaction or the intensity of reaction to purified protein derivative (PPD) has been observed in a group of lung cancer patients who were treated with 4800–4500 rads of radiation (47). However, Stefani et al. (63) found that the absolute numbers of T cells were markedly decreased after therapy. In addition, they found the percent and also numbers of B cells were decreased.

C. Cancer of Prostate and Bladder

Blomgren et al. (5) recently studied the peripheral blood T and B lymphocytes from 15 men and four women between the ages of 52 and 75 who were treated with external irradiation for cancer of prostate or bladder. All patients with prostatic cancer were treated with 5400 (30 × 180) rads in six weeks, but the patients with bladder cancer received various doses of irradiation. The total doses in the bladder cancer of each patient were between 3600 and 8400 rads. Using spontaneous rosette formation with sheep erythrocytes as identification of T cells and the formation of rosette formation with sheep erythrocytes coated with specific rabbit antibodies and complement to determine the B cells, these investigators found that there was a statistically significant decrease of about 22% of B cells. There were no significant changes in T cells in the nonpurified preparation of peripheral blood lymphocytes. They also found a significant decrease in the B cells, but not in the T cells in the purified peripheral blood lymphocytes preparation.

D. Hodgkin's Disease

Engeset et al. (22) studied the frequencies of the B lymphocytes of the peripheral blood of 23 patients, most of whom had stage III or IV Hodgkin's disease. Sixteen were studied before any treatment, and the others were studied 5–36 months after total lymph node irradiation with 3800–4000 rads. They found about one-half of the untreated patients were lymphopenic, but the fraction of the B cells was about the same as the controls. Although the lymphocyte counts were higher in the treated patients than the untreated patients, the difference was not statistically significant. They found a significantly higher percentage of B lymphocytes in the irradiated group than the untreated patients. These investigators considered Ig-positive lymphocytes may be more radioresistant than the Ig-negative lymphocytes, which are probably T lymphocytes. An alternative explanation to this would be that there is a more complete postirradiation regeneration of B than T lymphocytes. This cannot be given general validity because the thymus had been included in the field, and most of the patients had been splenectomized. In addition, Hodgkin's patients may have an abnormal lymphocyte response to mitogen.

E. Seminoma of Testis

The peripheral blood lymphocytes of patients with seminoma of the testis were selected for studies by Heier et al. (38) because: (a) there is a relatively good prognosis of this disease whereby the late effects of radiation can be studied; (b) thymus gland is not included in the radiation field in some patients; and (c) these patients have solid tumors of nonlymphoid organ. These investigators divided these patients into three groups: Group A consisted of men who were studied before, during and immediately after radiotherapy; Group B were patients who had been treated up to ten years ago; and Group C were similar to the type of patients as Group B but who also received mediastinum irradiation. These investigators found that lymphopenia developed with a decrease in the frequency of B cells, but the frequency of T cells remained unchanged or increased in patients after irradiation. They found a gradual increase of the total lymphocytes after radiation and by 5–10 years the total lymphocytes had returned to normal level. They also found that there were no differences among the total lymphocytes of Groups B and C patients. Although they noted that the percent of Ig-positive lymphocytes was higher in the irradiated patients than normal between six months and five years after irradiation, it was normal at tenth year. There was a higher frequency of Ig-positive cells in Group C than Group B. They interpreted their data as to indicate that the shift in B:T lymphocyte ratio induced by radiotherapy is not permanent but is normal after 5–10 years and that irradiation of the thymus in adults does not influence the main pattern of the recovery of these cells.

F. Comments

It is not possible to make a definite conclusion from the different reports cited above that the B or the T lymphocytes are more sensitive to radiation. These reports were from different laboratories using various techniques to determine B and T cells. Also, all the patients studied have various types of cancer. There are reports that the frequencies of B and T lymphocytes in cancer patients are different from the normals. Furthermore, there is suggestive evidence that the frequencies of these sub-populations of lymphocytes varies greatly depending on the stage of the patient's disease (36). Therefore, the change in the frequencies of the B and T lymphocytes in these patients following irradiation to their cancer may be the end result of the radiation effects upon the blocking antibody. This caused some mobilization of either T or B cells for the defense against their cancer. In spite of these shortcomings, these reports indicate irradiation can alter human B and T lymphocytes in the peripheral blood.

G. Thymus Irradiation in Infancy and Childhood

My interest in thymus irradiation and lymphocytes began when we attempted to culture the peripheral blood lymphocytes of a group of

Dr. Hempelmann's patients whose thymus glands were irradiated during infancy for presumed thymus enlargement. The peripheral blood of a number of these individuals in a subgroup with a high risk of developing radiation-induced neoplasms was cultured with PHA in 1964 with the hope of finding some chromosomal abnormalities as a late effect of irradiation. Chromosomal abnormalities have been demonstrated by Buckton *et al.* (10) in a group of patients with ankylosing spondylitis who were treated with X-ray many years before these cytogenetic studies. No mitosis was seen in our cultures. This was attributed to a technical artifact (unpublished data). In a subsequent attempt to culture the PHA stimulated peripheral blood lymphocytes of these thymus-irradiated subjects in 1971, we harvested part of the culture after 3-day and the other half after 7-day incubation. It became apparent that there were higher mitotic rates and greater numbers of metaphases among the 7-day than the 3-day cultures. Although the mitotic rate in the normal lymphocytes usually decreased with prolonged culturing (32), we observed an increased mitotic rate with prolonged culturing in patients with chronic lymphocytic leukemia (CLL). It has been shown that the lymphocytes in CLL may be B lymphocytes (73). It is possible that the lymphocytes obtained from the thymus-irradiated patients responded *in vitro* to PHA in the same way as CLL (26). Therefore, it seems likely that the lymphocytes in the thymus-irradiated patients are predominantly B lymphocytes. Thus, radiation to the thymus gland may have caused a selective injury to the T lymphocytes on these subjects. Confirmation of this observation would have great impact in experimental and clinical oncology.

The frequencies of B and T lymphocytes were determined in a group of 14 adults between the ages of 28 and 41 who were treated with X-ray to their thymus glands during infancy (59). They consisted of eight men and six women who had received 270 to 564 R. They were treated at the ages of 2 days to 2 1/2 years old. The B lymphocytes were determined by the direct fluorescent methods using fluorescein-isothiocyanate-conjugated goat antihuman globulin. The T cells were determined by using the spontaneous rosette-forming lymphocytes with sheep erythrocytes. In addition, the responses to PHA and PWM were also determined using mitotic rate as the degree of response to these mitogens. Lymphocytes were separated from other cells by passing them through a fiber glass column at room temperature.

There were no differences between the total number of lymphocytes per mm^3, but there were significant ($P < 0.005$) differences between the relative and absolute number of T cells per mm^3 among the previously irradiated and the control subjects. There was also a decrease in the B lymphocytes in this group of patients, but the difference was less significant ($P < 0.10$). Our observations of the decrease in T and B lymphocytes in these patients whose thymus glands were irradiated some 28–41 years previously using the direct method were further supported by the indirect methods. We found the mean mitotic activity of the PHA- and PWM-stimulated thymic irradiated lymphocyte cultures was less than the controls.

Thymus glands are extremely radiosensitive. Therefore, it is possible that our observations of significantly lower absolute numbers and percentages of B and T lymphocytes in the peripheral blood of the thymus-irradiated individuals were due to the damage of the thymus gland sustained during thymic irradiation in infancy. This damage lead to an inability to support T cell development. However, in our chromosomal analyses of the metaphases obtained from the PHA-stimulated peripheral blood lymphocyte cultures, we found a significantly higher frequency of abnormal cells and chromosomal breakages in the thymus-irradiated subjects (35). Since irradiation can cause chromosomal breakages that last for a long time, it is reasonable to conclude that the chromosomal abnormalities found in these patients were due to their original radiation some 23 to 41 years ago. Long-lived lymphocytes are believed to be T cells which can be stimulated to undergo mitosis by PHA. The chromosomal patterns of these patients were analyzed from the PHA stimulated cultures, therefore, these abnormal lymphocytes probably were the long-lived T lymphocytes that were injured during the original irradiation. An alternative explanation could be that radiation produced or activated a substance that is capable to effect human T cells for a long time (33).

VII. CONCLUSION

This chapter demonstrated that: (a) an association between irradiation and cancer exists, (b) radiation causes mutation in somatic cells and (c) radiation alters cell-mediated immunity. One can conclude that the mechanism of the radiation-induced cancer is through its mutagenic and cell-mediated immunosuppressive effects. This could be supported by the observations that many of the current carcinogenic chemicals also have these two properties. Since most of the somatic mutation effects of irradiation have been demonstrated as chromosomal aberrations in the PHA-stimulated lymphocytes and PHA appears to stimulate the T lymphocytes, it is conceivable that the cell-mediated immunosuppressive effects of irradiation are the phenotypic expression of the irradiation-induced somatic mutation in T lymphocytes.

GLOSSARY

Allogenic (allograft or homograft):   Tissue graft between members of a genetically heterogenous population but same species.

B Cells: A subpopulation of lymphocytes derived from bone marrow which are
thymus independent and depend on bursa of Fabricius in chicken and can be
identified by their surface immunoglobulin.

Bursopoietin: Extract from bursa which is capable of inducing differentiation of
both B and T cells. At a low concentration, it produces greater B cell differentiation than T cells (7).

Dinitrochlorobenzene (DNCB):   This substance is frequently used as an antigen to
test the patient for anergy.

Genotype: Genetic constitution of an organism.

Graft-versus-Host Reaction (GVHR):   In transplantation biology, it is not only that
host reacts against donor cells, but donor cells can react with the host cells.
This occurs in the transplantation of hematopoietic cells, notably the immune
competent cells of bone marrow and lymphoid organs.

Heterogenic (xenogenic or xenograft):   Grafts between different species.

Homograft: See *Allogenic.*

Mutation: A permanent change of genetic material which could be a point mutation (single gene) or chromosome structure (many genes) changes.

Philadelphia (or Ph¹) Chromosome: Abnormal chromosome resulting from a deletion of the long arm (q) of a normal chromosome 22, with the deleted part
most commonly translocated to the long arm of a chromosome 9. It is seen in
patients with chronic myelocytic leukemia.

Phytohemagglutinin (PHA):   Substance obtained from the kidney beans which is
capable of stimulating normal T cells to undergo blastoid transformation and
mitosis *in vitro.*

Pokeweed Mitogen (PWM):   Substance from pokeweed (phytolocca americana)
that is capable of stimulating both B and T cells to undergo blastoid transformation and mitosis *in vitro.*

Purified Protein Derivative (PPD):   Used as an antigen to test skin hypersensitivity of patient with tuberculosis.

Pyknotic: The nucleus stains intensely and appears shrunken with loss of struc-
tured details. This usually leads to death of cells.

Rad: Unit quantity of radiation that deposits 100 ergs per gm of tissue.

Roentgen: Unit quantity of ionizing radiation that will produce in 1 ml (0.001295
gm) of dry air at 0°C and 760 mm Hg pressure, ions carrying 1 electrostatic
unit of electricity of either sign.

Syngeneic (syngeneic graft or isograft):   The donor and recipient are of the same
inbred strain and are genetically identical.

T Cells: A subpopulation of lymphocytes which are derived from the bone marrow and are thymus dependent. They can be identified by their ability to form
spontaneous rosettes with sheep erythrocytes.

Thymosin: Hormone-like substance produced by the epithelial cells of the thymus gland which exhibits specific biological activity to elicit lymphocytosis *in vivo* and *in vitro.*

Transit Cell Pool: A population of radioresistant stem cells in the thymus which are capable of partially restoring the thymus in mice after heavy irradiation (45).

ACKNOWLEDGMENT

This work was supported in part by Research Grant CA 14876 from the National Cancer Institute, USPHS.

REFERENCES

1. Bender, M. A. 1957. X-ray induced chromosome aberrations in normal diploid human tissue cultures. *Science* 126: 974–975.

2. Bender, M. A., and Gooch, P. C. 1962. Persistent chromosome aberrations in irradiated human subjects. *Radiat. Res.* 16: 44–53.

3. Bender, M. A., and Gooch, P. C. 1963. Persistent chromosome aberrations in irradiated subjects. II. Three and one-half year investigation. *Radiat. Res.* 18: 389–396.

4. Blomgren, H., Glas, U., Melen, B., and Wasserman, J. 1974. Blood lymphocytes after radiation therapy of mammary carcinoma. *Acta Radiol.* 13: 185–200.

5. Blomgren, H., Wasserman, J., and Littbrand, B. 1974. Blood lymphocytes after radiation therapy of carcinoma of prostate and urinary bladder. *Acta Rad. Ther. Phy. Biol.* 13: 357–367.

6. Boveri, T. 1929. *The Origin of Malignant Tumors,* pp. 1–119. Williams and Wilkins Co., Baltimore.

7. Brand, A., Gilmour, D. G., and Goldstein, G. 1976. Lymphocyte-differentiating hormone of bursa of Fabricius. *Science* 193: 319–321.

8. Brill, A. B., Tomanaga, M., and Heyssel, R. M. 1962. Leukemia in man following exposure to ionizing radiation: A summary of the findings in Hiroshima and Nagasaki, and a comparison with other human experience. *Ann. Intern. Med.* 56: 590–609.

9. Bruton, O. C. 1952. Agammaglobulinemia. *Pediatrics* 9: 722–727.

10. Buckton, K. E., Jacobs, P. A., Court-Brown, W. M., and Doll, R. 1962. A study of the chromosome damage persisting after X-ray therapy for ankylosing spondylitis. *Lancet* 2: 676–682.

11. Carter, R. E., Cronkite, E. P., and Bond, V. P. 1954. The effect of neutrons on thymic and circulating lymphocytes in the mouse. *Amer. Natural.* 88: 257–267.

12. Conrad, R. A., Dobryno, B. M., and Suton, W. W. 1970. Thyroid neoplasia as late effect of exposure to radioactive iodine in fallout. *JAMA* 214: 316–324.

13. Coons, A. H., Leduc, E. H., and Connolly, J. M. 1955. Study on antibody production. I. A method for the histological demonstration of specific antibody and its application to a study of the hyperimmune rabbit. *J. Exp. Med.* 102: 49–59.

14. Court-Brown, W. W. and Doll, R. 1957. Leukaemia and aplastic anemia in patients irradiated for ankylosing spondylitis. Her Majesty's Stat. Off. London, 1957.

15. Court-Brown, W. W., and Doll, R. 1965. Mortality from cancer and other courses after radiotherapy for ankylosing spondylitis. Brit. Med. J. 2: 1327–1332.

16. Craig, J., Gitlin, D., and Jewett, T. 1954. Response of lymph nodes of normal and congenitally agammaglobulinemic children to antigen stimulation. Amer. J. Dis. Child. 88: 626.

17. Culliton, B. J. 1976. Breast cancer: Second thoughts about routine mammography. Science 193: 555–558.

18. Doida, Y., Hoke, C., and Hempelmann, L. H. 1971. Chromosome damage in thyroid cells of adults irradiated with X-rays in infancy. Radiat. Res. 45: 645–656.

19. Duffy, B. J., and Fitzgerald, P. J. 1950. Thyroid cancer in children and adolescence. Report on 28 cases. Cancer 3: 1018–1032.

20. Dukor, P., Miller, J. F. A. P., House, W., and Allman, V. 1965. Regeneration of thymus grafts. I. Histological and cytological aspects. Transplantation 3: 639–668.

21. Engel, E., Flexner, J. M., Engel-De Montmollin, M., and Frank, H. E. 1964. Blood and skin chromosomal alterations of a clonal type in a leukemic man previously irradiated for a lung carcinoma. Cytogenetics 3: 228–251.

22. Engeset, A., Froland, S. S., Bremer, K., and Høst, H. 1973. Blood lymphocytes in Hodgkin's disease: Increase of B-lymphocytes following extended field irradiation. Scand. J. Haemat. 11: 195–200.

23. Gavosto, F., Pileri, A., and Pegoraro, L. 1965. X-rays and Philadelphia chromosome. Lancet 1: 1336–1337.

24. Goh, K. O. 1965. Human Cytogenetics: An experimental and clinical approach to clinical medicine, in Year Book Med. Publishers, Inc., Disease-a-Month Monography Series, 1965, pp. 1–47. Chicago.

25. Goh, K. O. 1966. Smaller G chromosome in irradiated man. Lancet 1: 659–660.

26. Goh, K. O. 1967. Pseudodiploid chromosomal pattern in chronic lymphocytic leukemia. J. Lab. Clin. Med. 69: 938–949.

27. Goh, K. O. 1968. Total-body irradiation and human chromosomes: Cytogenetic studies of the peripheral blood and bone marrow leukocytes seven years after total-body irradiation. Radiat. Res. 35: 155–170.

28. Goh, K. O. 1968. Autoradiographic studies in chronic myelocytic leukemia, in R. L. Hayes, F. A. Goswitz, and B. E. P. Murphy (eds.), Radioisotopes in Medicine: In Vitro Studies 1968, pp. 695–715. AEC Symposium Series, No. 13, Conf. 671111.

29. Goh, K. O. 1968. Large abnormal acrocentric chromosome associated with human malignancies: Possible mechanism of establishing clone of cells. Arch. Intern. Med. 122: 241–248.

30. Goh, K. O. 1971. Total-body irradiation and human chromosomes. II. Cytogenetic studies of the cultured bone marrow cells seven years after total-body irradiation. Amer. J. Med. Sci. 262: 43–49.

31. Goh, K. O. 1973. Total-body irradiation and human chromosomes. III. Cytogenetic studies in patients with malignant hematologic diseases treated with total-body irradiation. *Amer. J. Med. Sci.* 266: 179–186.

32. Goh, K. O. 1975a. Phytohemagglutinin committed lymphocytes: The mitotic activity of the phytohemagglutinin stimulated lymphocytes. *Proc. Soc. Exp. Biol. Med.* 148: 1122–1125.

33. Goh, K. O. 1975b. Total-body irradiation and human chromosomes. V. Additional evidence of a transferable substance in the plasma of irradiated persons to induce chromosomal breakages. *J. Med.* 6: 51–60.

34. Goh, K. O. 1975c. Total-body irradiation and human chromosomes. IV. Cytogenetic follow-up studies 8 and 10 1/2 years after total-body irradiation. *Radiat. Res.* 62: 364–373.

35. Goh, K. O., Reddy, M. M., and Hempelmann, L. H. 1976. Chromosomal aberrations in lymphocytes of normal adults long after thymus irradiation. *Radiat. Res.* 67: 82–85.

36. Goh, K. O., and Reddy, M. M. 1976. B and T lymphocytes in man. II. Circulating B and T lymphocytes in cancer patients. *J. Med.* 7: 297–305.

37. Good, R. A. 1954. Absence of plasma cells from bone marrow and lymph nodes following antigenic stimulation in patients with agammaglobulinemia. *Rev. Hemat.* 9: 502.

38. Heier, H. E., Christensen, I., Froland, S. S., and Engeset, A. 1975. Early and late effects of irradiation for seminoma testis on the number of blood lymphocytes and their B and T subpopulations. *Lymphology* 8: 69–74.

39. Hempelmann, L. H., Pifer, J. W., Burke, G. J., Terry, R., and Ames, W. R. 1967. Neoplasms in persons treated with X-rays in infancy for thymic enlargement. A report of the third follow-up survey. *J. Natl. Canc. Inst.* 38: 317–341.

40. Hempelmann, L. H., Hall, W. J., Phillips, M., Cooper, R. A., and Ames, W. R. 1975. Neoplasms in persons treated with X-rays in infancy: Fourth survey in 20 years. *J. Natl. Canc. Inst.* 55: 519–530.

41. Henshaw, P. S., Snider, R. S., and Riley, E. F. 1951. Aberrant tissue developments of rats exposed to beta rays. Late effects of p32 beta rays, *in* R. E. Zirkle (ed.), *Effects of Beta Radiation 1951*, pp. 227–228. McGraw-Hill, New York.

42. Honda, T., Kamada, N., and Bloom, A. D. 1969. Chromosome aberrations and culture time. *Cytogen.* 8: 117–124.

43. Ishihara, T., and Kumatori, T. 1969. Cytogenetic studies on fishermen exposed to fallout radiation in 1954. *Jap. J. Genet.* 44: 242–251.

44. Ishimaru, T., Hoshino, T., Ishimaru, M., Okada, H., Tomiyasu, T., Tsuchimoto, T., and Yamamoto, T. 1971. Leukemia in atomic bomb survivors. Hiroshima and Nagasaki, 1 October 1950–30 September 1966. *Radiat. Res.* 45: 216–233.

45. Kadish, J. L., and Basch, R. S. 1975. Thymic regeneration after lethal irradiation: Evidence for an intra-thymic radioresistant T cell precursor. *J. Immun.* 114: 452–458.

46. Kamada, N. 1969. The effects of radiation in chromosomes of bone marrow cells. III. Cytogenetic studies on leukemia in atomic bomb survivors. *Acta Haemat. Jap.* 32: 249–274.

47. Kauppila, A., Raunio, V., and Taskinen, P. J. 1976. Immunosuppressive effect of radiotherapy on patients with lung cancer. Ann. Clin. Res. 8: 98–103.

48. Lewis, C. L., and Paterson, E. 1976. Leukopenia after postmastectomy irradiation. JAMA 235: 747–748.

49. MacKenzie, I. 1965. Breast cancer following multiple fluoroscopies. Brit. J. Cancer. 19: 1–8.

50. March, H. C. 1944. Leukemia in radiologists. Radiol. 43: 275–278.

51. March, H. C. 1950. Leukemia in radiologists in a 20-year period. Amer. J. Med. Sci. 220: 282–286.

52. Metcalf, D. 1956. The thymic origin of the plasma lymphocytosis stimulating factor. Brit. J. Cancer 10: 442–457.

53. Miller, J. F. A. P. 1962. Role of the thymus in transplantation tolerance and immunity, in G. E. W. Wolstenholme and M. P. Cameron (eds.), Ciba Foundation Symposium on Transplantation 1962, pp. 384–397. J. and A. Churchill Ltd., London.

54. Modan, B., Baidatz, D., Mart, H., Steinitz, R., and Levin, S. G. 1974. Radiation-induced head and neck tumours. Lancet 1: 277–279.

55. Mole, R. H. 1975. Ionizing radiation as a carcinogen: practical questions and academic pursuits. Brit. J. Radiol. 48: 157–169.

56. Moriyama, I. M., and Kato, H. 1973. JNIH-ABCC Life Span Study Report 7: Mortality Experience of A-bomb Survivors, 1970–1972, 1950–1972, Atomic Bomb Casualty Commission Technical Report 15–73, Hiroshima, Japan.

57. Myrden, J. A., and Hiltz, J. E. 1969. Breast cancer following multiple fluoroscopies during artificial pneumothorax treatment of pulmonary tuberculosis. Canad. Med. Ass. J. 100: 1032–1034.

58. Osoba, D., and Miller, J. F. A. P. 1963. Evidence for a humoral thymus factor responsible for the maturation of immunological faculty. Nat. 199: 653–654.

59. Reddy, M. M., Goh, K. O., and Hempelmann, L. H. 1976. B and T lymphocytes in man. I. Effect of infant thymic irradiation on the circulating B and T lymphocytes, radiation and the lymphatic system (CONF—740930), ERDA Symposium Series 37, National Technical Information Service, U.S. Dept. of Commerce, pp. 192–196. Springfield, Va. 22161.

60. Sheline, G. E., Lindsay, S., McCormack, K. R., and Galante, M. 1962. Thyroid nodules occurring late after treatment of thyrotoxicosis with radioiodine. J. Clin. Endocrinol. Metab. 22: 8–18.

61. Shellabarger, C. J., and Schmidt, R. W. 1968. Mammary neoplasia after in vitro X-irradiation of mammary tissue. Nature 218: 192–193.

62. Simpson, C. L., Hempelmann, L. H., and Fuller, L. M. 1955. Neoplasia in children treated with X-rays in infancy for thymus enlargement. Radiol. 64: 840–845.

63. Stefani, S., Kerman, R., and Abbate, J. 1976. Immune evaluation of lung cancer patients undergoing radiation therapy. Cancer 37: 2792–2796.

64. Stjernsward, J., Jondal, M., Vanky, F., Wigzell, H., and Sealy, R. 1972. Lymphopenia and change in distribution of human B and T lymphocytes in peripheral blood induced by irradiation for mammary carcinoma. Lancet 1: 1352–1356.

65. Takada, A., Takada, Y., Huang, C. C., and Ambrus, J. L. 1969. Biphasic pattern of thymus regeneration after whole-body irradiation. *J. Exp. Med.* 129: 445–457.

66. Takada, A., and Takada, Y. 1973. Proliferation of donor marrow and thymus cells in the myeloid and lymphoid organs of irradiated syngeneic host mice. *J. Exp. Med.* 137: 543–546.

67. Thomas, J. W., Coy, P., Lewis, H. S., and Yuen, A. 1971. Effect of therapeutic irradiation on lymphocyte transformation in lung cancer. *Cancer* 27: 1046–1050.

68. Tough, I. M., Buckton, K. E., Baikie, A. G., and Court-Brown, W. M. 1960. X-ray induced chromosomal damage in man. *Lancet* 2: 849–851.

69. Ulrich, H. 1946. The incidence of leukemia in radiologists. *N. Engl. J. Med.* 234: 45–46.

70. United Nations Scientific Committee on the Effects of Atomic Radiation. *Ionizing Radiation.* Vol. II, *Levels and Effects.* United Nations, New York, 1972.

71. Van Cleave, C. D. 1968. Late somatic effects of ionizing radiation. Division of Technical Information, USAEC, pp. 117–120. Washington, D.C.

72. Wanebo, C. K., Johnson, K. G., Sato, K., and Thorslund, T. W. 1968. Breast cancer after exposure to atomic bombings of Hiroshima and Nagasaki. *N. Engl. J. Med.* 279: 667–671.

73. Wilson, J. D., and Nossal, G. J. V. 1971. The T or B cell nature of chronic lymphocytic leukaemic lymphocytes. *Lancet* 2: 1153–1154.

74. Wood, S. E., Campbell, J. B., Anderson, J. M., and Kelly, F. 1974. Lymphocyte response after radiotherapy. *Lancet* 1: 863.

75. Ziegler, K. 1906. *Experimentelle und Klinische Untersuchungen über die Histogenese der Myeloischen Leukamie.* Gustave Fischer, Jena.

INDEX